Training and Supervision in Specialized Cognitive Behavior Therapy is two magnificent resources in one. Experienced clinicians will find tips that one rarely finds in current literature. Supervisors will find a superb and, so far, unique guide to support training for new clinicians. Richly detailed and wonderfully clear, each chapter weaves the experience of CBT from client, clinician, and supervisor perspectives. This book pioneers a new genre in psychotherapy literature. It is vital reading for CBT practitioners.

—**Joseph Blader, PhD,** Meadows Foundation & Semp Russ Professor of Child Psychiatry, Departments of Psychiatry & Behavioral Sciences and Pediatrics, Joe R. and Teresa Lozano Long School of Medicine, University of Texas Health Science Center at San Antonio

This is a very useful book for learning the key concepts and techniques for providing supervision and consultation on evidence-based interventions written by expert clinical researchers in psychotherapy. Each intervention includes discussion of key mistakes made by learners and how to overcome them—especially helpful for new clinicians. Also included is how to provide this supervision of treatments with special populations and in special settings.

—**Betsy D. Kennard, PsyD, ABPP,** Professor of Psychiatry, University of Texas Southwestern Medical Center, Dallas

This book should be on the shelf of every early career mental health professional who is learning how to supervise. For each evidence-based intervention, experts highlight the key concepts and techniques trainees need to know, common trainee mistakes and obstacles in supervision, and methods of addressing these mistakes and obstacles. The substantive takeaways from the book are specific, insightful, research-based, and culturally relevant.

—**Elissa J. Brown, PhD,** Child HELP Partnership at St. John's University, Queens, NY

Clinical supervision is a fundamental professional responsibility, but its real-world practice is often difficult. In their new book, *Training and Supervision in Specialized Cognitive Behavior Therapy: Methods, Settings, and Populations*, eminent scholars and clinicians Drs. Eric Storch, Jonathan Abramowitz, and Dean McKay remedy this problem through a science-informed and accessible text. Storch et al. and their expert contributors provide both naive and sophisticated readers with valuable supervisory know-how that I will repeatedly rely on, and I think you will too!

—**Robert D. Friedberg, PhD, ABPP,** Professor, Head of Pediatric Behavioral Health Emphasis, Palo Alto University, Palo Alto, CA

W0229964

Training and Supervision in

SPECIALIZED COGNITIVE BEHAVIOR THERAPY

Training and Supervision in

SPECIALIZED COGNITIVE BEHAVIOR THERAPY

Methods,
Settings,
and Populations

Edited by Eric A. Storch,
Jonathan S. Abramowitz,
and Dean McKay

AMERICAN PSYCHOLOGICAL ASSOCIATION

Published by
American Psychological Association
750 First Street, NE
Washington, DC 20002
https://www.apa.org

Order Department
https://www.apa.org/pubs/books
order@apa.org

In the U.K., Europe, Africa, and the Middle East, copies may be ordered from Eurospan
https://www.eurospanbookstore.com/apa
info@eurospangroup.com

Typeset in Meridien and Ortodoxa by Circle Graphics, Inc., Reisterstown, MD

Printer: Gasch Printing, Odenton, MD
Cover Designer: Gwen J. Grafft, Minneapolis, MN

Library of Congress Cataloging-in-Publication Data

Names: Storch, Eric A., editor. | Abramowitz, Jonathan S., editor. |
  McKay, Dean, 1966- editor.
Title: Training and supervision in specialized cognitive behavior therapy :
  methods, settings, and populations / edited by Eric A. Storch, Jonathan S.
  Abramowitz, and Dean McKay.
Description: Washington, DC : American Psychological Association, [2022] |
  Includes bibliographical references and index.
Identifiers: LCCN 2022011010 (print) | LCCN 2022011011 (ebook) |
  ISBN 9781433835803 (paperback) | ISBN 9781433835834 (ebook)
Subjects: LCSH: Cognitive therapy. | BISAC: PSYCHOLOGY / Movements /
  Cognitive Behavioral Therapy (CBT) | PSYCHOLOGY / Education & Training
Classification: LCC RC489.C63 T69 2022 (print) | LCC RC489.C63 (ebook) |
  DDC 616.89/1425--dc23/eng/20220622
LC record available at https://lccn.loc.gov/2022011010
LC ebook record available at https://lccn.loc.gov/2022011011

https://doi.org/10.1037/0000314-000

Printed in the United States of America

10 9 8 7 6 5 4 3 2 1

To all of my students. And to Ellie, Noah, and Maya—my favorite learners.
—ERIC A. STORCH

To all my supervisors; especially my parents, Ferne and Les Abramowitz—
my favorite teachers.
—JONATHAN S. ABRAMOWITZ

For my mentors who bestowed on me, with boundless generosity,
the opportunity to learn the nuances of supervision and consultation.
—DEAN McKAY

CONTENTS

CONTRIBUTORS

Jonathan S. Abramowitz, PhD, Department of Psychology, University of North Carolina, Chapel Hill, NC, United States

Moses Appel, MA, Student Counseling Services, Hofstra University, Hempstead, NY, United States

Donald H. Baucom, PhD, Department of Psychology and Neuroscience, University of North Carolina, Chapel Hill, NC, United States

Brian E. Bunnell, PhD, Department of Psychiatry and Behavioral Neurosciences, Morsani College of Medicine, University of South Florida, Tampa, FL, United States

Zeeshan Butt, PhD, Phreesia, Inc., Raleigh, NC; Department of Psychiatry & Behavioral Sciences, Feinberg School of Medicine, Northwestern University, Chicago, IL, United States

Mercedes Carswell, PhD, VA Atlanta Health Care System, Atlanta, GA, United States

Stacey B. Daughters, PhD, Department of Psychology and Neuroscience, University of North Carolina, Chapel Hill, NC, United States

Carter H. Davis, MA, Department of Psychology, Utah State University, Logan, UT, United States

Raymond DiGiuseppe, PhD, St. John's University, New York, NY; The Albert Ellis Institute, New York, NY, United States

Kristene A. Doyle, PhD, ScD, The Albert Ellis Institute, New York, NY, United States

Nicholas R. Farrell, PhD, NOCD, Chicago, IL, United States

Christopher A. Flessner, PhD, Department of Psychological Sciences, Kent State University, Kent, OH, United States

Rex Forehand, PhD, Department of Psychological Science, University of Vermont, Burlington, VT, United States

Kristin A. Gansle, PhD, Department of Communication Disorders and Special Education, Old Dominion University, Norfolk, VA, United States

Theresa R. Gladstone, BA, Department of Psychological Sciences, Kent State University, Kent, OH, United States

Livia Guadagnoli, PhD, Department of Chronic Diseases, Metabolism, and Ageing, KU Leuven, Leuven, Belgium

Emerson Hardebeck, MA, Department of Clinical Psychology, Antioch University, Seattle, WA, United States

Audrey Harkness, PhD, Department of Public Health Sciences, University of Miami, Miami, FL, United States

Michael Hickey, PhD, The Albert Ellis Institute, New York, NY, United States

Deborah J. Jones, PhD, Department of Psychology and Neuroscience, University of North Carolina, Chapel Hill, NC, United States

Robert J. Kohlenberg, PhD, ABPP, (deceased) Center for Science of Social Connection, Department of Psychology, University of Washington, Seattle, WA, United States

Jennifer Krafft, MA, Department of Psychology, Utah State University, Logan, UT, United States

Joseph La Torre, MTS, School of Psychology, University of Ottawa, Ottawa, ON, Canada

Robert L. Leahy, PhD, American Institute for Cognitive Therapy, New York, NY, United States

Rachel C. Leonard, PhD, Rogers Behavioral Health, Oconomowoc, WI, United States

Nicholas Long, PhD, University of Arkansas for Medical Sciences, Little Rock, AR; Arkansas Children's Hospital, Little Rock, AR, United States

Mary Plummer Loudon, PhD, The Seattle Clinic, Seattle, WA, United States

Dean McKay, PhD, Department of Psychology, Fordham University, Bronx, NY, United States

Robert J. McMahon, PhD, Simon Fraser University, Burnaby, BC; BC Children's Hospital Research Institute, Vancouver, BC, Canada

Jonathan Mitchell, PhD, Wellness Center, University of South Florida, St. Petersburg, FL, United States

Paige Morrison, PsyD, Department of Psychiatry and Behavioral Sciences, Baylor College of Medicine, Houston, TX, United States

George H. Noell, PhD, Department of Psychology, Old Dominion University, Norfolk, VA, United States

John E. Pachankis, PhD, School of Public Health, Yale University, New Haven, CT, United States

Amanda Palo, PhD, Department of Psychiatry and Behavioral Sciences, Baylor College of Medicine, Houston, TX, United States

Catherine E. Paquette, MPS, Department of Psychology and Neuroscience, University of North Carolina, Chapel Hill, NC, United States

Julie M. Petersen, MA, Department of Psychology, Utah State University, Logan, UT, United States

Elizabeth Raposa, PhD, Department of Psychology, Fordham University, Bronx, NY, United States

Elizabeth D. Reese, MA, Department of Psychology and Neuroscience, University of North Carolina, Chapel Hill, NC, United States

Bradley C. Riemann, PhD, Rogers Behavioral Health, Oconomowoc, WI, United States

Michael Rogers, PhD, Counseling Center, University of South Florida, Tampa, FL, United States

David H. Rosmarin, PhD, ABPP, Department of Psychiatry, McLean Hospital/Harvard Medical School, Belmont, MA, United States

Alison Salloum, PhD, LCSW, School of Social Work, College of Behavioral and Community Sciences, University of South Florida, Tampa, FL, United States

Jessica Spofford, PhD, Department of Psychiatry and Behavioral Sciences, Baylor College of Medicine, Houston, TX, United States

Eric A. Storch, PhD, Department of Psychiatry and Behavioral Sciences, Baylor College of Medicine, Houston, TX, United States

Sarah Sullivan-Singh, PhD, The Seattle Clinic, Seattle, WA, United States

Mavis Tsai, PhD, Center for Science of Social Connection, Department of Psychology, University of Washington, Seattle, WA, United States

Michael P. Twohig, PhD, Department of Psychology, Utah State University, Logan, UT, United States

Jason J. Washburn, PhD, Department of Psychiatry & Behavioral Sciences, Feinberg School of Medicine, Northwestern University, Chicago, IL, United States

Danielle M. Weber, MA, Department of Psychology and Neuroscience, University of North Carolina, Chapel Hill, NC, United States

Monnica T. Williams, PhD, School of Psychology, University of Ottawa, Ottawa, ON, Canada

Emily P. Wilton, MA, Department of Psychological Sciences, Kent State University, Kent, OH, United States

Training and Supervision in

SPECIALIZED COGNITIVE BEHAVIOR THERAPY

Introduction to Supervising and Consulting With Trainees and Clinicians in Cognitive Behavioral Therapies

Eric A. Storch, Jonathan S. Abramowitz, and Dean McKay

Supervision and consultation have been central components of ongoing professional training and practice in clinical psychology for decades, ranging from informal consultation in case conferences (Meehl, 1973) to individual and directed supervision (Loganbill et al., 1982) to small group discussions (Holloway & Johnston, 1985). Prevailing models of supervision and consultation have emphasized the process, in a manner resembling traditional direct therapeutic modalities based on psychodynamic theories (e.g., described in Frawley-O'Dea & Sarnat, 2001). While other psychotherapeutic modalities have emphasized processes in the conduct of supervision and consultation, there has been comparably less attention paid to the mechanics in cognitive behavior therapy (CBT). It is remarkable that this has not been the focus of greater attention. Most practitioners recognize CBT as a specialized approach to practice. For example, it has been represented as a specific specialization from the American Board of Professional Psychology for over 40 years. There are additional specialization credentials available within CBT (e.g., from the Academy for Cognitive Therapy).

Over the last half-century there has been a proliferation of CBT interventions for numerous types of psychological problems across the lifespan.

Research reported in this publication was supported by the Eunice Kennedy Shriver National Institute of Child Health and Human Development of the National Institutes of Health under Award Number P50HD103555 for use of the Clinical Translational Core facilities. The content is solely the responsibility of the authors and does not necessarily represent the official views of the National Institutes of Health.

https://doi.org/10.1037/0000314-001
Training and Supervision in Specialized Cognitive Behavior Therapy: Methods, Settings, and Populations, E. A. Storch, J. S. Abramowitz, and D. McKay (Editors)

These interventions have demonstrated robust efficacy ranging from more moderate yet clinically meaningful effects (e.g., attention-deficit/hyperactivity disorder; Cortese & Coghill, 2018) to dramatically impressive results (e.g., anxiety, van Dis et al., 2020; obsessive–compulsive disorder, McKay et al., 2015). As these interventions have been established, attention has shifted to actualizing dissemination and real-world implementation. One method of doing this has involved the increasing number of published manuals that are readily available to credentialed clinicians. Although helpful for detailing the elements of these interventions, as applied to specific *DSM* (*Diagnostic and Statistical Manual of Mental Disorders*) diagnostic categories, such one-size-fits-all treatment manuals often have shortcomings, one of which is that they typically do not address co-occurring problems and other clinical complexities, which tend to be the rule rather than then exception in clinical practice. Indeed, manuals often reinforce the misunderstanding that CBT is a single method of treatment. It is not. Rather, CBT is a highly diverse collection of evidence-based interventions whose efficacy is dependent on proper implementation with the appropriate goals (i.e., changing thinking and behavior) in mind.

To this end, clinical supervision and consultation form the cornerstone of training—at all levels—in how to implement efficacious interventions with high fidelity. In recognition of the rich diversity of interventions that CBT comprises, this book gathers experts on different approaches and describes methods of training, supervision, and consultation employing these treatment modalities. Although excellent training protocols exist, comprehensive texts that provide guidance on how to train and supervise clinicians in various approaches within the broader CBT theoretical context are few in number and scope. As many clinicians who are already experts in CBT are also frequently called upon to engage in consultation, this book serves as a valuable resource and contributes to the effective dissemination of CBT, as well as increasing the likelihood that the methods of this approach will be delivered with proper fidelity.

Divided into two broad parts, this book is notable in its scope and coverage. Part I, Techniques of Cognitive Behavior Therapy, focuses on several broad methods of interventions in CBT. Chapters written by leading scholars tackle supervisory aspects of exposure therapy, cognitive therapy, rational–emotive behavior therapy, acceptance and commitment therapy, dialectical behavior therapy, functional analytic psychotherapy, comprehensive behavior intervention for tics, behavioral activation, and parent management training. Part II covers special populations (i.e., CBT with underrepresented groups, behavioral activation for depression) and settings (i.e., community clinics, practitioners in independent practice). In this part, supervision of trainee clinicians in a variety of settings (e.g., community clinics, college counseling centers, private practice) and across various populations is addressed (e.g., children, religious patients, LGBTQ+ individuals). The division of this book into these two broad sections is in recognition of the highly specialized nature of CBT for its variety of approaches and applications to unique groups.

Across all chapters, the nuances of effective supervision are described in a structured framework that includes (a) an overview of the intervention, (b) key concepts for trainees to learn, (c) characteristics of training cases, (d) common trainee mistakes and how to address them, (e) ethical issues, and (f) overcoming common obstacles in supervision. It is our hope that this volume provides guidance on how to successfully supervise trainee clinicians, whether they are emerging professionals or experienced individuals developing a new skill set.

REFERENCES

Cortese, S., & Coghill, D. (2018). Twenty years of research on attention-deficit/hyperactivity disorder (ADHD): Looking back, looking forward. *Evidence-Based Mental Health, 21*(4), 173–176. https://doi.org/10.1136/ebmental-2018-300050

Frawley-O'Dea, M. G., & Sarnat, J. E. (2001). *The supervisory relationship: A contemporary psychodynamic approach*. Guilford Press.

Holloway, E. L., & Johnston, R. (1985). Group supervision: Widely practiced but poorly understood. *Counselor Education and Supervision, 24*(4), 332–340. https://doi.org/10.1002/j.1556-6978.1985.tb00494.x

Loganbill, C., Hardy, E., & Delworth, U. (1982). Supervision: A conceptual model. *The Counseling Psychologist, 10*(1), 3–42. https://doi.org/10.1177/0011000082101002

McKay, D., Sookman, D., Neziroglu, F., Wilhelm, S., Stein, D. J., Kyrios, M., Matthews, K., & Veale, D. (2015). Efficacy of cognitive-behavioral therapy for obsessive-compulsive disorder. *Psychiatry Research, 227*(1), 104–113. https://doi.org/10.1016/j.psychres.2015.02.004

Meehl, P. E. (1973). Why I do not attend case conferences. In P. E. Meehl (Ed.), *Psychodiagnosis: Selected papers* (pp. 225–302). University of Minnesota Press.

van Dis, E. A. M., van Veen, S. C., Hagenaars, M. A., Batelaan, N. M., Bockting, C. L. H., van den Heuvel, R. M., Cuijpers, P., & Engelhard, I. M. (2020). Long-term outcomes of cognitive behavioral therapy for anxiety disorders: A systematic review and meta-analysis. *JAMA Psychiatry, 77*(3), 265–273. https://doi.org/10.1001/jamapsychiatry.2019.3986

TECHNIQUES OF COGNITIVE BEHAVIOR THERAPY

1

Supervision of Exposure Therapy

Jonathan S. Abramowitz, Eric A. Storch, and Dean McKay

Despite its efficacy and effectiveness, exposure therapy remains underutilized by frontline clinicians, who often cite factors such as the presence of comorbid disorders, concerns about provoking anxiety in clients, and fears of dropout as reasons they avoid using exposure therapy (e.g., van Minnen et al., 2010). In addition, recent developments in the understanding and application of fear extinction to exposure therapy have led to advances in the implementation of exposure techniques to optimize outcome (Craske et al., 2014). In this chapter, we provide tools and suggestions for supervising novice therapists in the use of exposure therapy with the aim of addressing the issues just described. Although our focus is on adults, we note that clinicians working with children and adolescents often share many of the expectations and challenges discussed in this chapter; therefore, many of the same principles apply.

Exposure therapy, the repeated and systematic confrontation with feared stimuli, is a central component of cognitive behavior therapy (CBT) for anxiety and related disorders. The use of exposure derives from a conceptualization of clinical anxiety in which individuals have learned to overestimate the likelihood and severity of danger associated with a generally safe situation or stimulus (e.g., Abramowitz et al., 2019). In response to their fear, they engage in avoidance and other types of safety-seeking behaviors (e.g., compulsive rituals, coping strategies) aimed at escaping from distress and preventing feared outcomes. These behaviors are reinforced by the immediate reduction in distress they engender and thus become habits. In the longer term, however, they maintain

https://doi.org/10.1037/0000314-002
Training and Supervision in Specialized Cognitive Behavior Therapy: Methods, Settings, and Populations, E. A. Storch, J. S. Abramowitz, and D. McKay (Editors)

fear by robbing the individual of opportunities to correct the dysfunctional thinking patterns (Craske et al., 2008, 2014).

In line with this conceptualization, successful treatment must provide the person with opportunities to learn that their overestimates of threat are exaggerated and that avoidance and safety-seeking behaviors are unnecessary. Exposure therapy therefore begins with education about this conceptualization. Initial sessions also include a functional assessment of fear cues and avoidance and safety-seeking behavior. This information is then used to develop a list of items the individual will confront during exposure trials.

Exposure trials themselves involve repeated confrontation with feared stimuli, which may occur in real life (in vivo; e.g., actual exposure to uncomfortable social situations, public bathrooms, driving far from home), in imagination (e.g., recounting memories of traumatic events, thinking of fear-provoking thoughts), or interoceptively (e.g., provoking feared body sensations, such as a racing heart). During exposure, the client's degree of anxiety may be monitored and the process of *habituation*—the natural decline of anxiety within and between exposure sessions—may be observed. Exposure continues with therapist supervision and for homework between sessions until all stimuli on the exposure list have been confronted and the client has learned that these stimuli are generally safe—that is, *fear extinction* has occurred.

KEY CONCEPTS FOR TRAINEES TO LEARN

The traditional understanding of how exposure therapy works derives from emotional processing theory (EPT), which emphasizes habituation as an indicator of fear extinction (Foa & Kozak, 1986). From this perspective, exposure trials are designed to maximally elicit fear and then sustained long enough for within- and between-session decreases in arousal to occur (e.g., Bjork & Bjork, 1992). Research, however, indicates that habituation is not a strong predictor of long-term outcome (Jacoby & Abramowitz, 2016). Indeed, treatment gains are sometimes observed in the absence of habituation, and poor outcomes may be observed among those for whom habituation does occur.

Accordingly, Craske et al. (2008, 2014) introduced inhibitory learning theory (ILT) to (a) reconceptualize the mechanisms of exposure and (b) inform strategies for capitalizing on these mechanisms of change. ILT is grounded in research on learning and memory (e.g., Bjork & Bjork, 1992) suggesting that exposure does not "erase" or cause "unlearning" of fear, but rather allows for the learning of new safety-based information (e.g., elevators are safe) that competes with the existing threat-based (fear) associations (e.g., elevators are dangerous). The extent to which the new nonthreat information is learned in ways that inhibit the older threat-based thinking and then generalized across contexts, determines the extent of fear extinction and thus the efficacy and durability of exposure therapy.

Research also points to the role of *experiential avoidance*—the tendency to resist uncomfortable internal experiences, such as anxiety and its related physical sensations (i.e., the fight-or-flight response), in the maintenance of clinical anxiety (Hayes et al., 1996). Accordingly, rather than trying to reduce or eliminate anxiety, it is more productive to enhance the client's ability to accept and tolerate this universal (and harmless) experience. This complements the aim of enhancing inhibitory learning, since clients learn through exposure that anxiety itself is safe.

To summarize, theory and research on learning suggest that rather than relying on habituation as an indicator of the success of exposure therapy, one is better off using (a) observations of performance at posttreatment or follow-up and (b) tolerance of anxiety as signs that new nonthreat information has been consolidated in such a way as to extinguish fear. This shift from habituation to tolerance and long-term performance as indices of learning has implications for the methods clinicians and trainees can use to optimize the outcome of exposure.

KEY TECHNIQUES FOR TRAINEES TO LEARN

The basics of conducting exposure therapy can be learned through reading texts (e.g., Abramowitz et al., 2019), didactic teaching, and observing therapy sessions. In this section, however, we highlight concepts that many novice therapists find challenging and that therefore often arise in supervision.

Providing the Rationale for Exposure

Trainees are encouraged to develop the exposure treatment plan based on "what the client needs to learn." As examples, clients with social anxiety need to learn that negative evaluation is not as dreadful as they think. Those with panic attacks need to learn that arousal-related body sensations do not lead to physical or mental catastrophe. Those with posttraumatic stress disorder (PTSD) or obsessive–compulsive disorder (OCD) need to learn (among other things) that their intrusive memories and thoughts are safe and manageable, rather than predictors of danger.

Accordingly, novice clinicians can be taught to describe the goal of exposure to their clients as "learning new information by facing one's fears." Therapists should also convey that the goal is learning anxiety tolerance, rather than anxiety reduction. As we like to say, the aim is to get better at having anxiety, not to get better at making it go away. Consistent with this "bring it on" stance, when exposure stimuli trigger intense levels of anxiety, rather than rely on habituation to reduce subjective fear, trainees will help clients see such situations as opportunities to cultivate distress tolerance.

Developing the Exposure List

The *exposure list* is a catalog of the feared situations that will be confronted to help the client learn new information relevant to their fear predictions.

Thus, rather than being guided by questions such as "What are you afraid of?" the choice of exposure stimuli should be driven by the question "What does the client need to learn?" In other words, it is the client's fear prediction that drives the choice of exposure items. Someone afraid that experiencing "intense" anxiety for a given amount of time will lead to having a stroke, for example, must engage in an exposure trial in which this level of anxiety occurs for at least the specified amount of time, so that she can learn that this does not lead to a stroke. In selecting items for the exposure list, the trainee works collaboratively with the client to (a) assess the stimuli that provoke exaggerated fear-based predictions of negative consequences, (b) understand the parameters of these fear predictions themselves, and (c) create a list of all safety-seeking behaviors. Before any exposure trials begin, we recommend that supervisors review trainees' case conceptualizations as well as assessment data and exposure lists.

Maximizing Expectancy Violation

Exposure trials should optimize the mismatch between what the client believes will happen and what actually occurs when a stimulus is confronted. In fact, the more clients are surprised that the feared outcome of exposure does not occur, the more inhibitory learning takes place (Rescorla & Wagner, 1972). This is easily observed in the treatment of spider phobia, for example. When a client holds a tarantula for a prolonged amount of time and expects to be bitten but is not, she gains experiences that powerfully violate her expectations of harm, leading to the development of new nonthreat appraisals of such spiders.

As an alternative to tracking subjective units of discomfort (SUDS) during exposure, therapists can track changes in expectations of danger—a technique called *expectancy tracking* (Craske et al., 2014). This involves specifying a danger-based prediction before the exposure trial begins and asking the client to rate their belief in the prediction as time passes during and after exposure. The trial ends when the threat-based expectations have shifted (independent of SUDS level). After the exposure trial, time is spent consolidating what was learned by further discussing the discrepancy between what was expected and what actually occurred.

Combining Fear Cues

Traditionally, therapists expose their clients to one fear cue at a time, gradually working their way up a hierarchy of feared stimuli. Rescorla and Wagner (1972), however, suggested that fear extinction (and inhibitory learning) is maximized when expected feared outcomes fail to occur in the presence of multiple fear cues, rather than just a single cue (deepened extinction; Rescorla, 2006). For example, a therapist might incorporate both *in vivo* exposure to driving and interoceptive exposure to arousal-related body sensations (e.g., racing heart) for a client with a fear of driving who is afraid intense anxiety will impair her ability to drive.

Eliminating Safety-Seeking Behaviors and Cues

A core component of exposure is the elimination of safety behaviors such as compulsive rituals and other anxiety-reduction cues and strategies. This *response prevention* aspect of treatment facilitates the safety learning by removing any superfluous explanation for the nonoccurrence of predicted danger. Safety-seeking behaviors and cues may be subtle (e.g., shrewd reassurance seeking, thought suppression, wearing religious charms) and are therefore sometimes overlooked by trainees.

Maximizing Variability

Finally, research (Jacoby et al., 2019) suggests that although learning in diverse contexts slows the short-term acquisition of new information, it considerably strengthens long-term retention as well as the generalization of learning to varied and novel contexts. It is therefore important to maximize variability in exposure trials. This means helping the client to practice exposure to slightly different stimuli (e.g., different types of dogs) under different conditions (e.g., day, night), and in different settings (e.g., alone, with a therapist, with a parent). Mood states also represent an important context for exposure. If, for example, clients practice exposure only when feeling "good," they will not have the opportunity to learn that they can in fact manage distress even when they are having a "bad day." This could contribute to the return of fear if a prolonged period of stress arises for the client at some point. Long-term fear extinction thus depends on learning safety in an array of external and internal contexts.

CHARACTERISTICS OF A GOOD (AND POOR) TRAINING CASE

There are a number of factors to consider when thinking about an instructive training case for novice exposure therapists. First, trainees will benefit from working with clients who have strong incentives to overcome their fear and are therefore open to confronting fear-provoking stimuli. Clients who attend sessions regularly also set the stage for a beneficial training experience. Conversely, those who are unwilling to work collaboratively with the therapist or those who easily balk at the idea of confronting fear stimuli will be more of a challenge. The efficacy of therapeutic exposure relies on the therapist's skills as well as the client's willingness to actively engage in exposure trials both within and between sessions.

A second consideration is that, especially early in training, it will be most instructive for novice therapists to work with clients who easily articulate somewhat clear and immediate feared consequences. This is the case for many individuals with specific phobias, who, for example, overestimate the probability of being bitten by dogs, stung by bees, or stuck in an elevator. Clients with panic attacks who fear that such attacks will lead to sudden death, and those with OCD who fear that they will lose control and act on unwanted thoughts or become ill immediately upon touching "contaminated" surfaces, are also appropriate for training purposes. Such clients are "straightforward" because their fear predictions can be easily tested during exposure trials (i.e., expectancy violation is easily demonstrated). On the other hand, some presentations of anxiety (e.g., some obsessional problems; health anxiety) involve feared outcomes that are longer-term (e.g., "I will develop cancer in 10 years from exposure to pesticides"; Jacoby & Abramowitz, 2016, p. 32) or even unknowable (e.g., "I will go to hell because I had a blasphemous thought"; Jacoby & Abramowitz, 2016, p. 32). Designing exposures to violate such expectancies becomes complicated since the fear might concern the experience of uncertainty, anxiety, or other less concrete stimuli (Abramowitz et al., 2019). This is not to say that such fears are exclusionary criteria for training cases, yet they do present challenges that can interfere with the supervisee's ability to practice foundational exposure therapy skills.

Finally, clients who become highly emotionally dysregulated during exposure sessions can prevent the supervisee from practicing exposure skills since the majority of the session may be spent trying to calm the client. Those who are severely depressed or suicidal also do not make for good training cases, in that much of the session may be dedicated to managing negative cognitions or suicide assessment and safety planning. It's also important to note that clients with active psychotic symptoms, mania, and active substance use disorders are not appropriate for exposure therapy regardless of the therapist's experience.

COMMON MISTAKES THAT TRAINEES MAKE (AND HOW TO FIX THEM)

In this section, we discuss a range of pitfalls that clinicians in training commonly stumble upon, as well as how supervisors can work with clinicians to amend these mistakes. Interestingly, many of these pitfalls arise from a trainee's desire to minimize the client's anxiety during exposure.

Failing to Properly "Sell" Exposure

Providing an articulate and convincing rationale for exposure to the client is a task with which many therapists-in-training struggle. A strong knowledge of cognitive behavioral theory, however, helps alleviate this problem. Therapists who have a firm grasp of this conceptual approach to clinical anxiety are much more adept at eloquently explaining to fearful individuals why they should deliberately confront their fears, which helps ensure buy-in. Socializing a client to the conceptual model involves synthesizing the information collected during assessment and, in a transparent and collaborative way, placing the client's difficulties within the theoretical framework. Doing so helps the client under-stand how exposure therapy can be beneficial even if confronting feared stimuli seems counterintuitive (if not challenging). Supervisors will want to make sure that their trainees spend adequate time discussing with their clients that the aim of exposure is to learn new information about the safety and tolerability of feared stimuli.

A discussion of how exposure sessions will unfold also helps clients to understand the process. Therapists can explain that anxiety is expected, espe-cially when starting to confront the feared situation. But if the client remains exposed, without trying to fight the anxiety, these feelings will either begin to subside on their own, or they will remain present and the client will discover that they are manageable, even if unpleasant. This learning, however, occurs only if the exposure exercise is carefully designed and the client repeats it in different situations (e.g., office, home). Finally, it is critical to explain that the therapist's role is to provide support and coaching during exposure tasks. Sometimes, these tasks might seem risky or involve doing things that most people wouldn't ordinarily do. The client, however, must understand that the purpose of exposure is not to practice doing what most people do, but rather to do things that will lead to learning new information about safety to improve the client's life functioning.

Reluctance to Push Clients to Face Their Fears

Some well-meaning trainees will be uncomfortable with exposure because it increases rather than soothes distress. They may be reluctant to subject clients to temporary discomfort, even if it has longer term benefits, preferring instead to equip them with "anxiety coping skills," such as relaxation or breathing exercises. Of course, this perspective is empathic in that it comes from a genuine desire for the client to feel better. However, an emphasis on minimizing short-term anxiety aims empathy at the wrong target. Indeed, to enduringly reduce fear, anxious clients need to learn that feared stimuli (and the feelings of anxiety they provoke) are acceptably safe and tolerable and do not require the use of safety-seeking behaviors. Thus, durable anxiety reduction requires a certain type of learning that necessitates a challenging journey. Well-meaning and empathic clinicians who teach coping strategies may ironically deprive their clients of opportunities for a life with less clinical anxiety. Exposure therapists, on the other hand, prize their patients' long-term well-being over their imme-diate discomfort.

We therefore encourage supervisors to help trainees view their work as similar to that of a physical therapist, dentist, or physician. These health care providers often conduct temporarily painful procedures in the service of their patients' long-term health. Although the pain of some medical procedures may be aversive, patients are typically willing to accept it in the interest of their longer term well-being. Similarly, the majority of anxious clients are willing to accept the aversive experience of anxiety during exposure to overcome their fears in the long run. As we have discussed, exposure therapy requires patients to "lean into anxiety" and "invest in anxiety now for a calmer future" so they can learn (among other things) that fear itself is safe and manageable. According to the available research and our clinical experience, this is an investment most anxious individuals are willing to make.

Overreliance on Habituation

Another mistake that trainees commonly make is to rely too strongly on habituation as an indicator of a successful exposure trial. This might take the form of reinforcing the client's perception that the goal of exposure is to confront feared stimuli until anxiety goes down, informing clients that the exposure session is over when anxiety is reduced by a certain amount, or "rooting" for habituation during exposure trials. Yet, as we've pointed out, "habituation is neither a reliable predictor of exposure therapy outcome (short- or long-term) nor tantamount to . . . [fear extinction]. In other words, there is disconnect between fear expression during learning and fear learning itself (Craske et al., 2008)" (Jacoby & Abramowitz, 2016, p. 30).

In fact,

> dependence on habituation as an indicator of improvement . . . could have unintended negative consequences. Emphasizing the importance of fear reduction during . . . [exposure], for example, implies that anxiety itself is inherently bad, and that treatment is only successful if one is anxiety-free. This may perpetuate a "fear of fear" mindset and lead patients to interpret inevitable (and normal) unexpected surges of fear (either within or outside of exposure trials) as signs of failure . . . [Some clients] might also use exposures to *control* their anxiety (i.e., "I know I can do this exposure *because* my anxiety will come down"), which is contrary to the aim of *confronting* and learning to tolerate anxiety and fear as normal and nonthreatening experiences. (Jacoby & Abramowitz, 2016, p. 30)

Accordingly, although habituation is a normal part of exposure trials, trainees should dispel client beliefs that anxiety reduction is either as an important goal of exposure or an indicator of success. Instead, as we have discussed, trainees should emphasize learning that anxiety is safe and manageable as the goal.

Overreliance on Gradual Exposure

On a similar note, trainees often rely too heavily on the idea that exposure must be approached gradually in a hierarchical fashion (a tenant of EPT). Although a hierarchy-based approach fosters habituation and short-term fear reduction in the presence of exposure stimuli, it might inadvertently impede longer term fear extinction (and thus treatment outcome more generally) by failing to extinguish the fear of anxiety itself (Jacoby et al., 2019). This might occur for a number of reasons. First, the use of a fear hierarchy can cultivate an overreliance on habituation (as noted previously) by suggesting that anxiety must habituate during "easier" exposures before more anxiety-provoking tasks can be attempted. Second, it reinforces a "fear of fear" by implying (erroneously) that less intense anxiety is "safer" or "more tolerable" than more intense anxiety (e.g., "You're not ready to confront the most feared items yet"). Thus, when inevitable surges of anxiety occur following treatment, they might be interpreted as danger signals, ultimately contributing to relapse. Finally, feared stimuli do not tend to appear in a hierarchical fashion outside the therapy session, but rather in a random and variable manner; thus, gradual exposure is not a good match to "real-world" confrontations with feared stimuli.

Accordingly, although a gradual (hierarchy-based) approach to exposure in most instances will work just fine, trainees may consider conducting exposure without regard to fear levels (Jacoby et al., 2019). This variability in fear intensity can help the client learn that anxiety, at any level of intensity, is safe and manageable. It may also bolster the client's self-confidence. Further, it creates greater flexibility wherein clients might, for example, confront fears that most quickly reduce functional interference. We suggest the term *exposure list* (as opposed to hierarchy), which does not preclude a gradual approach but does free therapists and clients from strictly adhering to a hierarchy when planning exposures. Indeed, whereas gradual exposure may seem more acceptable to patients, this approach might not maximize long-term outcomes.

Misuse of Cognitive Therapy

Finally, many trainees (as well as seasoned clinicians) believe that using cognitive therapy (CT) to make exposure more "palatable" is necessary to "prepare" clients for facing their fears. Yet recall that extinction learning is strengthened when the difference between what patients predict and what actually happens during exposure trials is maximized. Therefore, techniques that minimize this discrepancy before (or during) exposure may attenuate extinction learning. Accordingly, CT, which is used to correct overestimates of likelihood (e.g., "They are unlikely to laugh at me") and severity (e.g., "Being laughed at is unpleasant but not the end of the world") of feared outcomes may actually hinder inhibitory learning if implemented prior to or during exposures. That is, paradoxically, CT may reduce negative expectancies prior to exposure and subsequently lessen the mismatch between prediction and reality.

This is not to say that therapists should avoid discussing mistaken cognitions during exposure. We do, however, recommend a different way of weaving CT into exposure by using it (a) before an exposure to help identify feared outcomes; (b) during exposure to remind the client of fear-based predictions; and (c) after an exposure to help process shifts in beliefs, expectations, and other mistaken cognitions and consolidate what has been learned. Specifically, after the exposure trial, clients can be asked to recount evidence that they gained that disconfirms fear-based thinking, and to generate healthier cognitions (i.e., rational responses) regarding the feared stimulus. Using CT in this way also prevents clients from using cognitive techniques as anxiety-reduction (reassurance-seeking) strategies, as is sometimes the case for individuals with OCD (Abramowitz & Jacoby, 2015).

ETHICAL ISSUES IN THE APPLICATION OF EXPOSURE THERAPY

Exposure therapy is the clear first-line treatment for clinical anxiety. Nevertheless, relatively few therapists provide this treatment, and most individuals with clinical anxiety do not receive exposure. One reason for this is a set of negative therapist beliefs about exposure, including that (a) clients have difficulty tolerating the distress that exposure provokes, (b) anxious clients are at risk for decompensating during exposures, (c) exposure is associated with high dropout rates, and (d) exposure works poorly for "complex" cases (Deacon, Farrell, et al., 2013). Accordingly, trainees might believe that exposure is unethical, intolerable, and dangerous.

These beliefs, however, do not have empirical support and are inconsistent with the experience of well-trained exposure therapists. In fact, there may be ethical (and perhaps even legal) concerns associated with not using (or not referring clients for) exposure therapy and instead using less effective or unsupported interventions. Of course, exposure therapy is not risk-free; indeed, it may provoke greater emotional discomfort than other forms of psychological treatment. However, by properly negotiating informed consent, objectively determining acceptable risk, properly managing potentially negative outcomes, remaining aware of boundary crossings and avoiding inappropriate boundary violations, and receiving appropriate training and supervision, trainees can significantly decrease risks to their clients. Indeed, the large disconnect between the effectiveness of exposure therapy, on the one hand, and the infrequency with which it is used, on the other, is of greater concern than are the risks associated with competently conducted exposure therapy.

COMMON OBSTACLES IN SUPERVISION AND WAYS OF OVERCOMING THEM

By far, the most common obstacle in supervision of exposure therapy is the trainee's reluctance to push the client to do difficult exposures that are likely to evoke intense fear. This might be driven by ethical concerns, as we have discussed, but may also be the result of the trainee's own discomfort with anxiety. Specifically, therapists who believe that anxiety itself is dangerous (i.e., they have elevated anxiety sensitivity) are more likely to run into difficulty challenging clients to persevere through more difficult exposure trials (Meyer et al., 2014). Accordingly, supervisors can directly assess and address the common misconceptions about exposure that we discussed previously, including misconceptions about the experience of anxiety itself.

For example, supervisors may let trainees know that despite its intense nature, exposure therapy is perceived favorably by many clients (Olatunji et al., 2009) and is extremely unlikely to lead to the kind of negative outcomes feared by some (Deacon, Lickel, et al., 2013). Additional techniques for reducing trainee concerns about the risks and tolerability of anxiety itself, such as education about the fight–flight response and perhaps even a trial of interoceptive exposure, can be implemented as part of training in the theory and practice of exposure (Farrell et al., 2013). Such strategies may be especially important for those trainees who are older, have a master's degree, and endorse concerns about the experience of anxiety itself (Meyer et al., 2014).

CONCLUSION

In this chapter, we have drawn on our own training experiences, missteps, and concerns when delivering exposure therapy in the hope of helping supervisors and those learning to apply exposure therapy in the treatment of clinical anxiety. One of the most meaningful realizations working with a wide range of clinically anxious individuals is how much stronger and more resilient these clients are than we ever expected. What do we mean by this? As implied earlier, it is easy for a therapist to view anxious individuals as psychologically fragile, like a flickering candle flame needing to be protected from the wind. Yet, it is useful to remember that anxious clients already possess a great deal of strength and courage. They acknowledge their problem and are actively seeking help. With this personal resilience and therapist support, clients are often able to successfully approach the stimuli that provoke fear.

Implementing exposure with anxious individuals can certainly be challenging, but it is also inherently rewarding. As exposure therapists, our role is to coach and cheerlead our clients through the difficult task of approaching the situations, stimuli, thoughts, memories, or bodily sensations that provoke anxiety and fear in order to help them learn that these stimuli are safe and do not require any superstitious avoidance or safety-seeking. When such learning takes place, it leads to improvements in domains of life functioning that were stifled by fear. Serving in this role as a therapist requires both scientific knowledge and artistry—a high degree of understanding, skill, and effort. In our experience, working with such clients is often a highly rewarding experience, teaching us about human resilience, strength, and bravery in the face of adversity.

REFERENCES

Abramowitz, J. S., Deacon, B. J., & Whiteside, S. P. H. (2019). *Exposure therapy for anxiety, Principles and practice* (2nd ed.). Guilford Press.

Abramowitz, J. S., & Jacoby, R. J. (2015). *Obsessive–compulsive disorder in adults.* Hogrefe Publishing.

Bjork, R. A., & Bjork, E. L. (1992). A new theory of disuse and an old theory of stimulus fluctuation. In A. F. Healy, S. M. Kosslyn, & R. M. Shiffrin (Eds.), *Essays in honor of William K. Estes, Vol. 2. From learning processes to cognitive processes* (pp. 35–67). Lawrence Erlbaum Associates.

Craske, M. G., Kircanski, K., Zelikowsky, M., Mystkowski, J., Chowdhury, N., & Baker, A. (2008). Optimizing inhibitory learning during exposure therapy. *Behaviour Research and Therapy, 46*(1), 5–27. https://doi.org/10.1016/j.brat.2007.10.003

Craske, M. G., Treanor, M., Conway, C. C., Zbozinek, T., & Vervliet, B. (2014). Maximizing exposure therapy: An inhibitory learning approach. *Behaviour Research and Therapy, 58,* 10–23. https://doi.org/10.1016/j.brat.2014.04.006

Deacon, B. J., Farrell, N. R., Kemp, J. J., Dixon, L. J., Sy, J. T., Zhang, A. R., & McGrath, P. B. (2013). Assessing therapist reservations about exposure therapy for anxiety disorders: The Therapist Beliefs About Exposure Scale. *Journal of Anxiety Disorders, 27*(8), 772–780. https://doi.org/10.1016/j.janxdis.2013.04.006

Deacon, B. J., Lickel, J. J., Farrell, N. R., Kemp, J. J., & Hipol, L. J. (2013). Therapist perceptions and delivery of interoceptive exposure for panic disorder. *Journal of Anxiety Disorders, 27*(2), 259–264. https://doi.org/10.1016/j.janxdis.2013.02.004

Farrell, N. R., Deacon, B. J., Dixon, L. J., & Lickel, J. J. (2013). Theory-based training strategies for modifying practitioner concerns about exposure therapy. *Journal of Anxiety Disorders, 27*(8), 781–787. https://doi.org/10.1016/j.janxdis.2013.09.003

Foa, E. B., & Kozak, M. J. (1986). Emotional processing of fear: Exposure to corrective information. *Psychological Bulletin, 99*(1), 20–35. https://doi.org/10.1037/0033-2909.99.1.20

Hayes, S. C., Wilson, K. G., Gifford, E. V., Follette, V. M., & Strosahl, K. (1996). Experiential avoidance and behavioral disorders: A functional dimensional approach to diagnosis and treatment. *Journal of Consulting and Clinical Psychology, 64*(6), 1152–1168. https://doi.org/10.1037/0022-006X.64.6.1152

Jacoby, R. J., & Abramowitz, J. S. (2016). Inhibitory learning approaches to exposure therapy: A critical review and translation to obsessive–compulsive disorder. *Clinical Psychology Review, 49,* 28–40. https://doi.org/10.1016/j.cpr.2016.07.001

Jacoby, R. J., Abramowitz, J. S., Blakey, S. M., & Reuman, L. (2019). Is the hierarchy necessary? Gradual versus variable exposure intensity in the treatment of unacceptable obsessional thoughts. *Journal of Behavior Therapy and Experimental Psychiatry, 64,* 54–63. https://doi.org/10.1016/j.jbtep.2019.02.008

Meyer, J. M., Farrell, N. R., Kemp, J. J., Blakey, S. M., & Deacon, B. J. (2014). Why do clinicians exclude anxious clients from exposure therapy? *Behaviour Research and Therapy, 54,* 49–53. https://doi.org/10.1016/j.brat.2014.01.004

Olatunji, B. O., Deacon, B. J., & Abramowitz, J. S. (2009). The cruelest cure? Ethical issues in the implementation of exposure-based treatments. *Cognitive and Behavioral Practice, 16*(2), 172–180. https://doi.org/10.1016/j.cbpra.2008.07.003

Rescorla, R. A. (2006). Deepened extinction from compound stimulus presentation. *Journal of Experimental Psychology: Animal Behavior Processes, 32*(2), 135–144. https://doi.org/10.1037/0097-7403.32.2.135

Rescorla, R. A., & Wagner, A. R. (1972). A theory of Pavlovian conditioning: Variations in the effectiveness of reinforcement and nonreinforcement. In A. H. Black & W. F. Prokasy (Eds.), *Classical conditioning II: Current research and theory* (pp. 64–99). Appleton-Century-Crofts.

van Minnen, A., Hendriks, L., & Olff, M. (2010). When do trauma experts choose exposure therapy for PTSD patients? A controlled study of therapist and patient factors. *Behaviour Research and Therapy, 48*(4), 312–320. https://doi.org/10.1016/j.brat.2009.12.003

2

Cognitive Therapy Supervision

Robert L. Leahy

The cognitive model advanced by A. T. Beck during the 1970s and after has had a significant influence on the treatment of depression (Hollon et al., 2021), bipolar disorder (Chiang et al., 2017), panic disorder (D. M. Clark et al., 1994), social anxiety disorder (D. M. Clark et al., 2003), posttraumatic stress disorder (Ehlers & Clark, 2000), generalized anxiety disorder (Arntz, 2003), substance abuse (McHugh et al., 2010), and personality disorders (Leahy et al., 2012). Similar to Ellis's (1994) emphasis on the relationship between thoughts and emotions, Beck's cognitive model proposes that thoughts can lead to emotions and behavior, and that individuals prone to a variety of psychopathology have predispositions to process and interpret information in a negative way (A. T. Beck et al., 1979; J. S. Beck, 2011; D. A. Clark & Beck, 2010). Thus, the emphasis in the cognitive model is on examining the specific thought patterns of the client.

In addition, Beck's model argues for specificity of thought content and unhelpful coping strategies for each of the major categories of psychopathology. For example, depression is characterized by the *negative triad* (negative beliefs about self, experience, and the future) and coping by avoidance, passivity, and rumination; anxiety is characterized by threat focus and the inability to cope with potential danger (panic disorder, generalized anxiety, social anxiety disorder) with avoidance and reassurance-seeking as coping strategies; anger is associated with perceived humiliation, disrespect, and frustration in achieving goals with coping by attack and attempts to dominate; and the various

https://doi.org/10.1037/0000314-003
Training and Supervision in Specialized Cognitive Behavior Therapy: Methods, Settings, and Populations, E. A. Storch, J. S. Abramowitz, and D. McKay (Editors)

personality disorders reflect dominant "schemas" or categories that determine how experiences are interpreted. For example, each personality disorder reflects a specific personal schema: narcissistic personality reflects the belief that one is a special and unique person; compulsive personality reflects an emphasis on order and responsibility; avoidant personality reflects the belief that one is incompetent; and dependent personality reflects the belief that one is helpless (A. T. Beck et al., 2015; Leahy et al., 2012).

The goal of psychological treatment is to alleviate symptoms but also to empower the client with the skills to utilize the cognitive model on one's own to identify, challenge, modify, and test their negative thinking and strategies. Thus, the longer term goals are not simply to relieve symptoms but also to acquire the skills that the therapist uses, so that the client becomes their own therapist. It is the difference between feeling better and being better able to cope. Throughout therapy the clinician should evaluate which techniques the client is using between sessions and how the client can anticipate problematic situations or setbacks and have a strategy of script to employ.

Cognitive therapy focuses on socializing the client to the cognitive model through bibliotherapy, instruction, and explanation; identifying cognitive biases such as automatic thoughts, assumptions, and schemas; examining the evidence for these unhelpful patterns; and setting up behavioral experiments to test out the beliefs that may impede progress. The emphasis is on the Socratic method, which is a mode of inquiry that involves questioning the client and assisting in the examination of the possible internal contradictions or problematic searching for evidence, and the biases underlying the specific thoughts, choices, emotions, and behavior.

KEY CONCEPTS FOR TRAINEES TO LEARN

Just as we encourage our clients to set goals and have an agenda, the supervisor and trainee should have specific goals for supervision. These goals include (a) learning the cognitive model, (b) using a wide variety of techniques, (c) developing a case conceptualization, (d) understanding and utilizing the model for a variety of specific diagnostic categories, (e) identifying roadblocks and overcoming them in therapy, and (f) applying the cognitive model to how the client and therapist view and respond to the therapeutic relationship. Without goals and ongoing evaluation of progress in supervision, there is a great risk of training becoming a series of episodes where fires are extinguished only to emerge once again. Moreover, supervision should be supportive but should also allow for direct feedback from both supervisor and supervisee, just as we would expect in an effective therapeutic relationship.

Clinicians within the cognitive tradition will often find that their understanding and use of the model undergoes a series of "stages" in depth and sophistication. The "naïve" early approach often simply reflects the understanding that thoughts often lead to emotions and behavior, and the novice will often rely on only a few techniques. As one gains experience, the clinician may find that they are able to develop a case conceptualization that goes beyond the fundamental "cognitive architecture" of automatic thoughts, assumptions, and schemas. Further development in training may lead to a broader, integrative view of current and past events where repeated patterns of unhelpful choices, behaviors, and vulnerabilities are identified—this entails a deeper case conceptualization (Kuyken et al., 2009; Persons, 2012). And even further development as a clinician can lead to a recognition of the role of the therapeutic relationship and the clinician's own biased predispositions to respond to certain problems in an unhelpful manner (Kazantzis et al., 2017; Leahy, 2001). The following are some of the key concepts and techniques that trainees can hope to learn in supervision.

Ongoing Evaluation

The cognitive model stresses the ongoing evaluation of behaviors, thoughts, and emotions, often utilizing self-report questionnaires (e.g., Beck Anxiety Inventory [A. T. Beck et al., 1988], Beck Depression Inventory II [BDI; A. T. Beck et al., 1996]), progress toward specific goals (e.g., increasing positive interactions, overcoming procrastination), and feedback from clients. However, it is not uncommon for therapists not to use measures of change or ask for feedback. The difficulty with a lack of ongoing evaluation for depression, for example, is that the nature of depressive pessimism is the difficulty in seeing improvement even when there has been objective improvement. For example, a client may begin treatment with a BDI of 34 (indicating significant depression) and after eight sessions may have a BDI of 17 (mild depression). The pessimistic interpretation the client might have is "I am still depressed" because they still endorse some of the items on the inventory. However, if there is ongoing evaluation, the clinician can have the client examine the changes on a variety of symptoms and also examine whether the client has a general tendency toward a negative filter of discounting the positive. Without objective measures it would be difficult to illustrate this. Thus, a 50% decrease in symptom level is certainly progress. The negative filter that can be illustrated by ongoing evaluation allows us to ascertain if the therapy is helpful and, in some cases, highlight specific symptoms that still need to be addressed. Thus, a decline of 50% on the BDI may include items of hopelessness that are still endorsed. The therapist can ask if discounting positives adds to hopelessness.

Agenda Setting

A hallmark of the traditional cognitive model is that the patient and therapist collaborate in setting an agenda for each session. This is to ensure some follow-up and continuity between sessions, to encourage the patient to think about what they wish to focus on, and to avoid therapy becoming disorganized with tangential conversations. Some clinicians are reluctant to set agendas, perhaps indicating that they do not wish to constrain the free expression that the patient may desire. In some cases, the client may not have an agenda. Rather than defer to "no agenda," the clinician can ask if this is a pattern in their lives—not having goals or relying on others to direct them. Clients with no agenda in therapy may be individuals who are not proactive or planful in daily life or who view therapy as a place to ventilate and receive validation. Expression of feelings and thoughts are important parts of therapy, but the goal in each session is to move forward in understanding unhelpful patterns and modifying them.

Automatic Thoughts, Assumptions, and Schemas

A fundamental part of the cognitive model is to help the patient identify unhelpful patterns of thinking, classify these thoughts into categories of cognitive "distortions," identify underlying rules, imperatives, and assumptions (e.g., "I must get the approval of everyone"), and identify schemas or core beliefs about self and others (e.g., self is incompetent, others are judgmental). Early on in supervision the trainee may have difficulty distinguishing between a feeling and a thought. For example, one can feel anxious, but the thought— "I am going to die from cancer"—is the focus in the cognitive model. Further, it is not uncommon for trainees to focus on the truth or falsity (or probability) of an automatic thought—for example, "He doesn't like me" (mind reading)— and overlook the more important assumption—"If someone doesn't like me, it is unbearable."

Case Conceptualization

The foregoing "cognitive architecture" (automatic thoughts, assumptions, schemas) is identified and linked together in an internally consistent pattern. For example, the schema that "I am incompetent" is linked to the assumption "I must be perfect to be accepted," which leads to the automatic thoughts "People think I am incompetent" (mind reading), "I am a failure" (labeling), and "My past success doesn't count because I do fail at some things" (discounting positives). These patterns of thinking can then be linked to earlier childhood experiences (e.g., a critical father) and unhelpful patterns of coping (e.g., avoiding challenging tasks).

KEY TECHNIQUES FOR TRAINEES TO LEARN

Cognitive therapy includes a wide range of techniques and conceptualizations that can be used in supervision. There is no one technique or one conceptualization, and it is helpful for trainees to realize that there are many ways of helping clients cope with emotions and thoughts. In this section, I review some of the more useful approaches, but we should keep in mind that cognitive therapy is a flexible approach.

Learn and Apply Cognitive Therapy Techniques

The goal is for the patient to learn the techniques that are practiced in session, so that the patient can "become their own therapist." The therapist can illustrate specific techniques in session—for example, identify the automatic thoughts, examine the degree of belief and emotion associated with that thought, examine the costs and benefits of believing the thought, examine the evidence for and against the thought, ask how the patient would think of another person who thought the same way, explore why there is a double-standard, collect evidence related to the thought, and other techniques. The goal is not simply symptom relief; it is the acquisition of the skills and understanding that can help prevent relapse.

Assigning Self-Help Homework

Cognitive therapy entails the practice and generalization of self-help. Each session should involve a demonstration of techniques and conceptualizations that are then assigned as homework of self-help between sessions. The therapist should not assume that the patient completely understands the techniques, so demonstrating them and correcting them, if need be, should be part of every session. In addition, the therapist can anticipate reluctance or difficulty in using these techniques—first, by asking the patient if they can foresee a problem with self-help and, second, offering some common reasons for not doing homework. The therapist can then troubleshoot with the client about reluctance or difficulty in doing self-help homework. The practice of homework will only work if it is carried out, and many of the patient's habitual negative thoughts are likely to surface. These include beliefs about incompetence ("I don't know how to do this"), hopelessness ("Nothing will work, so why bother"), externalization of problems ("Other people cause my problems, why should I change?"), and fear of negative evaluation ("The therapist will ridicule me if I don't do a perfect job"). These "reasons not to do homework" often reveal more general patterns in the patient's life and can be the focus of traditional cognitive therapy techniques.

Evaluating Homework

Continuity across sessions is an essential component of cognitive therapy and homework that is assigned but not reviewed is not likely to be practiced in the future. If the patient gets the idea that the homework is not important to the therapist, they are likely to assume it is not worth doing. Several factors interfere with reviewing homework. One is that the therapist does not structure the agenda in a continuous fashion, but rather surrenders the entire session to the patient. Reviewing the previous session, summarizing the points, asking for feedback, and reviewing self-help homework should be consistently part of every agenda, except for real emergencies. Second, the therapist may not want to make the patient uncomfortable about reviewing self-help homework—as if fragilizing the patient will help them build resilience. The reality is that therapy is often uncomfortable for patient and therapist and that tolerating and then examining the reasons for discomfort can be helpful in uncovering long-standing patterns of avoidance.

Asking for Feedback

Each session should involve two points at which the therapist always asks for feedback: the beginning and ending of the session. At the beginning, the therapist should ask for feedback about the previous session. This allows the therapist to learn what is working and what is not working, explore mutual misunderstandings and frustrations, and address difficulties. The ending of the session should also involve asking for feedback for the same reasons. It may be that the therapist fears asking for "negative feedback" because it will under-mine their self-confidence. This leads to missing what is going on with the patient, who may feel disengaged, annoyed, hopeless, or misunderstood. Indeed, it would be useful to openly explore if the patient would feel reluctant about giving negative feedback. For example, one concern a patient might have is that the therapist will become defensive and angry and might terminate the patient. The therapist should be prepared to receive negative feedback—even unfair criticism—since this is simply more information; if correct, negative feedback can help the therapist modify what they are doing, and, if incorrect, it can help the therapist observe how the patient may interpret relationships that matter.

Examining Your Own Thoughts and Assumptions

One of the most effective ways to learn cognitive therapy is to apply it to oneself. Therapists have their own set of automatic thoughts, assumptions, and schemas that may affect the success of therapy (Leahy, 2001). For example, the therapist may view the client's suicidal ideation as "catastrophic," as opposed to a symptom that often accompanies depression and anxiety. Other exam-ples of automatic thought biases include personalizing (viewing the client's response as a personal insult), discounting positives (not realizing that some improvement is still improvement), labeling (reducing the client to a diagnostic category), overgeneralizing (seeing a pattern where there is really variation), and emotional reasoning (equating one's own anxiety with a bad outcome). Improvement in therapy is typically gradual, not linear, and there are likely to be setbacks as events and variation of mood are manifested. I have found it helpful to write down the therapist's automatic thoughts and examine them using the traditional cognitive therapy techniques. In addition, maladaptive assumptions can also be examined. These include the view "I should cure all my patients," "If the patient does not improve, then I am a bad therapist," and "My patients should always like me and appreciate my efforts." Other personal schemas may also impede therapy, such as the view that the therapist is a special person and should be viewed that way, concerns about abandonment, beliefs that one should be able to be autonomous, and demanding standards for the self and patients.

Specific Techniques

Many cognitive therapists—including novices and experienced therapists—fall into the pattern of using a few techniques rather than drawing on a wide range of techniques that may be available. Leahy (2017), for example, described over 100 techniques with specific examples, dialogues, and problems. In Table 2.1 we can see examples of a number of helpful techniques that may be used. Supervisors might suggest that therapists vary their routine if they generally tend to rely on a restricted range of cognitive techniques.

TABLE 2.1. Cognitive Therapy Techniques

Technique	Example
1. Distinguish between thoughts, feelings, and facts	Indicate that a feeling (anxious, sad) is different from a thought ("I am a failure") that can be tested against the facts—for example, "Have you failed at everything?"
2. Identify automatic thoughts and categorize them	Identify thoughts associated with problematic behavior of feelings and categorize them. For example, Mind Reading, Fortune Telling, Catastrophizing, Labeling, Discounting the Positive, etc.
3. Rate belief in thought and intensity of emotions	How much do you believe you are a failure and how sad do you feel, using a scale from 0–100?
4. Examine costs and benefits of believing a thought	What are the costs to you and benefits of believing this thought? How would things be different for you if you believed it less?
5. Identify maladaptive assumptions	What are your "if–then" thoughts, your "rules," and your "shoulds"? For example, "I should succeed at everything," or "If I don't succeed at a task, I am a failure."
6. Use vertical arrow	Look at the implication of a string of your thoughts. For example, "If I don't do well, then I am a failure, then I will fail at everything, then no one will want to be with me, then my life will have no meaning."
7. Identify core beliefs and schemas about self and others	What are the core issues that arise for you? For example, the need to be special, the belief that you are incompetent, the idea that you are responsible for everything.
8. Examine the evidence for and against the thought	Identify and weigh the evidence for and against your thought. For example, what is the evidence that you are a failure, what is the evidence you are not a failure?
9. Use semantic technique	What does this label mean? What does it mean to be a failure and not a failure?
10. How would someone else see it?	Would other people have a different view of these events? Why is your view different from theirs?

(continues)

TABLE 2.1. Cognitive Therapy Techniques (*Continued*)

Technique	Example
11. What advice would you give a friend who believed this?	What would you tell your best friend if they were saying this? Why would you be more generous or less generous with a friend than you are with yourself? Is there a reason for your double standard?
12. Monitor activities, thoughts, and feelings	Keep track of your activities, thoughts, and feelings for a week and notice if there is a pattern.
13. Set up an experiment and collect information	Set up a series of experiments, and see if your predictions are accurate. For example, if you think that you are a failure, try a variety of tasks for a week and see if you obtain any success.
14. Act against the thought	Engage in behavior that is the opposite action of your thought. Act as if you are not a failure. Act as if you are confident.
15. View events along a continuum	Rather than view things as black and white or catastrophic, view events along a 0-to-100 continuum with the worst possible outcome at 100. Are you viewing things out of proportion?
16. Consider changing your goal	Rather than getting stuck on one goal where you are frustrated, consider changing your goal.
17. Consider changing expectations	Rather than expect something that is not happening, consider changing your expectation to match what is happening.
18. Get into a time machine	How will you feel about this next week, next month, next year? Why will your feelings change?
19. Aim for indifference	What if you became indifferent about this event? How would that help you? Have you become indifferent about things that bothered you?
20. Examine how your feelings have changed about past problems	Looking back to the past, why have your feelings changed so much? Could this also be true for what you are feeling now?

WHAT PATIENT CHARACTERISTICS MAKE FOR A GOOD TRAINING CASE (AND WHAT MAKES FOR A POOR TRAINING CASE)?

Training and supervision do not need to be like a Navy SEAL's survival of the fittest ordeal. We want trainees to learn and experience success, not fail to change a patient that no one has ever helped. Trainees will be like other therapists and have considerable difficulty with clients who have severe depression, abuse substances, lack motivation for change, or fail to engage in therapy for other reasons. Everyone has difficulty working with such individuals! The ideal training case is a patient with emotional discomfort who is motivated to change, has the capacity for insight into their difficulties, has few co-occurring psychological difficulties, does not have psychotic symptoms, and is able to attend therapy on a regular basis. The capacity for insight, understanding, and acceptance of the cognitive model and an optimistic view of psychological treatments will be most desirable for trainees to work with. This is not to say that the patients without these characteristics cannot be treated, but they are likely to have more success with a more experienced therapist as opposed to a trainee.

COMMON MISTAKES TRAINEES MAKE AND HOW TO FIX THEM

Anyone learning cognitive therapy is likely to make "mistakes" in using the wide range of techniques and conceptualizations that the model provides. In this section, I review seven common problems and how the supervisor may help the clinician.

Jumping on the First "Irrational Response"

The clinician may be eager to identify and modify "irrational" or "unhelpful" thoughts and may quickly focus on the first statement that the client makes. For example, the client may say, "I don't think she likes me," and the clinician immediately identifies this as "mind reading." The problem with too quick a response like this is that the "automatic thought" may be true and may lead the client to think that the clinician is naïve or simply practicing "the power of positive thinking." This undermines the credibility of the therapy. In addition, focusing too quickly on the "cognitive distortion" of the first statements may impede the therapeutic relationship and lead to missing out on the opportunity to explore the deeper meaning. That is, "What would it mean if she didn't like you?" This question can lead to identifying maladaptive assumptions and schemas of a more general and pervasive nature.

Sounding Like an Interrogator

Beginning cognitive therapists can sometimes come across like an aggressive prosecutor cross-examining a witness they are trying to catch in a lie or contradiction. This is not the Socratic method that Beck has advanced, but rather a method of legal disputation. The session should not sound like browbeating. Still, eager and enthusiastic novices are sometimes determined to prove that the patient is wrong. For example, I recall supervising a new therapist who was clever and articulate. We conducted a role play wherein I took the role of a patient who was often inhibited and self-critical, and he played the therapist. He badgered me with one rational response after another, pointing out how illogical and irrational I was. I asked him, "How do you think the patient would have felt about this interaction?" He looked at me bewildered: "I never thought about that. I have no idea." I said, "Well, if the patient is self-critical and inhibited and you are telling him how illogical he is, he's likely to feel humiliated and defeated . . . and perhaps even more self-critical. It's likely he won't return." The Socratic method is not a debate in which the therapist scores points and the patient loses points. Rather, it is best thought of as "guided discovery" that progresses at a slower pace, allowing for reflection on the part of the patient (Waltman et al., 2021).

Not Going Deeper Beyond the First Thoughts

Once an automatic thought is identified, the clinician can dig deeper, using the *downward arrow* technique: "Let's say she actually doesn't like you . . . what would that mean to you?" This can lead to a string of implications that reveal general assumptions. For example,

> If she doesn't like me, I must be boring. If I am boring, then no one will like me. If no one likes me, I am a total loser. I will end up alone. I will always be depressed. Life won't be worth living.

Thus, the downward arrow reveals in this case the assumption "If I don't get people to like me, then I am a loser" and "If one person doesn't like me, then no one will." These general assumptions underpin and give power to the negative thoughts. After all, everyone has people who do not like them, but that does not mean no one will like them.

Not Examining Whether the Rational Response Is Relevant

A frequent mistake that trainees make is that they focus on "alternative responses" that sound "positive" as evidence or arguments against the automatic thought. But the rational response should be relevant to disputing or proving that the automatic thought is not reasonable, rational, or factual. For example, a client came up with the following "rational response" to the thought "I will fail the exam": "I am a good person. I try hard. People like me." Each of these statements could be true, but none of them are relevant to the automatic thought about failing an exam. More relevant responses would be the following:

> I have done well on other exams. I have studied, and I can study more. There is no evidence I will fail. I don't have to get a perfect score to pass the exam. Even if I don't do well, it will not be catastrophic.

One way of looking at this is to ask, "Has the rational response put the lie to the automatic thought? Has it really decreased the credibility of that thought?"

Not Eliciting Thoughts

The trainee may be eager to jump to the solution and may tell the client what they are "probably thinking" and dictate to the client the "correct" response. For example, in conducting a role play with a supervisee, we were able to identify how the trainee dogmatically guessed at the client's thoughts and even the underlying assumptions, without exploring how the client actually was thinking. This can often lead to missing what may appear to be the idiosyncratic thoughts and implications that the client may have.

Not Going for the Ultimate Downward Arrow

This is a variant of the previous problem of not going deeper. The trainee may stop using the downward arrow when they reach a negative thought like, "Then that would mean I am a loser." But, one can go even further with this thought and ask, "What would be the worst thing about being a loser?" This might lead to other consequences and implications that are not readily apparent, such as, "I would disappoint my parents" or "If I am a loser, I'm not perfect; and if I'm not perfect, then life is not worth living." Thus, the ultimate fear is that one is not perfect, that the only meaningful experiences must involve perfection, that one should never disappoint one's parents. Digging deeper using the downward arrow may reveal a wide range of core beliefs or schemas that can make the therapy far more meaningful and of deeper relevance.

Not Looking for Lifelong Patterns

Increasingly, as clinicians focus on staying in the moment and quickly using techniques, there is less emphasis among many people practicing cognitive behavior therapy (CBT) to explore lifelong patterns. We know now that many patients will experience recurrence of major depressive disorder (Burcusa & Iacono, 2007) or anxiety disorders (Scholten et al., 2013). It is almost as if some therapists believe that they are practicing emergency medicine rather than also looking for chronic diathesis. This is especially common among novices who may not have enough life or clinical experience to recognize that there are patterns in the lives of some troubled people. For example, a trainee who was eager to do well in "curing" patients seldom obtained enough life history to explore any patterns in the lives of most of his clients. This led him to practice a short term, somewhat effective but not entirely long-lasting therapy. Thus, clients might have some symptom relief but later would relapse to their old patterns. The supervisor, who has more clinical experience, should be attentive to this myopic approach and direct the trainee toward exploring other patterns of problematic behavior. For example, a client whose anger and depression were often triggered by criticism from authority figures and romantic partners had been initially focused on "automatic thoughts," such as personalizing, mind reading, and catastrophic thinking. This approach worked up to a point, but the patterns continued in other areas of his life. When the clinician explored the history of these patterns—going back to the client's earlier marriage that ended in divorce and conflicts with his boss in two previous jobs—what emerged was a core schema of not being good enough, being humiliated by others, and needing to dominate and defeat others to avoid "losing" and "being a loser."

Getting Stuck on Too Few Techniques

Clinicians are creatures of habit who can easily fall into habitual ways of responding to their clients. For example, the novice therapist may find themselves relying on a handful of techniques, not realizing that there may be literally hundreds of ways of approaching the dilemmas that the client is facing (Leahy, 2017). It often remains an empirical question as to which techniques will be helpful for a particular client. The supervisor can also be limited to a few habitual strategies of change. Both supervisor and trainee should consider the following question: "What other techniques might I use? How would someone from a different CBT orientation approach this?" Cognitive therapy is part of a larger approach—CBT—and the clinician should be flexible to draw on techniques from mindfulness, ACT, behavior activation, dialectical behavior therapy (DBT), and metacognitive therapy. And the clinician should familiarize themselves with the wide range of techniques within the cognitive therapy model.

Not Recognizing What Is Not on the Agenda

The traditional cognitive model emphasized the idea that the client should set the agenda, with the therapist also adding "set items" such as reviewing the previous session, reviewing homework, and assigning self-help. However, what may be as important at times is what is not placed on the agenda. The agenda-driven model runs the risk of missing issues such as shame, reluctance to discuss substance abuse, anger control, or other uncomfortable topics. Taking a life history and searching for difficult patterns and issues may instruct the therapist as to what is not being said. Since avoidance is a key strategy of coping for anxious and depressed clients, their reluctance to talk about certain topics will find its way to agenda-setting. The supervisor may also be limited at times by an emphasis on the client setting the agenda. Thus, there is implicit collaboration of avoidance in the therapy. The supervisor can indicate to the trainee that this is a risk of too rigid adherence to agenda setting. Statements that might be helpful are the following:

> Sometimes it is natural to avoid topics that are uncomfortable. We all are ill at ease about something. This might affect what we talk about in sessions. I would like you to think about which issues you might be uncomfortable talking about. The reason that this is important is that we cannot solve problems unless we know about them and share them.

In addition, the supervisor can suggest that there may be valuable insights that can be gained by understanding which topics are "hidden" and why. For example, the client may feel embarrassed talking about sex or substance abuse or might fear that the therapist will judge them or that discussing the topic will lead to things going out of control. This allows the therapy to become more meaningful, touching on the very "secrets" that the client believes are necessary to hold onto. One cannot build trust by holding on to secrets that are never discussed.

ETHICAL ISSUES IN TREATMENT APPLICATION

New therapists are often eager to share their experiences in supervision with supervisors, colleagues, and friends. This can sometimes lead to violations of confidentiality. For example, the supervised may disclose too much identifying information to the supervisor, so that the client's identity and the identity of other people who are discussed are revealed. Even more problematic is the risk of the supervisee discussing clients with friends and other colleagues, where the client's confidentiality is once again sacrificed. This has become increasingly problematic on professional Listservs where therapists will give detailed information about a client in treatment. The test should be if someone heard or read this information—including the client—would they be able to identify who it is. The supervisor should be aware of these risks and periodically discuss confidentiality with supervisees.

Another potential ethical issue is to oversell the treatment to the client, making promises that cannot be kept. As new trainees are often eager to persuade the client and themselves of the value of the treatment, it is common for supervisees to instruct clients that "if you do this, then you can expect that." All interventions should be discussed in terms of tentative possibilities, relative advantages and disadvantages, and as one set of approaches among many. For example, cognitive restructuring does not always work, homework is not always useful, and people in treatment sometimes do not improve. It is advisable to present options as "experiments"—"Let's see what happens over the next few weeks if you do some of these things." In addition, supervisees should be open to considering other interventions both within the CBT camp and in the biomedical camp. For example, for refractory depression that does not respond to cognitive therapy, consultation with other professionals with expertise in the use of next line therapeutics (e.g., transcranial magnetic stimulation) might be indicated. The main issue is not to rigidly adhere to your approach only, since the client has come to us seeking effective treatment, not fidelity to a movement.

COMMON OBSTACLES IN SUPERVISION AND WAYS OF OVERCOMING THEM

Being a supervisee is often a difficult position for the novice who is learning a new approach from someone with ostensibly more power and experience. Some trainees find themselves intimidated and will often be reluctant to discuss cases where they are having a difficult time. They do not wish to seem incompetent and may use supervision as an attempt to impress the more "expert" supervisor. I have found it helpful to anticipate this reluctance by telling trainees the following:

> All of us are always learning and no one has perfect techniques and no one cures all their patients. I may learn as much from you as you learn from me. My style of doing therapy does not have to be your style. But I hope that you can trust this process and me, and that you will feel free to bring the most difficult problems so that we can brainstorm together. This all means bringing to our work what you consider "mistakes," since we will learn the most from what are mistakes or impasses.

Another obstacle in supervision is what I call the "hypomanic cognitive therapist." This is not a psychiatric diagnosis. Rather, it describes a communication style that some therapists may have early in training, where they try to implode the client with as many techniques as possible. Sessions can sound like an interrogation of a hostile witness in a felony trial. Helping trainees slow down their communication, give the client room to breathe and reflect, and set aside their sense of urgency can help the therapeutic relationship.

Although cognitive therapists are not often known for their attention to transference and countertransference, these are issues in any therapeutic relationship (Leahy, 2001). One aspect of this is what I have described as the "emotional schemas" of the therapist. This term refers to the beliefs that the therapist has about the client's emotions (Leahy, 2015). For example, a therapist with negative schemas might believe that the client's emotions will last forever, go out of control, don't make sense, completely define the identity of the client, and are dangerous. As a consequence, the therapist may feel they are walking on eggshells and cannot directly raise issues that arouse strong affect. The supervisor can inquire from the trainee whether they sometimes have these beliefs and does this lead to avoidance of more direct interventions such as challenging beliefs, engaging in behavioral experiences, or recalling traumatic memories. The supervisor can then validate, normalize, and make sense of these beliefs while also setting up behavioral experiments by the supervisor and collect information about the "danger" of emotions.

CONCLUSION

Perhaps the most important message to convey in supervision is that it is the clinician's job to develop a nonjudgmental curiosity about why the client's thoughts and feelings make sense to them. It may often seem like cognitive therapy can be disputatious and even invalidating, but it need not be. In fact, the cognitive approach reveals how depression, anxiety, and anger "make sense," given the client's construction of reality. Of course, the point is that there are different ways of seeing things, but curiosity about how the client sees things may help unlock a string of assumptions and schemas that would otherwise be overlooked. Never assume you know what someone else is thinking. That is a key part of the Socratic dialogue. Conveying this in therapy will make the experience for both client and therapist more relevant, more interesting, and more validating. Understanding someone is different from telling them how you think they think.

I have reviewed a number of the goals and pitfalls in supervision—learning how to conduct therapy is an exercise in acquiring knowledge, communicating, understanding, and persuasion. But it is also an exercise in humility. Too often, trainees vacillate between believing they know everything and fearing they know nothing. Indeed, being an effective therapist involves learning something new—primarily from your patients and from your own response to patients. The wise supervisor is able to communicate their own incompleteness—they are not gurus, saints, or perfect iconic figures. Just like our patients and our trainees, we will never have it "just right." Helping trainees realize that their struggle forward is the same journey that the supervisor is on—and will continue to follow. The supervisor is not qualitatively different from the trainee. We are all trainees and will remain so. It is like the castle in the distance where you think the answers are, but you can never reach—you can only hope to get closer to what you do not understand. In short, good supervision is reflecting that the journey will continue for both the trainee and the more experienced supervisor, and that the cognitive model is a vehicle that carries you forward but is not itself the destination. This is why when training people in cognitive therapy, I say, "This is one way of doing this. But the good news is that there are many ways. There is no final answer. And that is exciting—and perhaps a little frightening at times."

REFERENCES

Arntz, A. (2003). Cognitive therapy versus applied relaxation as treatment of generalized anxiety disorder. *Behaviour Research and Therapy, 41*(6), 633–646. https://doi.org/10.1016/S0005-7967(02)00045-1

Beck, A. T., Davis, D. D., & Freeman, A. (2015). *Cognitive therapy of personality disorders* (3rd ed.). Guilford Press.

Beck, A. T., Epstein, N., Brown, G., & Steer, R. (1988). Beck Anxiety Inventory [Database record]. *APA PsycTests.* https://doi.org/10.1037/t02025-000

Beck, A. T., Rush, A. J., Shaw, B. F., & Emery, G. (1979). *Cognitive therapy of depression.* Guilford Press.

Beck, A. T., Steer, R. A., & Brown, G. K. (1996). *Manual for the Beck Depression Inventory-II.* Psychological Corporation.

Beck, J. S. (2011). *Cognitive behavior therapy: Basics and beyond* (2nd ed.). Guilford Press.

Burcusa, S. L., & Iacono, W. G. (2007). Risk for recurrence in depression. *Clinical Psychology Review, 27*(8), 959–985. https://doi.org/10.1016/j.cpr.2007.02.005

Chiang, K. J., Tsai, J. C., Liu, D., Lin, C. H., Chiu, H. L., & Chou, K. R. (2017). Efficacy of cognitive-behavioral therapy in patients with bipolar disorder: A meta-analysis of randomized controlled trials. *PLOS ONE, 12*(5), e0176849. https://doi.org/10.1371/journal.pone.0176849

Clark, D. A., & Beck, A. T. (2010). *Cognitive therapy of anxiety disorders: Science and practice.* Guilford Press.

Clark, D. M., Ehlers, A., McManus, F., Hackmann, A., Fennell, M., Campbell, H., Flower, T., Davenport, C., & Louis, B. (2003). Cognitive therapy versus fluoxetine in generalized social phobia: A randomized placebo-controlled trial. *Journal of Consulting and Clinical Psychology, 71*(6), 1058–1067. https://doi.org/10.1037/0022-006X.71.6.1058

Clark, D. M., Salkovskis, P. M., Hackmann, A., Middleton, H., Anastasiades, P., & Gelder, M. (1994). A comparison of cognitive therapy, applied relaxation and imipramine in the treatment of panic disorder. *British Journal of Psychiatry, 164*(6), 759–769. https://doi.org/10.1192/bjp.164.6.759

Ehlers, A., & Clark, D. M. (2000). A cognitive model of posttraumatic stress disorder. *Behaviour Research and Therapy, 38*(4), 319–345. https://doi.org/10.1016/S0005-7967(99)00123-0

Ellis, A. (1994). *Reason and emotion in psychotherapy* (2nd ed.). Carol Publishing Company.

Hollon, S. D., DeRubeis, R. J., Andrews, P. W., & Thomson, J. A. (2021). Cognitive therapy in the treatment and prevention of depression: A fifty-year retrospective with an evolutionary coda. *Cognitive Therapy and Research, 45*(3), 402–417. https://doi.org/10.1007/s10608-020-10132-1

Kazantzis, N., Dattilio, F. M., & Dobson, K. S. (2017). *The therapeutic relationship in cognitive-behavioral therapy: A clinician's guide.* Guilford Press.

Kuyken, W., Padesky, C., & Dudley, R. (2009). *Collaborative case conceptualization: Working effectively with clients in cognitive-behavioral therapy.* Guilford Press.

Leahy, R. L. (2001). *Overcoming resistance in cognitive therapy.* Guilford Press.

Leahy, R. L. (2015). *Emotional schema therapy.* Guilford Press.

Leahy, R. L. (2017). *Cognitive therapy techniques: A practitioner's guide* (2nd ed.). Guilford Press.

Leahy, R. L., McGinn, L., & Davis, D. (2012). Cognitive therapy for personality disorders. In T. Widiger (Ed.), *Oxford handbook of personality disorders* (2nd ed., Part 5). Oxford University Press. https://doi.org/10.1093/oxfordhb/9780199735013.013.0034

McHugh, R. K., Hearon, B. A., & Otto, M. W. (2010). Cognitive behavioral therapy for substance use disorders. *Psychiatric Clinics of North America, 33*(3), 511–525. https://doi.org/10.1016/j.psc.2010.04.012

Persons, J. (2012). *The case formulation approach to cognitive-behavior therapy.* Guilford Press.

Scholten, W. D., Batelaan, N. M., van Balkom, A. J. L. M., Penninx, B. W. J. H., Smit, J. H., & van Oppen, P. (2013). Recurrence of anxiety disorders and its predictors. *Journal of Affective Disorders, 147*(1-3), 180–185. https://doi.org/10.1016/j.jad.2012.10.031

Waltman, S. H., Codd, R. T., III, McFarr, L. M., & Moore, B. A. (2021). *Socratic questioning for therapists and counselors: Learn how to think and intervene like a cognitive behavior therapist.* Routledge.

3

Supervision and Training in Rational Emotive Behavior Therapy

Kristene A. Doyle, Michael Hickey, and Raymond DiGiuseppe

Rational emotive behavior therapy (REBT), originally named *rational therapy*, was developed by Dr. Albert Ellis in 1955 and is one of the original forms of cognitive behavior therapy (CBT). Ellis was trained as a psychoanalyst and developed REBT when he became disenchanted with the results of his psychoanalytic practice (Ellis, 1962). Ellis was highly influenced by philosophy, and Stoicism in particular, when developing REBT. Consistent with Stoic philosophy, REBT posits that it is not the experiences from childhood that lead to emotional disturbance, but rather it is the attitude and life philosophy that one takes at an early age, which is often maintained throughout adulthood. REBT's philosophical roots are illustrated in a quote from Stoic philosopher Epictetus, who stated, "Men are disturbed not by things, but by the views which they take of them" (Dryden, 2002).

Based on this philosophical influence, Ellis developed the ABC model of REBT. A represents an *activating event*, which is something that an individual encounters and can be a situation, a thought, or an emotion. B represents an individual's *beliefs* and attitudes about the activating event, and C is the emotional and behavioral *consequences* resulting from the individual's beliefs when confronted with an activating event. According to REBT theory, emotional and behavioral disturbance result from *irrational beliefs* (IBs), defined as rigid, illogical, dysfunctional, and inconsistent with reality. IBs lead to unhealthy negative emotions (UNEs; e.g., depression, anxiety, unhealthy anger, shame, hurt, guilt, jealousy, unhealthy envy) and maladaptive behavior, and interfere

https://doi.org/10.1037/0000314-004
Training and Supervision in Specialized Cognitive Behavior Therapy: Methods, Settings, and Populations, E. A. Storch, J. S. Abramowitz, and D. McKay (Editors)

with goal achievement. The four IBs include (a) demandingness; (b) frustration intolerance; (c) awfulizing/catastrophizing; and (d) self-, other-, and life-condemnation. *Demandingness* is the dogmatic expectation that individuals, events, and life should or must be exactly the way a person wishes them to be. *Awfulizing* involves exaggerating the negative consequences of something to an extreme and is often referred to as "end of the world" thinking. *Frustration intolerance* (FI) refers to believing that things should come easily and/or the belief that one cannot stand or tolerate discomfort. The IB of *condemnation* refers to the global rating of oneself, others, or life based on any given factor (e.g., behavior, failures, achievements, etc.) and operates under the implication that the worth of human beings can be rated (DiGiuseppe et al., 2014). Thus, a core tenet of REBT is that unconditional self, other, and life acceptance promotes psychological well-being.

Among the cognitive behavior therapies, REBT uniquely posits a theory of emotion that involves a qualitative as opposed to a quantitative change in emotion (Ellis, 1962). Rather than reducing the intensity of the emotion, REBT emphasizes the importance of a qualitative shift from unhealthy to healthy negative emotions. This change occurs by having the client challenge and question their IBs and replace them with *rational beliefs* (RBs), which are defined as flexible, logical, functional, and consistent with reality. RBs result in healthy negative emotions (HNEs; e.g., sadness, concern, healthy anger or annoyance, disappointment, regret, healthy envy) and promote adaptive behavior and goal attainment (David et al., 2009).

Since its beginning, REBT has been used to treat numerous emotional problems and psychological disorders (Ellis, 1962). A recent meta-analytic review (David et al., 2018) provided strong support for REBT as an effective transdiagnostic psychotherapy.

KEY CONCEPTS FOR TRAINEES TO LEARN

REBT shares several concepts with all psychotherapies (DiGiuseppe, 2021). The first of these is that common factors contribute to the effectiveness of all psychotherapies. Some common factors include forming a therapeutic alliance, unconditionally accepting the client, providing the client a safe, confidential, empathetic relationship with the psychotherapist, and presenting the client with a rationale of the presenting problem and for the therapy itself. Many trainees new to REBT jump in to dispute clients' IBs and fail to attend to the common factors.

Trainees have to learn the ABC model of emotional experience. Each time a client experiences a disturbing emotion or performs a dysfunctional behavior, the sequence of experiences is fitted to this ABC model. It is impossible to proceed in any discussion of REBT if the trainee cannot differentiate these aspects of clients' experiences.

REBT distinguishes between (a) cognitions that represent the possible future or the past occurrence of adverse events (e.g., "I am likely to fail the exam") and (b) beliefs that are imperatives or evaluations of those possible occurrences (e.g., "If I failed the exam, it would mean that I am a failure!") and targets the latter, focusing on imperative beliefs that adverse events must not occur (demandingness), the extreme evaluations of the events (awfulizing), one's ability to cope with the events (frustration intolerance), or the worthlessness of the people involved in the events (global evaluations of human worth). This strategy of not challenging cognitive errors about the likelihood of adverse events and instead challenging IBs is called the *elegant* or *philosophical solution*. The *inelegant* or *practical solution* challenges distortions about probability or likelihood of negative events. The philosophical solution is considered preferable because it provides the client with a coping strategy, even if the undesirable events occur.

It is imperative for trainees to understand that REBT has a unique view of human emotions. It does not adhere to the common idea that emotions differ along a single continuum from weak to strong and that reducing the intensity of the emotion leads to less disturbance. Instead, REBT posits that humans can have at least two different emotional reactions within the same family of emotions, UNEs and HNEs. IBs lead to UNE, and RBs led to HNEs. Healthy negative emotion acknowledges that an adverse event has occurred and mobilizes the person to appropriately focus on the problem and consider an adaptive response to it. An REBT practitioner treating a patient with depression works with that individual to develop RBs that would facilitate sadness rather than depression.

REBT also makes a distinction between emotion disturbance and meta-disturbance. In *metadisturbance*, a person's internal experience (their thoughts, images, or emotions) become the activating event about which they have IBs that cause further disturbance about the disturbance. REBT posits that therapists target the metadisturbance first because a discussion about ABCs can trigger the IBs about that disturbance, cause more disturbance, and distract the client from attending to the first ABCs.

KEY TECHNIQUES FOR TRAINEES TO LEARN

In this section, we discuss the main clinical strategies and interventions that we look for trainees to learn and apply. In addition, we have included an evaluation form that we use with our supervisees to assess REBT technical skill development (see Figure 3.1).

Establishing Goals and Tasks of Therapy

Many clients are more interested in changing or escaping the activating event or adversity (i.e., the practical solution), rather than working on their cognitive reactions to the event (i.e., the emotional solution). REBT therapists typically strive to first work on the *emotional solution* and then engage in practical

FIGURE 3.1. Student Evaluation Form

_____
(NAME)

STUDENT EVALUATION FORM

SKILL AREA For each item, mark "✓" or "x"	Session 1	Session 2	Session 3	Session 4
Identified a specific problem				
Asked for a specific example of the problem				
Asked about the Critical A				
Identified specific emotional & behavioral C's				
Discriminated between healthy & unhealthy C's				
Established agreement on the goals & tasks of the session				
Assessed and identified irrational belief(s)				
Discriminated between rational and irrational B's				
Established B-C connection				
Debated IBs (functional, empirical, logical, semantic, friend, philosophical)				
Established Full Rational Belief				
Relevant homework was negotiated				
RATE PARTICIPANT 1 TO 5 (See scale at bottom):				
Overall performance in the session				
COMMON ERRORS: (Put letter in appropriate box)				
P = Too passive				
C = Too confrontational				
L = Too much lecturing				
A = Let client discuss A's in too much detail				
A-C = Used A-C language (e.g., It made you feel . . .)				
FACULTY INITIALS:				

✓ - Adequately achieved skill
x - Failed to achieve skill
1 - Excellent, outstanding (top 10% overall of Primary Certificate Practicum participants)
2 - Good, above average, satisfactory
3 - Fair, average, but still satisfactory
4 - Poor, needs to demonstrate improved skills
5 - Inadequate, should not be awarded certificate

problem-solving where applicable. Indeed, sometimes there is no practical solution for the client's problem. Moreover, clients will more successfully problem solve and implement a solution when they are not as emotionally activated. When clients enter therapy focused on changing the activating event, we recommend trainees engage them in *motivational syllogism*, which involves the following four steps:

1. socratically eliciting from the client all of the negative consequences of their present emotion and/or behavior;

2. teaching the client that an acceptable alternative emotion/behavior exists in the presence of the current activating event that will not have these negative consequences;

3. teaching the connection between beliefs and emotional/behavioral consequences; and

4. reinforcing the idea that to change dysfunctional emotion and maladaptive behavior requires changing cognitions.

Steps 1 and 2 address agreement on the goals of therapy, and Step 4 addresses agreement on the tasks of therapy.

Teaching the Binary Model of Emotions

REBT's conceptualization of emotions incorporates the binary model of emotional distress. According to this perspective, there is a qualitative distinction between dysfunctional and functional emotions, rather than a quantitative difference (Ellis & DiGiuseppe, 1993). Trainees teach their clients that concern is not simply "less" anxiety, but rather a qualitatively different emotion stemming from different belief systems (i.e., IBs vs. RBs). As a result, unlike other CBT approaches, REBT aims to replace dysfunctional emotions with functional (albeit still negative) ones (e.g., Hyland & Boduszek, 2012).

Inference Chaining and Hypothetico-Deductive Method of Assessment

When therapists assess for IBs about particular situations, clients often relate automatic thoughts and inferences. To address this issue, trainees are taught the technique of *inference chaining*, in which the client's inferences are linked to uncover the IBs being held. The client's inferences are assumed temporarily to be true, and through conjunctive phrasing and/or incomplete sentences, the therapist continues to ask questions such as "Let's assume that to be true, and then what?" or "What would that mean for you?" until one or more IBs are discovered. In the hypothetico–deductive method, trainees use REBT theory to formulate and present hypotheses to their clients about their emotional and/or behavioral disturbances, which can be confirmed, rejected, or modified.

Disputation/Cognitive Restructuring of Irrational Beliefs

The process of disputing IBs is a form of debating the unrealistic, illogical, and typically self-defeating nature of the client's thinking. This technique is an attempt to change the client's erroneous beliefs through the use of persuasion (DiGiuseppe et al., 2014). Several different types of disputation questions may be used during the cognitive restructuring process, including functional/ pragmatic, logical, empirical, philosophical, and semantic. The goal is to engage the client in scientific thinking while helping them to examine their own beliefs. Disputation in REBT is sometimes misunderstood or viewed as arguing with the client, largely due to an error on the trainee's part of failing to prepare the client for the disputation process (see the section on common mistakes later in this chapter).

Generating Full Rational Alternative Beliefs

Although disputation is an important technique for trainees to learn and exercise in REBT, we also emphasize the generation of replacement RBs. The idea behind this is that even though a client may recognize the self-defeating nature of their current IBs, if they do not have something to replace these with, they will continue to hold onto the IBs. RBs are nonabsolute evaluative cognitions typically worded as preferences, desires, wants, or wishes, leading to healthy, functional negative emotions, and adaptive behavior(s) in the presence of adverse activating events. An example of a full RB for the IB "People must respect me," would be "I want people to respect me, but there is no reason that they must." The goal of generating full RBs is to negate the IB and ensure clients are unable to "sneak" back in an IB.

Negotiating Homework Assignments and Identifying Obstacles to Completion

A common thread to all the CBT approaches is the use of homework to reinforce concepts and ideas discussed in therapy. Homework in REBT is no different, but it is a skill that trainees often need to learn. We aim to teach trainees how to negotiate with their clients in assigning tasks that are challenging but not overwhelming. Collaboration with the client is the key approach when doing so. Furthermore, the importance of identifying any practical or emotional obstacles that may interfere with carrying out the assignment is taught to trainees to increase the likelihood of completion and success.

PATIENT CHARACTERISTICS FOR A GOOD (AND POOR) TRAINING CASE WITH REBT

Several factors and patient characteristics contribute to a good training case with REBT. Therapists that are early in their training can benefit from working with clients who are motivated to change. Since REBT involves the patient taking emotional responsibility, clients who are open to exploring their belief systems and are willing to work collaboratively with their therapist tend to be optimal in assisting novice REBT practitioners in cultivating their skills. Contrarily, patients who are overly agreeable may make for a poor REBT training case because they may be overly passive, fearful of offending the therapist if they disagree with a hypothesis that is offered, or may have certain needs for approval that play out during the therapy session. More experienced REBT therapists may recognize this and address the IBs that are creating this dynamic, but therapists early in their training may have difficulty doing so.

Patients who are committed to the therapy process and attend their sessions regularly also set the stage for a good training experience for supervisees. Change in REBT is dependent not only on the skills of the therapist but also on the willingness of the patient to actively engage in homework assignments that help facilitate lasting, philosophical change.

Some patients seek therapy to get advice, solutions to practical problems, or even companionship. These cases may not be suitable for training in that REBT aims to work through the emotional problems that lead to barriers to goal achievement. Patients who are not reporting any emotional distress or refuse to explore how their emotions may be impacting their functioning typically do not provide a good training experience for new REBT therapists. Similarly, those who are extremely dysregulated during sessions may interfere with an REBT supervisees' ability to practice and enhance their skills because the majority of the session may be spent on trying to calm the patient. Finally, patients who are highly suicidal do not make for good training cases in that much of the session may be dedicated to suicide assessment and safety planning.

It is common for patients to want to spend time discussing their activating events and to, at times, become tangential in their thought processes. In these cases, supervisees can hone their skills of redirecting, focusing the patient, and establishing a goal orientation. However, in some cases, patients cannot be "reigned in" despite the best efforts of therapists to redirect and structure the session. Some such patients may be experiencing cognitive or neurological impairment, a manic episode, or even psychosis. While these factors are not necessarily exclusionary criteria for REBT training cases, they do present challenges that can interfere with the supervisee's ability to practice foundational REBT skills.

COMMON MISTAKES THAT TRAINEES MAKE AND HOW TO FIX THEM

Trainees in REBT (as well as seasoned practitioners) are prone to a number of common errors when practicing the various stages of therapy. For the purpose of clarity, we break down some of the more important errors seen in trainees as they learn and practice REBT.

Focusing Too Much on or Avoiding Expectations

To begin with, many trainees either spend too much time examining their clients' expectations of REBT or neglect to investigate this concept altogether. We have found that when failing to discuss clients' expectations of therapy (as well as of the therapist), it is more challenging to develop a strong working therapeutic alliance. However, the opposite can also be problematic—namely, spending too much time discussing a client's expectations of therapy. Furthermore, while it may be useful to discuss a client's previous history of receiving therapy, many trainees discuss this in too much depth, which takes time away from more important goals in therapy.

Assuming a Therapeutic Relationships Must Be Established Before Intervening

Another common erroneous assumption is that before one can intervene with a problem, a therapeutic relationship must be established. REBT holds a different perspective on this topic, proposing that relationships develop as a result of individuals working together. By helping a client in the first session with something that has brought them to treatment, whether it be teaching the connection between beliefs and emotions/behaviors (i.e., B-C connection), or discussing the concepts of irrational versus rational beliefs, clients will typically leave the first session with the sense that their REBT therapist has given them something to think about, apply the therapist's guidance to one of their other problems, and feel that this therapeutic approach can be helpful for them. What better way to build a relationship than by demonstrating to your client that you are actively listening to their problems and giving them tools in the first session?

Not Teaching Clients the Difference Between Thoughts and Emotions

Another common mistake REBT trainees make is failing to teach clients the difference between thoughts and emotions. Specifically, trainees often ask their clients how they felt when the particular event occurred. But clients sometimes couch their thoughts and beliefs as feelings, saying, "I felt like she shouldn't have done that." Emotions, however, are usually one word: depression, anger, guilt, or elation. One helpful strategy for reinforcing the difference between beliefs and emotions is to ask trainees what emotion(s) the client experienced when the event occurred, rather than what feeling(s) they had. Another strategy is to encourage trainees to respond with "So you thought she should not have done that, and when you had that thought, what emotion(s) did you experience?"

Struggling to Interrupt Talkative Clients

Many trainees often struggle with interrupting verbose clients. This might be based on trainees' own IB, such as "I must not interrupt my client because if

I do, it means I'm a rude, uncaring person," "I must always have my client's approval or else I'm a lousy therapist" or "I might miss something important and that would be awful." REBT trains supervisees to understand that inter-rupting is not only a necessary part of therapy, but it also demonstrates active listening. We recommend to trainees that they let clients know at the beginning of therapy that there will be times when interruptions are necessary, and the purpose is not to invalidate what the client is saying, but rather to keep the session on track and focused. Above all, interruptions are about tact. Although inoculating clients to interruptions often proves helpful, there are clients who will have a negative reaction to being interrupted. In such instances, we recommend an ABC analysis with the client about what is occurring at that specific moment in the session. Usually, the trainee and the client see that there are some IBs being held resulting in the unhealthy negative emotion in the session, often a microcosm of what occurs outside of the session with others in their lives. This strategy can be instructive for clients and allows the trainee to see in vivo the true IBs and emotional disturbance the client holds that may be problematic in their lives.

Avoiding All Confrontations

The term "confrontation" typically has a negative connotation (e.g., a spat with the cable company's customer service representative). Yet in REBT, con-frontation takes on a different meaning. When there are discrepancies between a client's verbal and nonverbal behaviors, or a discrepancy between a reported emotion (e.g., annoyed) and behavior (e.g., punched a wall and broke some plates), or between a belief (e.g., I just want people to like me) and an emotional consequence (e.g., depression, hurt, shame), we encourage trainees to confront their clients. This is not a hostile, aggressive intervention. Rather, it means being curious, or even confused, and asking the client for clarification and under-standing. Again, "confronting" a client about a discrepancy demonstrates active listening and can serve to further strengthen the therapeutic relationship.

Devoting Too Much Attention to Activating Events

Beginning therapists using REBT may also allow clients to discuss the activating event in too much detail, perhaps for fear of missing the "crucial" aspect of the problem, or because they want the client not to feel invalidated. Other times, allowing a client to give an exhaustive review of the event comes from trainees' interest in the "story," and wanting to see how it ends, typically due to their own curiosity. Yet this error reinforces the false connection between the acti-vating event/adversity and the emotional/behavioral consequences. Addition-ally, REBT makes a very clear distinction between feeling better and getting better. When clients discuss the activating event in great detail, they may leave the session feeling better, but return in subsequent sessions with the same problem. Getting better results from changing their cognitive reactions to the event. REBT corrects this error by encouraging trainees to have the client summarize in a few sentences the most distressing part of the activating event (i.e., the *critical A*) so they can work on the beliefs that are creating the disturbance (Neenan & Dryden, 2001).

Errors in Establishing Session Goals With Clients

An interesting error that many trainees make occurs when a client presents with a behavioral problem. To highlight this common error and strategies to correct it, we will use a specific example. Let us suppose a client comes to therapy with a problem of procrastination. Essentially, there are two different ABC formulas that can be applied to this problem. The first ABC formulation could be something like the following:

- A—Procrastinating on writing a book chapter
- B—I should not put off writing this chapter
- C—Anger towards self; ruminating about the chapter

In this formulation, the trainee would help the client change the unhealthy anger towards herself and replace it with healthy annoyance or frustration—in essence, helping the client become less disturbed about the behavioral problem of procrastinating.

A second formulation might be:

- A—Came home and thought about writing the chapter
- B—It's too uncomfortable to write this chapter
- C—Procrastinated and watched TV instead

Here, the trainee would help the client with the frustration intolerance that drives the behavioral problem of procrastinating and get the chapter done. The error trainees make is to assume the first ABC formula is the target intervention, rather than asking the client what it is they prefer to work on (i.e., what is the client's goal?). This failure to establish and agree on the goal of the session can lead to a rupture in the alliance or concern on the part of the client that the therapist does not understand the problem or has their own agenda. We encourage trainees to discuss with their clients who bring in behavioral problems (and all problems for that matter) what their therapy goal is, rather than making assumptions.

Trainees might also make errors when setting goals with clients and assume therapy is successful when their clients achieve intellectual insight regarding their problems, rather than encouraging and fostering emotional insight as well. Intellectual insight occurs when RBs are endorsed lightly and are intermittently held, whereas emotional insight involves RBs that are deeply and consistently held. This is the well-known conundrum of the head–gut problem, "I know it in my head, but I don't feel it in my gut." The way to move from intellectual insight to emotional insight is to encourage clients to rehearse forcefully the healthier RBs as frequently as possible. We make the analogy of going to the gym and picking up weights, and doing one repetition as intellectual insight versus multiple repetitions to build a stronger "rational muscle."

Moving to the Cognitive Restructuring Phase Without Preparations

When the therapeutic process moves to the cognitive restructuring phase, perhaps the biggest error we see trainees make is moving forward without the necessary preparation for this process. To address this, supervisors can spend time teaching the steps of identifying clear As, Bs, and Cs; establishing a realistic emotional or behavioral goal with the client; and ensuring the client understands and accepts the B-C connection. When these steps are taken, the process of examining self-defeating belief systems and becoming committed to replacing IBs with healthier RBs is self-evident. This process also eliminates the idea of disputation as arguing with clients.

Errors When Assigning Homework

Homework negotiation in REBT also comes with its own set of mistakes that trainees sometimes make, particularly when clients are told what to do for their homework, rather than the process being a collaborative one. Therapists sometimes overlook the importance of identifying practical and emotional obstacles that might interfere with homework completion. Trainees are encouraged to identify and address any IBs that might interfere with homework completion prior to the end of the session.

ETHICAL ISSUES IN TREATMENT APPLICATION

Supervisors have the responsibility to ensure not only that trainees develop competencies in delivering therapy but also that they deliver competent therapy to clients. Failure to meet these responsibilities represents the primary ethical conflict for REBT supervisors. Accordingly, we believe it is critical that supervisors observe their trainees at work, whether directly or by reviewing recordings of sessions.

REBT training distinguishes between strategies and techniques in therapy. *Strategy* refers to the supervisor and the supervisee understanding the client, developing a case conceptualization of the client's problem, and planning interventions based on the conceptualization. *Technique* refers to the skills and competencies with which the trainee delivers the treatment. Competent technique usually involves an integration of the strategy with empathy, acceptance, and warmth. The strategy is more comfortable for trainees to discuss because it is about the client. The strategy might also be more comfortable for the supervisor to discuss because it is interesting, intellectual, and involves less criticism of the trainee. Technique, on the other hand, may be uncomfortable to discuss because it can uncover errors made by trainees.

COMMON OBSTACLES IN SUPERVISION AND WAYS TO OVERCOME THEM

A frequent stumbling block we observe with supervisees who are learning and practicing REBT is a reluctance to address the elegant solution. Many supervisees have their own irrational beliefs and cognitive distortions about eliciting their client's worst-case scenarios. This is particularly evident when a client's problem involves a family member with a terminal illness or the client themself is confronting health issues that might lead to death. Supervisees often have a belief that "if I discuss the worst-case scenario with the client (e.g., death), that will be too unbearable for them and will only serve to upset them more." When we delve further into these issues with our supervisees, it is often the case that it is more the supervisee's discomfort regarding the topic of death than the client's anticipated discomfort. Identifying and challenging the supervisee's discomfort intolerance is crucial for both the therapeutic process as well as in assisting the client in achieving therapeutic goals. In fact, we have found that clients appreciate the elegant solution, as their catastrophizing and discomfort intolerance beliefs are precisely the beliefs that disturb them. By creating an environment where these beliefs can be addressed, clients benefit from REBT and are given permission to discuss their beliefs that are resulting in emotional and/or behavioral disturbance.

Another obstacle we often observe is when trainees refrain from reporting on the technical aspects of REBT, and instead provide an update on their client. A distinction should be made between the two approaches, as they both have merit. Case conceptualization is the cornerstone of informing treatment. However, we view the acquisition and execution of specific REBT technical skills to be just as important when working with a client. When trainees come to supervision reporting that each of their cases is "going well," with no concerns, we have red flags as supervisors. This is an important reason we require our supervisees to record their sessions: to enable supervisors to hear concretely what is occurring in a session and to be able to correct any mistakes before the trainee has their next session. In REBT supervision, we aim to foster an environment of support and safety, while at the same time teaching trainees to recognize that one of our key priorities is the development of clinical acumen.

CONCLUSION

Developing a sound relationship with supervisees is a parallel process to supervisees developing a sound therapeutic relationship with their clients. This includes agreement on (a) the goals and tasks of supervision, (b) expectations of supervisors, (c) the importance of creating a collaborative environment, and (d) the reality of human fallibility. As REBT continues to develop, so does the approach we take in conducting supervision with those we train. The flexibility that is espoused in the REBT model is the same flexibility we attempt to engender in our trainees during the process of supervision.

REFERENCES

David, D., Cotet, C., Matu, S., Mogoase, C., & Stefan, S. (2018). 50 years of rational-emotive and cognitive-behavioral therapy: A systematic review and meta-analysis. *Journal of Clinical Psychology, 74*(3), 304–318. https://doi.org/10.1002/jclp.22514

David, D., Lynn, S. J., & Ellis, A. (2009). *Rational and irrational beliefs: Research, theory, and clinical practice*. Oxford University Press. https://doi.org/10.1093/acprof:oso/9780195182231.001.0001

DiGiuseppe, R. (2021). REBT's place in modern psychotherapy: Similarities with all psychotherapies, with other forms of CBT, and unique characteristics. In W. Dryden (Ed.), *New directions in rational emotive behaviour therapy* (pp. 33–54). Routledge.

DiGiuseppe, R. A., Doyle, K. A., Dryden, W., & Backx, W. (2014). *A practitioner's guide to rational emotive behavior therapy* (3rd ed.). Oxford University Press.

Dryden, W. (2002). Rational emotive behaviour therapy. In W. Dryden (Ed.), *Handbook of individual therapy* (4th ed., pp. 347–372). Sage Publishing.

Ellis, A. (1962). *Reason and emotion in psychotherapy*. Lyle Stuart.

Ellis, A., & DiGiuseppe, R. (1993). Are inappropriate or dysfunctional feelings in rational–emotive therapy qualitative or quantitative? *Cognitive Therapy and Research, 17*, 471–477. https://doi.org/10.1007/BF01173058

Hyland, P., & Boduszek, D. (2012). A unitary or binary model of emotions: A discussion on a fundamental difference between cognitive therapy and rational emotive behaviour therapy. *Journal of Humanistics and Social Sciences, 1*(1), 49–61. http://eprints.hud.ac.uk/id/eprint/15915

Neenan, M., & Dryden, W. (2001). *Learning from errors in rational emotive behaviour therapy*. Wiley.

4

Training and Supervision in Acceptance and Commitment Therapy

Michael P. Twohig, Jennifer Krafft, Julie M. Petersen, and Carter H. Davis

Acceptance and commitment therapy (ACT) is a modern form of cognitive behavior therapy (CBT) that targets maladaptive psychological processes applicable to a wide range of clinical presentations. While ACT shares similarities with other forms of CBT, it is also unique in its philosophy and its ties to basic science, theory, intervention techniques, and therapeutic style. Awareness of these key features of ACT has important implications for how clinical supervision is carried out.

The way in which ACT conceptualizes behaviors, both external and internal (cognitions, emotions, sensations), is rooted in a philosophy of science known as *functional contextualism* (Hayes et al., 1988). At its core, functional contextualism posits that a behavior cannot be understood (and subsequently responded to in therapy) without considering the context in which it takes place. In other words, ACT does not target behaviors in isolation, nor does it assign them such labels as "good," "bad," "rational," or "irrational." Instead, from a functional contextual perspective, any analysis of behavior must incorporate that behavior's unique situational and historical context. The second key feature of functional contextualism is that the goal for any work (scientific or clinical) is predefined and outcomes are judged against that goal. For instance, clearly defining one's professional goals as a therapist or supervisor provides a way to evaluate the utility of a particular conceptualization and intervention and prevents creep to different goals or misunderstandings.

https://doi.org/10.1037/0000314-005
Training and Supervision in Specialized Cognitive Behavior Therapy: Methods, Settings, and Populations, E. A. Storch, J. S. Abramowitz, and D. McKay (Editors)
Copyright © 2022 by the American Psychological Association. All rights reserved.

In addition to this underlying philosophy, ACT is informed by the basic science of human cognition. Shocking findings from stimulus equivalence and rule-governed behavior opened the door to *relational frame theory* (RFT), which helps explain the ways that human cognition affects how we experience and respond to stimuli (Dougher et al., 2014). The key finding from RFT is that verbally able humans will respond to stimuli (internal or external) in terms of a wide array of relations with other stimuli (referred to as *relational responding*). There are unlimited ways in which we can relate to stimuli, such as bigger than, same as, hierarchical, and so on. Nothing is merely what we see or feel; cognition always adds something to it. Relational responding is central to ACT in that separate elements of the client's environment indicate what a stimulus is and how they should respond to it, from a relational responding perspective. This is important clinically because it allows the therapist to choose when to help a client see a stimulus differently (e.g., seeing that anxiety is not actually dangerous) or learn to respond to a stimulus differently (e.g., approaching anxiety rather than avoiding it). In RFT, we call these two aspects of the environment the *relational context* and the *functional context*. Therapists can choose to work on the relational context, the functional context, or both. Because research with human (Wilson & Hayes, 1996) and nonhuman participants (Fontes et al., 2018) has shown that responses are never completely extinguished (i.e., they will return under certain circumstances), ACT leans toward altering how we respond to stimuli rather than focusing on their meaning. This is evident in ACT's emphasis on mindfully watching and accepting internal events. We will respond to the content of stimuli, but we generally save that for the values part of ACT, where we work to add to the meaning of stimuli. For example, if a stimulus is scary, we try to add to that stimulus by saying, "It is scary, and that feeling of fear means you are moving toward something important."

Instead of focusing explicitly on relational responding and rule governance in client behavior, we instead target a simpler construct called *psychological inflexibility*. This is a midlevel term rather than a technical one, but it is useful in practice to describe someone who relationally and functionally responds in a rigid literal fashion. In essence, a person who is responding in an inflexible way is overly regulated by internal experiences such as thoughts, emotions, memories, expectations, and so on. Someone who is responding in a psychologically flexible way, on the other hand, may relationally respond to such experiences but have the skills to functionally choose simply to watch their reactions and keep moving in a valued direction. For example, a client might have the thought, "If I speak in front of my class, I'll throw up from anxiety." If responded to from a rigid (psychologically inflexible) stance, this thought is an accurate representation of the current contingency and would require immediate action (avoidance). If responded to flexibly, that client might notice it as a funny or interesting thought and choose to pursue things they care about, such as education, and speak while having those "frightening" thoughts. While this might feel like a lot of theory and "psychobabble," these few key ideas guide everything we do in ACT. Thus, from a supervision perspective, time should be spent reading about, teaching, and discussing these philosophical, theoretical, and empirical concepts as they inform the practice of ACT.

KEY CONCEPTS FOR TRAINEES TO LEARN

As described in the previous section, the use of ACT involves looking at all therapeutic events functionally. This includes statements from the client, nonverbal behavior, overt behaviors, what stories are shared, and so on. Successful ACT therapists learn to respond not to the content, but instead to the function. As this is a very generalized skill, we can only really illustrate with a handful of examples. If the client has a high or low score on a measure such as the Beck Depression Inventory (Beck et al., 1996), instead of noting this as a bad thing, ask the client how they experience their depression and what effect it has on them. If the client is a college student, ask what attending college does for them. If they dress blandly or flashily, ask how dressing that way serves them. Notice that we are not asking why they do something, as that will often lead to a rigid, literal story. We are instead looking for the function of each action. If they are loud or quiet in session, figure out what function that fulfills for them. If they say, "I hate myself," ask, "How long have you thought that?" and "What effect does that thought have on you?" Maybe the answer is as simple as, "My parents taught me I'm crap, so I listen to that thought." The successful use of ACT requires learning to see things functionally and not topographically. Accordingly, learning to identify and track psychological inflexibility is important.

Psychological inflexibility is defined as an overarching pattern of behavior that is overly controlled by rigid verbal regulation and a corresponding avoidance of or attachment to emotional experiences, such that opportunities for vital, meaningful living are lost. To engender therapeutic change, trainees learning ACT should develop skills to assess psychological inflexibility and its inverse (psychological flexibility), and to undermine inflexibility and encourage flexibility in therapy. Understanding the six component processes of psychological inflexibility and flexibility, as we describe next, is a useful starting point.

Six Processes of Change in ACT

There are six processes of change in ACT that all work together to build psychological flexibility. We generally think of four of them—acceptance, cognitive defusion, self as context, and flexible attention—as representing the acceptance and mindfulness side. The remaining two processes—values and committed action—have to do with personal values and behavior change.

First, *cognitive fusion* refers to viewing and responding to thoughts as if they were a literal description of reality. An example would be having the thought "I can't study. I'm too overwhelmed" and subsequently giving up on studying.

In place of cognitive fusion, ACT therapists foster *cognitive defusion*: the ability to notice the process of thinking, without it overly controlling behavior. Second, a particular form of fusion exists around self-evaluations called *self-as-content*. This way of behaving involves literally and rigidly responding to self-evaluations and working to protect them. This is particularly dangerous in instances when those self-evaluations pull one away from their values. For example, a professional might feel the need to be "right," when being open to new things is the best move in a situation. *Self-as-context* (i.e., being the context in which self-evaluations occur) involves openly and flexibly observing self-evaluations and choosing when to listen to them and when not to, all based on values.

Third, *experiential avoidance* refers to the related process of rigidly attempting to avoid unwanted emotions, often in ways that are ineffective for living an engaged life. In some presentations, experiential attachment (rigidly attempting to experience or maintain specific emotions) may also be an issue. Trainees must learn to facilitate *acceptance* (an open, curious stance) toward a full range of emotions instead. This can be particularly challenging, as clients often seek and begin therapy with the explicit expectation that the goal is to experience less unwanted emotion. As such, a course of ACT often begins by explicitly discussing this agenda, and helping clients examine whether they wish to continue focusing on emotional control or whether focusing on the alternative goal of increasing valued living while carrying along difficult thoughts and feelings would be more effective.

Fourth, another component of psychological inflexibility is *inflexible awareness*, often a tendency to focus on the past or future, or an excessive focus on one aspect of experience (e.g., thoughts, sensations) over other stimuli. Trainees correspondingly learn to encourage *flexible attention* to a full range of internal and external stimuli, often practiced through mindfulness exercises.

The final two components are closely related to the aim of living a values-consistent life. Trainees encourage clients to identify and describe personally meaningful *values*, while facilitating patterns of behavior (*behavioral commitments*) that fit these values. When clients are psychologically inflexible, they may have limited awareness of what is meaningful to them. They may have disconnected from it over time, or they may be stuck in patterns of behavior that are guided by fusion and avoidance rather than values. Trainees should learn these processes and the wide range of behaviors that can exemplify them, in order to begin developing the ability to assess and treat clients from an ACT framework.

Fostering Psychological Flexibility

Learning how to foster psychological flexibility is an essential part of learning ACT, and trainees should learn the therapeutic stance of ACT conceptually and practically. ACT is fundamentally behavior analytic, so therapists must attend to the function of their client's behaviors and their own behaviors. For one client, taking a day off work may be a values-consistent step that requires defusing from perfectionistic judgments; for another, it may be about avoiding social anxiety. Learning to not be reactionary, and to really dig into the function of each action is important.

ACT is also an experiential therapy, with a strong emphasis on helping the client notice and learn from their own experience. As such, ACT therapists are circumspect about didactic methods. Importantly, ACT involves modeling, eliciting, and reinforcing psychological flexibility in a moment-by-moment manner, and thus, trainees must attend to their own psychologically flexible and inflexible behaviors, as well as considering how their clients' steps towards flexibility can be effectively reinforced. For example, one client told me (Twohig) that she was thinking about suicide. Instead of immediately assessing for risk (that happened later), I asked what it was like to have those thoughts. The remainder of the session was spent practicing defusion from and acceptance of suicidal thoughts in the context of the client's values and what she wanted from life. At the end of therapy, the client told me that this had been the best part of therapy, because she had been scared of her suicidal thoughts, and I had modeled that such thoughts were OK. The client specifically said, "You showed me the thoughts were OK, as long as I didn't act on them." This is one example of the experiential nature of ACT.

KEY TECHNIQUES FOR TRAINEES TO LEARN

Once trainees have a conceptual understanding of ACT processes, beginning to recognize these processes in specific clients is crucial. In practice, trainees do this using self-report measures that have been validated for this purpose. There are many such instruments listed in books and articles about ACT (Hayes et al., 2012; Twohig, 2012). Trainees also track these processes informally throughout every session and constantly think about which processes should to be addressed in order to promote psychological flexibility.

An unlimited set of techniques can be used to undermine psychological inflexibility and foster psychological flexibility (Stoddard & Afari, 2014). ACT frequently uses metaphors and experiential exercises, given the focus on helping clients directly contact their experience and not promote fusion. For example, the "passengers on the bus" metaphor may be used to help clients to notice their unwanted thoughts and feelings and focus on values by describing these internal experiences like unpleasant passengers that board a bus they are driving toward their values (Hayes et al., 2012). Many mindfulness exercises are useful for fostering psychological flexibility, although it is important to frame their purpose as an opportunity to practice awareness and acceptance, rather than finding relaxation. Common metaphors and experiential exercises can be found in numerous books, articles, and videos on ACT, and are likely to be useful for trainees new to ACT. As trainees become more competent in ACT, they may find it both natural and helpful to generate their own metaphors and exercises. A growth exercise for supervision is to purposefully create client-specific exercises and metaphors rather than relying on ones the therapist is comfortable with.

Depending on the therapist and client, ACT may also be very conversational. Process-focused questions and observations (e.g., "When you did that, was it about feeling better or doing what matters? What thoughts and emotions showed up? How did you respond to them? That's cool, that seems new") can be very useful. There are also many opportunities to model psychological flexibility in conversation. For instance, when a client speaks in a fused manner (e.g., "I've already tried everything"), you can model defusion ("That might be right. And if we both fully buy into that thought, that you've tried everything, what would it mean for our work together? How might we act then?"). This is central from a supervision and training standpoint. We find that many trainees are overly focused on saying the right words versus being in the moment and having the right function.

The behavioral roots of ACT lead to a stance in which ACT therapists change the client's *context* through their own behavior (what they encourage, model, and reinforce), rather than intervening with the client in a top-down manner. It may be useful to attend to how trainees describe their ACT work—the trainee who says "We talked about acceptance" or "I described defusion" is likely further from an ACT-consistent stance than the one who says, "I guided the client to notice the impact of avoidance" or "I reinforced defusion in-session."

First, trainees should intervene based on a specific case conceptualization. Case conceptualizing takes practice and guidance from supervisors. The ways in which the six processes interact given the client's characteristics is idiographic. This is where the art of practicing ACT comes into play (as opposed to the science). Practice and supervision will help improve case conceptualization and planning. Second, ACT therapists attend to the ongoing behavior of their clients, in and between sessions, and intervene based on what is most likely to move the client toward their specified goals. In doing so, it is essential to track the actual effects of intervening as well. For example, if the trainee encourages a client to open up to anxiety and talk about something difficult in session, but the client is then even less flexible after that (e.g., engaging in a lot of storytelling, questioning the value of therapy), it may be valuable to approach acceptance from a different angle or shift to a different process, such as values. Reaching an intermediate to advanced skill level in ACT means learning to use ongoing, moment-by-moment assessment to flexibly guide treatment, rather than following a protocol.

WHAT MAKES A GOOD OR A POOR ACT TRAINING CASE?

The first key issue when selecting a case that will work well for training is to confirm that psychological inflexibility is important in the clinical presentation. Because ACT focuses on promoting psychological flexibility and growing values-based behavior, if psychological inflexibility is not part of the presenting problem, then ACT is not a good fit for the client. As a result, this will be a poor training case.

A very clear example is a client with a learning disability who is primarily seeking therapy to help manage such a skill deficit. The fact that a client lacks the repertoire to engage in a skill usually is not because they are psychologically inflexible. Skills such as those that allow one to compensate for a learning disability, for example, can be taught outside of teaching psychological flexibility. Of course, it is still possible that learning psychological flexibility could be helpful, for example in handling the client's fears of failing or being different, but this may or may not be primary.

A more common poor training case is someone who is already fairly psychologically flexible at intake. This can be assessed with a number of psychological flexibility measures (as mentioned previously in this chapter). If someone is already psychologically flexible, there will be less opportunity for the clinician to practice fostering flexibility. Such individuals might be better cases for more advanced trainees who are able to work on the finer points of psychological flexibility. Sometimes we will have high-functioning clients who are clear on their values and engaging in meaningful life activities but low on the other four processes of change. High-achieving professionals can sometimes present this way. These can be acceptable initial clients, as they are less complex, but it limits the chances to work on all six processes of change.

A third characteristic of a poor ACT training case is one in which it is difficult to clarify the inner experiences that the client is struggling with. For example, I (Twohig) worked with a teenaged girl who was engaging in substance abuse. She knew that using substances was a problem but had no idea why she used (i.e., what using gave her or took away from her). I did a poor job at figuring out the function of her actions, which in turn made it a challenge to know what phenomena to target when teaching acceptance and defusion. Therapy would have been much smoother if we had known the function of her actions. Looking back on that case, using substances relieved feelings of stress and fear, and that made her feel accepted (or took away feelings of loneliness). Thus, therapy should have targeted psychological flexibility around stress, fear, and loneliness. Maybe starting with an anxiety or depression case would be easier because the likely key inner experience will be anxiety or depression; the therapist will not have to dig to conceptualize what the client needs to become psychologically flexible toward.

It is also important to assess whether the client is interested in or open to ACT, and to looking at their struggles in this way. This is very rarely an issue, but providing informed consent about the goals of ACT-based therapy is helpful to eliminate this potential barrier. As mentioned previously, clients often come to therapy with goals to improve their emotional control and reduce internal symptoms (e.g., stopping anxiety or controlling their anger). Because ACT emphasizes acceptance over challenging or changing internal experiences, it is important to ensure that the client is open and willing to take a different approach—and this may require some reframing. Importantly, the ACT approach does not need to be immediately accepted and utilized by the client, but they should express interest and willingness to engage in new (or perhaps reworded) therapy goals. Thus, a client who is strongly fused with a desire to control their internal experiences (e.g., someone who wants to get rid of their intrusive traumatic memories) is likely not a good starting case for a student ACT therapist.

Several other characteristics may indicate a poor ACT training case. First, clients struggling with metaphoric language (e.g., a client on the autism spectrum) may not be the best fit as a starter case due to ACT's heavy reliance on metaphors. Low insight, while likely difficult for all trainees, may also be especially challenging for a first ACT case. For example, if a client with obsessive–compulsive disorder has poor insight regarding their intrusive violent thoughts, it may be especially difficult to facilitate acceptance and defusion. Furthermore, for clients who have extreme difficulty tolerating internal experiences (e.g., emotion dysregulation in borderline personality disorder), a different approach may be indicated. For example, it may be hard for a trainee to facilitate acceptance if the client is easily dysregulated and struggles with the simple presence of strong emotion, let alone acceptance.

Therefore, a good initial case for an ACT trainee would likely be an individual who had a relatively clear internal experience about which they demonstrate psychological inflexibility (e.g., anxiety, urges to use substances). They would have struggled with this internal experience for a while so that they understand it and have some understanding of how hard it has been to control. They will be more open to learning ACT techniques if they have experienced how poorly emotional control works. Openness to ACT might even come from someone who has struggled for a long time or failed at other therapies. Finally, to make it easier on the trainee, it will likely be helpful if the client can follow and appreciate exercises and metaphorical language. ACT has been done with people diagnosed on the autism spectrum, but they might be more difficult initial cases.

COMMON MISTAKES THAT TRAINEES MAKE AND HOW TO FIX THEM

The most common error that we see students or professionals make is that they teach ACT rather than do ACT. Seasoned professionals or younger therapists who are already good at other therapies—especially empirically supported ones—have a habit of being didactic about ACT: "Today we are going to talk about defusion." Doing ACT, on the other hand, involves talking about struggles that the client had over the week and finding the spots where the client experienced fusion. The therapist then helps the client see their fusion and the impact it has had on their life, and subsequently incorporates a defusion exercise. A line we use in teaching is, "It is worth 10 points if the client figures it out, and 1 point if you tell them." Thus, supervisors can train therapists to help the client see these processes through discussion, examples, metaphors, and exercises.

New therapists sometimes allow their fear and uncertainty to block them from doing ACT, which often leads them to teach ACT in a didactic way. They get so concerned with saying the right things that they miss the wonderful events happening right in front of them. For example, clients may say to a trainee, "Am I your first client?" Instead of recognizing this as a fused statement, the therapist will usually answer, "No, I've had lots of training. This is the main area I work in." That is, the trainee also engages in fusion and avoidance. A much more useful answer to this question might be, "Please tell me what is behind that question." The answer might be, "I'm just worried I won't get better." With that answer, the trainee can respond with an ACT-consistent, function-based answer such as "Has that thought blocked you in the past?" and a response like that can lead to a nice ACT-based discussion.

Another way of thinking about learning to use ACT is that ACT is much more like dancing, music, or sports. None of those activities work well when done from a very verbal, conceptual place. A trainee can be cognitive about learning therapy when reading, practicing, watching video, or in class, just like an athlete can be very purposeful when in practice. But in the session or in the game, the trainee should be present and respond in the moment. Be prepared to mess up. Do not be pushed around by fears of messing up. Maybe messing up actually leads to more growth.

ETHICAL ISSUES IN TREATMENT APPLICATION

The most basic ethical issues to consider with ACT trainees are (a) consent to treatment and (b) boundaries of competence. Consent to ACT is of the utmost importance. As discussed previously, it is an ethical imperative that the client understands and consents to a treatment approach focusing less on symptom reduction and more on releasing control attempts in order to live a valued life. It may be necessary to reframe clients' goals to provide an illustrative example before consent (e.g., changing the goal "I want to stop feeling anxious in social situations" to "I want to work on engaging in social situations that are important to me even when I feel anxious"). Furthermore, because the therapist is still in training, the supervisor and trainee should be sure that the therapist-in-training is acting within the appropriate bounds of competence with regard to the implementation of ACT (American Psychological Association, 2016).

Self-disclosure also presents an important ethical issue in the application of ACT. At its best, ACT lessens the typical power dynamic of the therapeutic relationship by acknowledging the shared challenges of living as a thinking and feeling human being. Self-disclosure in ACT can be used similarly to traditional CBT—to enhance therapeutic alliance and normalize client experience—or as a way to model ACT processes (e.g., defusion; Tsai et al., 2010). For example, self-disclosure can be effective when doing values work by providing examples of how the trainee is living their values within the therapy room, or in modeling cognitive defusion by noting feelings of stuckness or frustration in session.

However, self-disclosure in ACT must still be utilized judiciously in order to ensure it does not affect the treatment process by burdening a client or damaging a boundary (Behnke, 2015; Tsai et al., 2010).

The ACT processes of values and contact with the present moment also bring special ethical considerations to the forefront of training and supervision. There is need for careful awareness and ethical considerations around cultural context in values work. It is common and normal for values conflicts to arise within a therapeutic context. While some have argued that Western therapies such as ACT may not align with clients from other cultural contexts (Jadaszewski, 2017), there is also growing evidence for the effectiveness of acceptance and mindfulness-based interventions across a variety of global settings (e.g., Castellanos et al., 2020; Shabani et al., 2019; Stewart et al., 2016). Multicultural sensitivity and awareness are key, and the emphasis should lie on achieving a functional outcome desired by the client, rather than forcing the client to follow a specific moral code or something else that may be specifically decreed by the trainee or supervisor's own cultural background (Jadaszewski, 2017). The trainee and/or supervisor should also consider consultation and/or referrals in the rare cases of genuine values conflicts that interfere with treatment or proper supervision.

Contact with the present moment may also involve careful ethical considerations. Concerns about the ethical use of mindfulness in psychological treatments has recently come to light with concerns about incorrectly using and/or altering the largely Buddhist tradition (Monteiro et al., 2015). Alternatively, some argue that the evidence for the positive effects of mindfulness makes its use ethical because such outcomes are in line with general Buddhist traditions of compassion and reducing suffering (Baer, 2015). Furthermore, the use of values alongside mindfulness, as in ACT, also allows for a more ethical application of mindfulness, as it is used to help a client lead a fulfilling life (Baer, 2015). In general, it is important to consider how to use mindfulness ethically as a trainee/supervisor. For example, it might be important to make the intention behind the use of mindfulness explicit and even engage in regular personal mindfulness practice (e.g., meditation, yoga, retreats) if you are going to ask a client to practice mindfulness (Monteiro et al., 2015). One may also consider teaching mindfulness in line with the ethics in which it was conceived (e.g., loving kindness, nonjudgmental stance). In sum, it is important to be careful about the use of mindfulness, and it is therefore recommended to be intentional and use your own values to guide how you act with a client.

COMMON OBSTACLES IN SUPERVISION AND HOW TO OVERCOME THEM

I (Twohig) have been supervising therapists in ACT for almost 15 years and believe that the biggest obstacle is that there is so much to learn and do at once in ACT. The therapist needs to track everything that is occurring in session, determine the function of those actions, continually update the conceptualization of the client in terms of the six ACT processes of change, be aware of what processes need addressing, and choose what to work on in each moment based on where the client wants to be. Sometimes the trainee will have plans of going in a certain direction within the session, but then the data collected within that session suggest the need to go in a different direction. In many ways, it is like learning to drive—there are numerous variables to track all at once.

As with driving (and most other skills), it takes a great deal of practice to learn how to track and work with all of these variables. Such practice can occur outside of the therapy session. For example, the trainee can practice detecting the six ACT processes by watching characters in television shows and thinking about how they might address that process in therapy. Practice can also involve taking any client statement and turning it into a teaching moment around any of the six processes. For example, if the client says, "I hate my life," the trainee might say, "Can you just notice your reaction to that thought?" for being present; "How does that thought grab you?" for defusion; or "How does that thought push you around?" for acceptance; or "How does that thought push you away from things you care about?" for values. With a lot of practice, this can become smooth and easy.

Finally, the best training method we have encountered is viewing and coding ACT therapy sessions. By coding, we mean coding the presence of these six ACT processes in the client and then separately coding the response by the therapist. Therapy sessions have great material. We have seen brand new therapists perform really well with their only real training being many hours of coding videos of ACT sessions. If you do not have access to genuine ACT therapy sessions, many mock sessions have been shared online by ACT trainers.

CONCLUSION

Learning to do ACT well takes time, as does staying talented at ACT. Mastering the art and science takes a great deal of work and practice. Supervisors might suggest trainees begin by reading conceptual or theoretical materials (Hayes et al., 2012; Luoma et al., 2007) followed by more practical manuals (Twohig et al., 2020), then watching videos of therapy sessions. After that, the trainee might be ready to work with a few clients (who meet the criteria for good training cases) while closely following a treatment manual (Twohig et al., 2020). Then, as comfort grows, the trainee can move on to doing treatment without a manual. Encourage trainees to be creative and to be okay with making mistakes and growing from them. Then, as their skills start to develop, trainees can learn about the smaller details of ACT: being more present, learning more theory, and digging into how to create one's own client-centered metaphors. Learning a new therapy is a huge task. We encourage ACT trainees to take it in steps.

REFERENCES

American Psychological Association. (2016). Revision of ethical standard 3.04 of the "Ethical Principles of Psychologists and Code of Conduct" (2002, as amended 2010). *American Psychologist, 71*(9), 900. https://doi.org/10.1037/amp0000102

Baer, R. (2015). Ethics, values, virtues, and character strengths in mindfulness-based interventions: A psychological science perspective. *Mindfulness, 6*(4), 956–969. https://doi.org/10.1007/s12671-015-0419-2

Beck, A. T., Steer, R. A., & Brown, G. K. (1996). *Manual for the Beck Depression Inventory-II.* Psychological Corporation.

Behnke, S. (2015). Ethics, self-disclosure and our everyday multiple identities. *Monitor on Psychology, 46*(3), 70. http://www.apa.org/monitor/2015/03/ethics

Castellanos, R., Yildiz Spinel, M., Phan, V., Orengo-Aguayo, R., Humphreys, K. L., & Flory, K. (2020). A systematic review and meta-analysis of cultural adaptations of mindfulness-based interventions for Hispanic populations. *Mindfulness, 11*(2), 317–332. https://doi.org/10.1007/s12671-019-01210-x

Dougher, M., Twohig, M. P., & Madden, G. J. (2014). Editorial: Basic and translational research on stimulus–stimulus relations. *Journal of the Experimental Analysis of Behavior, 101*(1), 1–9. https://doi.org/10.1002/jeab.69

Fontes, R. M., Todorov, J. C., & Shahan, T. A. (2018). Punishment of an alternative behavior generates resurgence of a previously extinguished target behavior. *Journal of the Experimental Analysis of Behavior, 110*(2), 171–184. https://doi.org/10.1002/jeab.465

Hayes, S. C., Hayes, L. J., & Reese, H. W. (1988). Finding the philosophical core: A review of Stephen C. Pepper's World hypotheses: A study in evidence. *Journal of the Experimental Analysis of Behavior, 50*(1), 97–111. https://doi.org/10.1901/jeab.1988.50-97

Hayes, S. C., Strosahl, K. D., & Wilson, K. G. (2012). *Acceptance and commitment therapy: The process and practice of mindful change* (2nd ed.). Guilford Press.

Jadaszewski, S. (2017). Ethically problematic value change as an outcome of psychotherapeutic interventions. *Ethics & Behavior, 27*(4), 297–312. https://doi.org/10.1080/10508422.2016.1195739

Luoma, J. B., Hayes, S. C., & Walser, R. D. (2007). *Learning ACT: An acceptance and commitment therapy skills-training manual for therapists.* New Harbinger Publications.

Monteiro, L. M., Musten, R. F., & Compson, J. (2015). Traditional and contemporary mindfulness: Finding the middle path in the tangle of concerns. *Mindfulness, 6*(1), 1–13. https://doi.org/10.1007/s12671-014-0301-7

Shabani, M. J., Mohsenabadi, H., Omidi, A., Lee, E. B., Twohig, M. P., Ahmadvand, A., & Zanjani, Z. (2019). An Iranian study of group acceptance and commitment therapy versus group cognitive behavioral therapy for adolescents with obsessive-compulsive disorder on an optimal dose of selective serotonin reuptake inhibitors. *Journal of Obsessive-Compulsive and Related Disorders, 22*, 100440. https://doi.org/10.1016/j.jocrd.2019.04.003

Stewart, C., White, R. G., Ebert, B., Mays, I., Nardozzi, J., & Bockarie, H. (2016). A preliminary evaluation of Acceptance and Commitment Therapy (ACT) training in Sierra Leone. *Journal of Contextual Behavioral Science, 5*(1), 16–22. https://doi.org/10.1016/j.jcbs.2016.01.001

Stoddard, J. A., & Afari, N. (2014). *The big book of ACT metaphors: A practitioner's guide to experiential exercises and metaphors in acceptance and commitment therapy.* New Harbinger Publications.

Tsai, M., Plummer, M. D., Kanter, J. W., Newring, R. W., & Kohlenberg, R. J. (2010). Therapist grief and functional analytic psychotherapy: Strategic self-disclosure of personal loss. *Journal of Contemporary Psychotherapy, 40*(1), 1–10. https://doi.org/10.1007/s10879-009-9116-6

Twohig, M. P. (2012). Acceptance and commitment therapy: Introduction. *Cognitive and Behavioral Practice, 19*(4), 499–507. https://doi.org/10.1016/j.cbpra.2012.04.003

Twohig, M. P., Levin, M. E., & Ong, C. W. (2020). *ACT in steps: A transdiagnostic manual for learning acceptance and commitment therapy.* Oxford University Press. https://doi.org/10.1093/med-psych/9780190629922.001.0001

Wilson, K. G., & Hayes, S. C. (1996). Resurgence of derived stimulus relations. *Journal of the Experimental Analysis of Behavior, 66*(3), 267–281. https://doi.org/10.1901/jeab.1996.66-267

5

Supervision in Dialectical Behavior Therapy

Elizabeth Raposa

Dialectical behavior therapy (DBT) is an evidence-based treatment for borderline personality disorder (BPD; American Psychiatric Association, 2006; Linehan, 1993), and it has been shown to lead to reductions in suicidal behavior, nonsuicidal self-injury (NSSI), and use of psychiatric crisis services relative to treatment as usual in this population (Kliem et al., 2010; Panos et al., 2014). Preliminary evidence also suggests that adaptations of traditional DBT may be effective in treating conditions often comorbid with BPD, such as posttraumatic stress disorder (Harned et al., 2012) and substance use disorders (Dimeff & Linehan, 2008). In practice, DBT is often applied with multiproblem clients presenting with a number of high-risk behaviors, including chronic suicidality, NSSI, history of treatment failure, and frequent use of psychiatric crisis services.

DBT blends traditional cognitive behavior therapy techniques with mindfulness approaches rooted in Eastern spiritual practices (Koerner, 2012; Linehan, 1993). Adopting a collaborative stance, the therapist enlists the client in identifying target behaviors for the intervention. These target behaviors are organized within a treatment hierarchy that designates life-threatening behaviors (e.g., suicide attempts, NSSI) as Level 1 targets, therapy-interfering behaviors (e.g., homework noncompliance) as Level 2 targets, and all other quality of life–interfering behaviors (e.g., substance use, bingeing/purging) as Level 3 targets. The therapist then coaches the client in ways to address the contingencies, skills deficits, or problematic cognitions and/or emotions that may be

https://doi.org/10.1037/0000314-006
Training and Supervision in Specialized Cognitive Behavior Therapy: Methods, Settings, and Populations, E. A. Storch, J. S. Abramowitz, and D. McKay (Editors)

maintaining these behaviors, using a blend of change-based (e.g., cognitive restructuring, in vivo exposure) and acceptance-based (e.g., mindfulness of current emotions, "urge surfing") techniques. Throughout the treatment, the focus on changing behavior is balanced with a radical acceptance of the unique circumstances that have given rise to the client's current behavior, as well as intentional validation of the client's emotional experiences. In blending techniques focused on acceptance and change, the DBT approach emphasizes a *dialectical* worldview, in which truth can be found in seemingly opposite or incompatible points of view (Koerner, 2012; Linehan, 1993). The use of both behavioral therapy and mindfulness practices embodies a core dialectic within DBT: an attitude of acceptance of the client exactly as they are, and at the same time, an often-urgent movement toward change.

Traditional DBT is highly structured and contains four modalities: individual psychotherapy, weekly DBT skills instruction (individual or group-based), between-session phone coaching sessions, and a consultation team for the therapist (Koerner, 2012; Linehan, 1993). DBT skills sessions address skill deficits in areas of mindfulness, distress tolerance, emotion regulation, and interpersonal effectiveness, and individual sessions involve application of those skills to target problems (Linehan, 2015). Between-session phone coaching helps clients to apply newly learned skills in all relevant contexts. The frequency of client target behaviors, emotions, and practice of new skills is tracked daily via client self-report on a DBT diary card. The traditional DBT structure also includes regular opportunities for supervision for all DBT therapists who are providing active treatment, not just trainees. A weekly therapist consultation team is a setting where therapists can be held accountable for effective treatment, as well as receive validation around the difficulties encountered in their work (Linehan, 1993; Sayrs, 2018). This consultation team embodies the same dialectical tensions as the therapist–client relationship. That is, members of the consultation team aim to elicit more effective therapeutic behaviors from each clinician through behavioral assessment and problem solving, while also providing acceptance and validation to limit burnout and keeping the clinician engaged in treatment.

In addition to the consultation team, it is also recommended that trainees new to DBT receive supervision targeted to their specific cases (Linehan, 1993). In fact, adequate training and supervision may be especially critical for effective dissemination of DBT. Alarmingly few mental health professionals report adequate training in treating suicide and NSSI, and many clinicians do not feel prepared to deal with the stressful threats of suicide and client hostility that often occur within BPD (Brodsky et al., 2017; Hellman et al., 1986; Linehan, 1993). As a result, BPD remains a condition some clinicians refuse to treat altogether (Linehan et al., 2000). Individual supervisors in DBT adopt the same frame and many of the same strategies as DBT clinicians do with their clients (Waltz et al., 1998). Traditional cognitive behavioral techniques are used to conduct behavioral analyses of the trainee's problematic behaviors in session. Together, the supervisor and clinician work to identify whether these behaviors are maintained by contingencies (i.e., reinforcing or punishing consequences of using a certain technique in-session), skills deficits, and/or ineffective cognitions (e.g., "This client is hopeless") or emotions (e.g., fear around conducting *in vivo* exposure with a sexual abuse survivor). Sometimes, trainees' behaviors are addressed using change-focused techniques such as cognitive restructuring, behavioral rehearsal, or imaginal exposure. At other times, the supervisor may encourage the practice of acceptance-based skills, such as radical acceptance of a difficult emotion through mindfulness practice or self-validation exercises. Throughout the process of supervision, the supervisor strives to balance the focus on urging change and drawing out more effective behaviors from the trainee with building an atmosphere of acceptance and explicit validation around the trainee's challenges.

Despite the clear need for rigorous training and supervision in DBT, empirical evidence for best practices within DBT supervision remains limited at this time (cf. Rizvi et al., 2016). This chapter therefore incorporates perspectives from treatment manuals and theoretical writings about DBT, which often describe strategies and goals for DBT supervision, in addition to utilizing findings from empirical studies that have evaluated various approaches to training and ongoing supervision within DBT.

KEY DBT CONCEPTS

The *biosocial model of the etiology of emotion dysregulation* is foundational to DBT case conceptualization. This model postulates that severe emotion dysregulation arises when an inherited predisposition to heightened emotional experiences is compounded by a chronically invalidating early family environment (Crowell et al., 2009; Linehan, 1993). According to the biosocial model, individuals with BPD and other problems of emotion dysregulation are often born with a tendency to experience emotions that flare up more easily, reach a higher peak intensity, and take longer to return to baseline than other individuals. This emotional vulnerability, often evidenced as impulsivity or extreme emotional sensitivity, becomes problematic when the individual has an early family environment that communicates to them that their emotional experiences are invalid responses to a situation. At the same time, this invalidating environment fails to equip the individual with skills to understand and regulate their intense emotional experiences. DBT clinicians should be able to use this model to conceptualize a client's target behaviors and skills deficits, and clearly describe this case formulation to clients during the pretreatment phase of DBT.

All DBT trainees should also be oriented to the basic ideas of *dialectical philosophy*, and the ways in which dialectics infuse the practice of DBT (Linehan, 1993). A dialectical perspective posits that there are opposing sides or forces within any situation and encourages clinicians and clients alike to consider perspectives they may be missing, while searching for a synthesis that incorporates the "kernels of truth" in each viewpoint. This principle informs the clinician's interactions with the client, as well as their interactions with supervisors and the therapist consultation team. Trainees should cultivate an awareness of moments when viewpoints have become polarized, as well as practice skills for moving away from extremes and searching for the truth in opposing viewpoints. Dialectical philosophy also involves an appreciation of the interconnectedness of all things—of individuals to one another, and of individuals to their surroundings—and the fact that change is transactional, with each individual constantly influencing their environment, and vice versa. These principles can help the trainee to consider the ways in which their behavior influences the client, their client's behavior influences their family environment, and so on. An appreciation for the interconnectedness of all things also provides a foundation for some of the core mindfulness exercises in DBT that aim to promote experiences of unity and groundedness. Finally, a dialectical perspective acknowledges that change is constant. Trainees must learn to practice (and teach) acceptance of change throughout the treatment, including adjustments to the therapist's personal limits, changes in hospital staff, or changes within the therapist–client relationship. The second edition of the *DBT Skills Training Manual* (Linehan, 2015) contains detailed suggestions for practicing skills based in dialectics that may be useful for DBT trainees looking to learn these ideas or teach them to clients.

Emerging from this dialectical philosophy, a set of three common *dialectical dilemmas* in BPD (see Table 5.1) are helpful guides in conceptualizing a client's behavioral patterns (Koerner & Linehan, 1997; Linehan, 1993). The therapist and client aim to arrive at a synthesis that balances these opposing patterns of extreme underregulation versus overregulation of emotion (Koerner & Linehan, 1997). It is important to note that these dialectical dilemmas remain largely untested in the empirical literature on BPD and DBT, and these three dialectical patterns are not intended to be universal or exhaustive in describing the behaviors typical of BPD (Linehan, 1993). Nevertheless, they can be helpful heuristics in making sense of the sudden and confusing shifts in behavior often evidenced by clients with BPD, while avoiding common pitfalls associated with a nondialectical approach to treatment (e.g., attempting to change painful emotions and inadvertently reinforcing patterns of client self-invalidation).

TRAINING KEY DBT TECHNIQUES

It is critical that all DBT trainees learn *risk management and crisis intervention* protocols before providing treatment. Many clinicians are trained to rely on clinical judgment for suicide risk and management, essentially integrating one's knowledge of the research evidence with one's previous clinical experiences to create a subjective judgment of risk (Ægisdóttir et al., 2006; Wingate et al., 2004). Yet, research has repeatedly indicated that clinical judgments alone are not particularly predictive of actual client behavior (e.g., Ægisdóttir et al., 2006; Grove & Meehl, 1996). Moreover, traditional approaches to managing increases

TABLE 5.1. Using Dialectical Dilemmas of Borderline Personality Disorder in Dialectical Behavior Therapy Case Formulation

Dialectical dilemma	Description	Goals for the training clinician
Emotional vulnerability vs.	Extreme emotional sensitivity and intensity and inability to regulate emotion states	Validate the client's affective experiences and inner wisdom while teaching skills for emotion regulation
Self-invalidation	Dismissing one's own emotional experiences and oversimplifying the ease of solving one's problems	Validate the difficulty of the client's life problems Be alert to client's behavioral reactions to therapist invalidation
Active passivity vs.	Approaching life's problems passively or helplessly and demanding that the environment fix problems	Validate the immense difficulty of the work needed to fix life problems while gently demanding skillful behavior from the client
Apparent competence	Behaviors that lead others to assume an individual is competent and able to handle problems (e.g., facial expressions indicating no distress when very distressed)	Carefully assess the client's ability to use skills across different contexts Use behavioral shaping to encourage small steps toward active problem-solving, rather than assuming a lack of ability
Unrelenting crises vs.	An inability to tolerate or fix short-term stressors contributes to a constant, often self-perpetuated, state of crisis	Coach the client in skills needed to tolerate distressing events without exacerbating problems Communicate confidence that client can survive painful events and emotions while teaching skills for regulating painful affect
Inhibited grieving	Involuntary tendency to avoid or escape painful emotional responses, rather than experiencing or integrating one's responses to difficult events	

in suicidality/NSSI often fail to incorporate interventions that directly treat these behaviors and result in long-term reductions in life-threatening behavior (Comtois & Landes, 2018). DBT trainees should therefore receive training in comprehensive, evidence-based tools for screening and responding to risk for suicide and NSSI, such as the Linehan Risk Assessment and Management Protocol (LRAMP; Linehan et al., 2012) or Linehan Suicide Safety Net (LSSN; Harned et al., 2017). Trainees should have a thorough knowledge of basic DBT crisis survival skills (see Linehan, 2015), and should be able to use these strategies across diverse treatment contexts, including individual sessions, phone coaching calls, and DBT skills groups.

Given the level of unrelenting crisis that often accompanies severe emotion dysregulation and chronic suicidality, it is also critical that trainees master the use of DBT *treatment structure*, including the treatment target hierarchy, diary card review, and time management within sessions and phone coaching calls (Ben-Porath & Koons, 2005; Koerner, 2012; Koons, 2011; Linehan, 1993). Particularly for trainees accustomed to more unstructured therapeutic modalities, it can be difficult to learn to work effectively within this structure. It is especially important that trainees be oriented to the rationale for each aspect of the DBT treatment structure. This allows the clinician to flexibly adhere to the principles underlying the treatment structure as needed, rather than rigidly following a set of rules in-session.

All DBT trainees should be familiar with the core sets of change- and acceptance-based strategies used within individual DBT sessions. It is critical that DBT trainees have at least basic training in the theory and application of *behavioral assessment and contingency management*. These techniques form the basis for the behavioral chain analyses and solution analyses that DBT clinicians use to identify and address the contingencies, skills deficits, or problematic cognitions/emotions that give rise to a target behavior (Rizvi & Ritschel, 2014). At the same time, DBT trainees should learn to use *validation* with intentionality throughout a session. Linehan (1993) has specified six levels of validation, arranged in order of increasing intensity, to assist clinicians with effectively communicating validation to the client (see also Carson-Wong & Rizvi, 2016). Many of these validation strategies will be familiar to clinicians trained in psychotherapies other than DBT, but not all will be. DBT trainees should rehearse ways that they can practice validation, even in response to particularly difficult client behaviors (e.g., hostile behavior toward the therapist, NSSI), and should rehearse strategies for flexibly moving between validation and change-based strategies.

Finally, DBT trainees should become familiar with all of the skills covered in the *four modules of DBT skills training*: mindfulness, emotion regulation, distress tolerance, and interpersonal effectiveness (Linehan, 2015). In order to be an effective DBT clinician, the trainee should be able to (a) quickly call to mind a number of specific skills (both change- and acceptance-based) that could address a key link on a behavioral chain assessment of a problem behavior; (b) effectively teach the client to apply one or more of these skills in a targeted way, using behavioral rehearsal as needed; and (c) anticipate and plan for potential problems that may arise when the client implements the new skill in a highly emotional and/or high-risk situation. The supervisor can facilitate this learning by encouraging the trainee to consider and practice each of the skills themselves, and by engaging in explicit conversations about how particular skills may be useful for addressing the trainee's own in-session behavior with the client.

For example, a clinician and their supervisor may note that the clinician has failed to address several significant instances of a client's NSSI (Level 1 target behavior), instead focusing on the client's severe bingeing/purging (Level 3 target behavior). After conducting a behavioral assessment, the supervisor may engage the trainee in the "pros and cons" skills from the emotion regulation module to remind themself about the advantages and disadvantages of adhering to the DBT treatment target hierarchy. The trainee might then practice a "Wise Mind" mindfulness exercise to connect with their own wisdom about more thoroughly assessing and addressing the client's NSSI and use the "opposite to emotion action" skill in-session to address the client's life-threatening behavior thoroughly, even as the trainee feels fear about doing so.

CHOOSING A DBT TRAINING CASE

In contrast to the process of learning many other psychotherapeutic modalities, achieving even a basic proficiency in DBT is more likely to require training cases that are particularly complex and severe in terms of the presenting problems. It is of course necessary to attend to the overall risk profile of the trainee's caseload, and to ensure that it maps onto the trainee's availability and current skill level. Nevertheless, DBT is designed to help clinicians manage complicated and life-threatening psychopathology, and to work effectively with clients who have often experienced numerous treatment failures in the past (Linehan, 1993). As such, the modality requires that trainees work with clients presenting with a range of features typically avoided in "training" cases, including life-threatening behaviors, frequent and acute behavioral crises, high utilization of psychiatric crisis services, and/or a history of failed treatment.

In addition to choosing an appropriate case, it is also important to consider the readiness of the trainee for DBT. As noted earlier, any DBT trainee should have at least basic training in behavioral therapy and mindfulness. Trainees should also be thoroughly oriented to the requirements of DBT and should express a willingness to tolerate the unique challenges of engaging with this therapeutic modality (Waltz et al., 1998). DBT clinicians must encourage clients to rehearse new skills while tolerating the client's immense and urgent emotional pain, without using strategies that may reduce short-term pain but impede the client's long-term stability (e.g., inpatient hospitalization). This requires a considerable emotional investment on the part of the clinician, and any effective training case will involve a trainee who is aware of these challenges and committed to making such an investment.

TROUBLESHOOTING COMMON CHALLENGES FOR DBT TRAINEES

This section details several common challenges encountered by DBT clinicians, including suggestions for how to prevent or address each challenge.

Distress Tolerance and Commitment to Long-Term Change

Many of the most common obstacles to effective treatment for new DBT trainees are related to the significant emotional burden of treating clients with BPD, including fear and anxiety around the clinical acuity of the case (Waltz et al., 1998). Encouraging the client to practice new skills in the face of rising urges for suicide, NSSI, and other high-risk behaviors requires that the clinician and client tolerate a large amount of distress in the short term in the service of gradually changing crisis behaviors in the long term. This can be incredibly challenging for the trainee, and at times, short-term solutions like inpatient hospitalization, rescinding requests for structured skills practice, or even ending/transferring treatment will seem like much more expedient approaches to keeping the client safe than proceeding with DBT. As noted previously, these difficulties can be prevented, to some extent, by orienting the trainee thoroughly in the demands of DBT and obtaining their firm commitment to the job before beginning treatment. Some supervisors may even find it useful to have a written "contract" with the trainee that outlines the unique aspects of DBT. These original commitments can be revisited throughout supervision, with the supervisor and therapist consultation team providing encouragement while holding the trainee accountable to DBT practices.

Negative Emotional Reactions to Clients

DBT often involves working with particularly difficult clients, many of whom have difficulty regulating their emotions and behavior (including within the therapy relationship) as well as a history of treatment disengagement and/or failure as they enter the DBT relationship (Hellman et al., 1986; Linehan, 1993). As such, it is natural that training therapists may find themselves feeling frustrated, angry, or resentful toward the client at various points during treatment. In these moments, the supervisor must find a way to empathically validate the experience of the trainee, while at the same time helping the trainee find a way to feel compassion and liking for the client. In DBT, this compassion and liking are often found by (a) defining the behaviors that are difficult for the trainee in concrete and specific terms (e.g., calling for phone coaching only after 10:00 p.m.; repeatedly saying that they want to report my incompetence to my supervisor) and (b) striving to understand the causes and contingencies that maintain the behavior using traditional behavioral assessment tools. This approach can help the trainee to arrive at a place of greater understanding and empathy for the client, while also yielding potential paths forward to address the problematic client behaviors and reduce the therapist's burnout.

Observing Personal Limits

In DBT, limits in the therapeutic relationship are defined through "real relationship negotiation, not a set of arbitrary rules" (Koerner, 2012, p. 199). This is liberating in some ways, allowing the trainee to make decisions about self-disclosure and phone consultation in a personally relevant way, rather than relying on codified rules or theories of therapeutic neutrality. Yet, at the same time, this approach requires trainees to be aware of and effectively observe personal limits. This may be a new set of skills for some trainees and can often be quite challenging. Trainees must learn to attend carefully to their own emotional reactions to client behaviors, and notice when increasing burnout may indicate overstretched limits. At the same time, they must communicate effectively about limits with their clients, initiating open and assertive conversations about the relationship, rather than relying on prescriptive rules. On top of all of this, the therapist and client will need to navigate inevitable inconsistencies in personal limits (Koons, 2011; Linehan, 1993). Not all clinicians working with the client will have the same personal limits, and the trainee's personal limits may also evolve over time—at times, a clinician may need to stretch their limits at a pivotal point in the treatment, and at other times, a clinician's personal limits may need to constrict (e.g., after the birth of a child). The supervisor should be attentive to the challenges of navigating personal limits and should initiate conversations with the trainee to foster awareness of their limits, while also engaging in skills building and behavioral rehearsal as needed to ensure that the trainee can have effective conversations about these limits with the client.

Dialectics of Treatment Structure

Few studies have directly studied DBT clinicians' adherence to the in-session structure of DBT (cf. DiGiorgio et al., 2010). However, previous research has highlighted more general difficulties with adherence to cognitive behavioral treatment structures (e.g., agenda-setting, pacing during sessions; Waltman et al., 2018), while also noting that adherence to structure may be a key predictor of clinical outcomes in cognitive behavioral therapies (Feeley et al., 1999; Shaw et al., 1999). Moreover, DBT couples a particularly complex structure with an exceptionally challenging clinical population. In the face of novel crises, the clinician may therefore find themselves ignoring certain aspects of this structure, perhaps ignoring the treatment hierarchy to address a resurgence of opioid use (Level 3 target) before thoroughly assessing and addressing new urges for suicide (Level 1), or failing to address the fact that a client has begun to frequently miss DBT skills group sessions or scheduled phone coaching calls. Indeed, clinicians are often punished for maintaining treatment structure— for example, by a client who becomes hostile every time the topic of her incomplete diary card is raised—and reinforced for departures from this structure. Complicating matters even further is the fact that a dialectical approach requires that trainees don't simply adhere to the structure of DBT with rigid inflexibility, refusing to notice when compassionate departures from the typical agenda may be necessary for relationship building and/or treatment progress.

Supervisors can assist DBT trainees by modeling adherence to a similar structure during supervision sessions: beginning and ending supervision sessions on time, setting a clear agenda, and following a transparent supervision structure that follows the treatment target hierarchy. Difficulties with cases that involve life-threatening (Level 1) issues should be discussed first, followed by issues with therapy-interfering (Level 2) and then quality-of-life interfering (Level 3) behaviors. Supervisors should also be attentive to the trainee's adherence to DBT treatment structure in their sessions with clients, always maintaining an awareness of the dialectical tension between losing structure and rigid inflexibility, and they should bring up any potential difficulties the trainee is exhibiting during discussion of therapy-interfering targets in supervision. As with any supervision target, supervisors should thoroughly assess these difficulties before problem solving with the trainee. Once the key factors contributing to problematic trainee or client behaviors have been identified, a solution analysis can be used to link a particular solution to each problematic component of the session. Throughout this process, the supervisor should model a dialectical approach, considering acceptance-based strategies like validation of the trainee's struggles, in tandem with change-based strategies like cognitive restructuring or contingency management.

Reliance on Intuition for Risk Management

As noted in an earlier section, all DBT trainees should receive basic training in evidence-based tools for screening and responding to risk for suicide/NSSI, including DBT crisis survival skills that can be applied with clients who are at acute risk for life-threatening behavior. Because it can be difficult to access and implement this training in highly emotional crisis situations, these skills should be "overlearned" to some extent. The supervisor may wish to use behavioral rehearsal of crisis intervention across diverse contexts during supervision or to review protocols and decision trees that help to streamline the crisis intervention process for trainees (Ben-Porath & Koons, 2005; Harned et al., 2017). Yet, even with these initial training procedures in place, it can be difficult for trainees to maintain a commitment to thorough and structured treatment of suicide and/or NSSI. For one thing, these life-threatening behaviors are so common (and often chronic) in DBT cases that it can be easy for a trainee to begin to treat these behaviors as "background noise" as they move on to more emergent issues in treatment. Moreover, interactions between the clinician and the client around life-threatening behaviors are subject to a host of contingencies. Bypassing structured conversations about risk behaviors can be negatively reinforced by reductions in the trainee's anxiety, a reduction in the client's negative emotions, or both. Trainees must also balance the need for structured risk assessment and management with the fact that some life-threatening behaviors may be maintained, in part, by positively reinforcing interactions with the clinician or other health care providers.

   The supervisor should be alert to the ways in which the trainee is shaped into less effective behavior around risk management and should assist the trainee with identifying skills to support more effective practices. Supervisors should obtain a commitment from the trainee to use evidence-based tools, rather than relying on intuitive or anecdotal assessments of client risk. If needed, the supervisor may wish to assess unhelpful cognitions or emotions that arise for the trainee when considering the implementation of risk management protocols (e.g., intense fear; thoughts like, "Standardized risk assessment protocols will damage my rapport with the client"). Unhelpful cognitions can be addressed with standard cognitive restructuring techniques and behavioral experiments, and difficult emotions like fear can be addressed through formal or informal exposure to crisis situations in supervision (e.g., role plays, watching taped sessions).

Problem-Solving Before Assessment

Trainees may show a tendency to implement skill-based solutions before thorough assessment of the factors maintaining a problematic behavior. Particularly as the clinician becomes more familiar with the typical patterns of severe emotion dysregulation in BPD, as well as more familiar with a particular client and their target behaviors, it can be tempting to rely on assumptions about what is driving a particular target. Yet, a fundamental premise of behavioral therapy involves idiographic analysis of a particular behavior—the solution analysis should always be tied to a prior behavioral chain analysis that highlights critical links from a prompting event to the problem behavior (Koerner, 2012; Linehan, 1993). Otherwise, a particular solution may not be targeting the factors that are most directly tied to this instance of the target behavior.

For example, consider a client that frequently engages in NSSI after intense arguments with her mother. Based on past cases and research evidence about NSSI, the clinician may assume that the self-injurious behavior is being maintained by a pattern of negative reinforcement—when the client engages in NSSI, she experiences relief from intense feelings of anger and shame. However, careful behavioral assessment of multiple instances of this client's NSSI may uncover other factors that are more critical to maintenance of this client's NSSI, such as a positively reinforcing response from the mother—expressions of warmth and caring that the client never receives from her mother other than when she engages in NSSI. Instead of (or in addition to) focusing on the emotional antecedents of the NSSI, the clinician and client can then work collaboratively on interpersonal effectiveness skills that directly target the mother's response to the client's NSSI.

Supervisors should be alert to instances in which the clinician is proceeding to problem-solving before thorough assessment and help to guide the clinician through behavioral assessment of the client's behavior. Often, a target behavior that is persisting even in the face of repeated, effective use of skills by the client is a good indicator that the solution has not been tied to the critical antecedents and consequences for that behavior. The supervisor can frame failures in treatment to acknowledge this fact:

> Ah, so she used the temperature TIPP skill [a distress tolerance skill] appropriately three different times, and still ultimately engaged in self-harm? We must be missing something important. Let's go back to your chain analysis—how does this behavior make sense for her in this situation?

The supervisor can also model this process in the supervisory relationship by taking advantage of opportunities to illustrate behavioral analysis of the trainee's behaviors before suggesting targeted solutions. Finally, the supervisor can frame and approach failed supervisory interventions in the same way— by returning to the search for the key factors contributing to the trainee's behavior in-session through behavioral assessment.

ETHICAL ISSUES IN DBT

A primary ethical concern for any treatment designed for individuals with BPD and/or chronic emotion dysregulation involves navigating the risk for suicide and NSSI, as well as other high-risk and impulsive behaviors (e.g., drug use, criminal behavior, risky sexual behaviors). DBT takes the stance that high-risk urges and behaviors should be managed, as much as possible, in an outpatient setting (Linehan, 1993). According to the DBT model, this approach benefits the client's progress by encouraging rehearsal of skills for managing problematic behaviors in real-life settings, while also avoiding the possibility that hospitalization is inadvertently reinforcing (and thereby exacerbating) the occurrence of dangerous behaviors.

In DBT, risk for self-harm is managed in a number of ways. A thorough history of suicidal and self-injurious behavior is taken early in the intake process, preferably using structured tools for completeness and documentation purposes (e.g., the Suicide Attempt Self-Injury Interview; Linehan et al., 2006). Moreover, frequent assessment with well-validated risk management protocols is built into the treatment. In fact, some research shows that training mental health workers in this risk management protocol, without implementation of the full DBT structure, might play an important role in reducing some self-harm behaviors (Linehan et al., 2015). There are a host of other DBT assessment and treatment strategies designed to reduce clients' risk for self-harm, including the target hierarchy and the focus on rehearsing distress tolerance skills specific to managing emotional crises. It is the responsibility of the supervisor, in conjunction with the consultation team, to ensure that the trainee is appropriately implementing these strategies throughout treatment, even when the trainee is not reinforced (or indeed, is punished) by the client and others for doing so.

Yet, even within a perfectly executed DBT treatment, there will be situations in which the trainee and supervisor remain concerned about the safety of treating the client in an outpatient setting. Supervisors and trainees should prepare for these situations by discussing the challenges of tolerating anxiety about the client's safety in the short term in order to benefit the client's learning and overall progress in the long term. In addition, supervisors should frequently review with the trainee any setting-specific rules or regulations about the hospitalization of suicidal clients, and the ways in which those interact with the DBT treatment plan. Ethical concerns about life-threatening behaviors should be discussed thoroughly in the therapist consultation team, and outside consultation with other DBT clinicians may also be sought.

A related ethical concern can involve making a decision about whether a target behavior should be designated as "life-threatening" (Level 1) and therefore prioritized first in treatment, versus addressing the behavior as a "quality of life–interfering" (Level 3), and therefore a lower priority target. Typically, only urges, affect, and behavior functionally related to the intention to physically harm the body (self-injury) or kill oneself (suicidal) are considered Level 1 targets (Koerner, 2012; Linehan, 1993). Other problematic behaviors, although they may be quite severe, take a lower priority in the treatment target hierarchy. This is true even when quality of life–interfering behaviors become quite dangerous, as is the case with heavy drug use that could result in overdose or a serious eating disorder that could cause medical complications.

With each of these behaviors, the supervisor can help the trainee to use chain analysis to thoroughly assess the client's intention when engaging in the behavior. For example, is the client using alcohol and driving recklessly with the goal of killing themselves in mind? Or is the client using alcohol to manage difficult emotions and impulsively engaging in dangerous behaviors without a clear intention of suicide in mind? Moreover, designating a behavior as a Level 3 target does not mean that it should not be considered a treatment priority. It can be addressed as the top-priority Level 3 target, and sessions can focus on assessing and problem solving around these dangerous behaviors. The treatment target hierarchy merely serves as a reminder to the trainee to assess and address (briefly or at length, depending on what is required) any life-threatening or therapy-interfering behaviors before engaging in this important Level 3 work.

Finally, trainees may also struggle with ethical concerns around the DBT approach to case management. DBT espouses a dialectical approach to case management that balances consultation to the client with direct intervention in the client's environment (Linehan, 1993; Miller et al., 1998). In most situations, DBT clinicians support the client in building and practicing skills to interact with their own environment (e.g., family members, parole officers, psychiatrists). As such, DBT clinicians make an effort to include the client in discussions about their case, and do not "pull strings" to alter the natural consequences of a client's behavior. For example, a client may report that their psychiatrist isn't taking their concerns seriously, and that meetings with the psychiatrist are ending with hostility on both sides and no desired changes in the prescribed medications. Rather than calling the psychiatrist directly to discuss potential medication changes, the clinician might coach the client in interpersonal effectiveness skills to more clearly and assertively state their concerns. If this does not work, the clinician may join the client at the next meeting with the psychiatrist, providing in-the-moment coaching to the client on how to skillfully express their concerns and wishes.

However, there are some cases in which the benefits of environmental intervention on the part of the clinician may outweigh the costs of depriving the client of an opportunity to learn effective skills use within their environment. Some trainees may struggle with this dialectical tension between consultation to the client and environmental intervention, particularly in interactions with other health care professionals. Many clinicians have been trained in models of case management that involve frequent conversations and decision making without the client being present. And it can seem more efficient for a clinician to make a quick call to a psychiatrist or inpatient clinician to ensure that a problem gets sorted out. The supervisor can help the trainee to notice and appreciate this dialectical tension and should assist the trainee in navigating the diverse ethical considerations (e.g., client long-term well-being, client short-term safety, hospital regulations) involved in deciding on the appropriate degree of environmental intervention.

TROUBLESHOOTING COMMON CHALLENGES IN DBT SUPERVISION

Many of the common obstacles in DBT supervision mirror the challenges encountered by the therapist in working with their clients, and often these obstacles can be traced to a dialectical failure of some kind (Waltz et al., 1998). For example, a supervisor may find themselves focusing solely on change-based strategies for eliciting more effective behavior from the trainee, while forgetting to adopt a dialectical approach to balancing acceptance and change within supervision. A sole focus on change, without validation of the considerable challenges inherent in doing DBT, may lead to feelings of dejection, resentment, or shame on the part of the trainee, and can interfere with the progress of supervision. Likewise, the supervisor and trainee may find themselves polarized in their opinions about how to move forward with a particular case. It can be tempting for the supervisor to assume that their position is inherently more "true" given their role as supervisor, rather than collaboratively searching for the wisdom in both perspectives and arriving at a solution that represents the synthesis of these polarized positions. This dialectical approach to supervision can prove especially challenging when the client is in crisis or extreme emotional pain and the trainee is eager for an absolute "right" way to fix the client's problems quickly. Supervisors must tolerate the distress of both the trainee and the client as they support the trainee's long-term learning process. At the same time, the supervisor must attend to their own personal limits, levels of burnout, and feelings toward the trainee and their clients.

Just as in DBT treatment, orienting and commitment strategies are essential to a successful supervision relationship (Waltz et al., 1998). Prior to beginning supervision, supervisors should review the basic approach of DBT treatment and supervision with the trainee and ensure that both the supervisor and trainee are committed to working within this therapeutic framework. In addition, it is recommended that supervisors and trainees regularly review the dialectical agreements of DBT therapist consultation (Linehan, 1993; Sayrs, 2018). These statements outline the basic commitments made by each member of the DBT team when engaging in supervision or consultation and can help both the supervisor and clinician to avoid common pitfalls within supervision. For example, these agreements contain reminders that all clinicians are fallible and should approach their own problematic behaviors in the least defensive way possible; that all clinicians are free to set their own personal and professional limits; and that all parties should search for a synthesis of opposing viewpoints, rather than assuming the existence of an absolute truth, when engaging in polarizing conversations.

Even under ideal circumstances, a supervisor may encounter challenges in their relationship with their trainee or their oversight of a particular case that they are unable to resolve on their own. Fortunately, DBT supervisors and trainees are provided with an extra layer of support through the therapist consultation team. Supervisors can model the DBT approach to case consultation for the trainee by discussing ongoing challenges with the consultation team, and nondefensively accepting the team's feedback for next steps. DBT supervisors may also wish to seek consultation from DBT colleagues outside of their own consultation team for difficult cases.

CONCLUSION

Supervision is fundamental to the practice of DBT, and indeed has been built into the comprehensive model of DBT for clinicians of all levels through therapist consultation teams. DBT supervision follows the same principles as DBT treatment, including a warm and genuine relationship between equals, a dialectical balance of acceptance and change (in considering the behavior of both the client and the trainee), a strong grounding in behavioral principles of assessment and skills-based intervention, and a commitment to tolerating short-term distress in the service of improving the lives of high-risk clients with challenging and complex psychopathology. Although empirical research on evidence-based principles for DBT supervision is still relatively limited, the theoretical writings on DBT treatment, supervision, and consultation teams, in combination with the empirical research on best practices for supervision in traditional cognitive behavior therapy, can be helpful resources for the DBT supervisor.

REFERENCES

Ægisdóttir, S., White, M. J., Spengler, P. M., Maugherman, A. S., Anderson, L. A., Cook, R. S., Nichols, C. N., Lampropoulos, G. K., Walker, B. S., Cohen, G., & Rush, J. D. (2006). The meta-analysis of clinical judgment project: Fifty-six years of accumulated research on clinical versus statistical prediction. *The Counseling Psychologist, 34*(3), 341–382. https://doi.org/10.1177/0011000005285875

American Psychiatric Association. (2006). *American Psychiatric Association practice guidelines for the treatment of psychiatric disorders: Compendium 2006.*

Ben-Porath, D. D., & Koons, C. R. (2005). Telephone coaching in dialectical behavior therapy: A decision-tree model for managing inter-session contact with clients. *Cognitive and Behavioral Practice, 12*(4), 448–460. https://doi.org/10.1016/S1077-7229(05)80072-0

Brodsky, B. S., Cabaniss, D. L., Arbuckle, M., Oquendo, M. A., & Stanley, B. (2017). Teaching dialectical behavior therapy to psychiatry residents: The Columbia psychiatry residency DBT curriculum. *Academic Psychiatry, 41*(1), 10–15. https://doi.org/10.1007/s40596-016-0593-0

Carson-Wong, A., & Rizvi, S. (2016). Reliability and validity of the DBT-VLCS: A measure to code validation strategies in dialectical behavior therapy sessions. *Psychotherapy Research, 26*(3), 332–341. https://doi.org/10.1080/10503307.2014.966347

Comtois, K. A., & Landes, S. J. (2018). Crisis management and treating suicidality from a behavioral perspective. In S. C. Hayes & S. G. Hofmann (Eds.) *Process-based CBT: The science and core clinical competencies of cognitive behavioral therapy* (pp. 415–426). New Harbinger.

Crowell, S. E., Beauchaine, T. P., & Linehan, M. M. (2009). A biosocial developmental model of borderline personality: Elaborating and extending Linehan's theory. *Psychological Bulletin, 135*(3), 495–510. https://doi.org/10.1037/a0015616

DiGiorgio, K. E., Glass, C. R., & Arnkoff, D. B. (2010). Therapists' use of DBT: A survey study of clinical practice. *Cognitive and Behavioral Practice, 17*(2), 213–221. https://doi.org/10.1016/j.cbpra.2009.06.003

Dimeff, L. A., & Linehan, M. M. (2008). Dialectical behavior therapy for substance abusers. *Addiction Science & Clinical Practice, 4*(2), 39–47. https://www.ncbi.nlm.nih.gov/pmc/articles/PMC2797106/

Feeley, M., DeRubeis, R. J., & Gelfand, L. A. (1999). The temporal relation of adherence and alliance to symptom change in cognitive therapy for depression. *Journal of Consulting and Clinical Psychology, 67*(4), 578–582. https://doi.org/10.1037/0022-006X.67.4.578

Grove, W. M., & Meehl, P. E. (1996). Comparative efficiency of informal (subjective, impressionistic) and formal (mechanical, algorithmic) prediction procedures: The clinical–statistical controversy. *Psychology, Public Policy, and Law, 2*(2), 293–323. https://doi.org/10.1037/1076-8971.2.2.293

Harned, M. S., Korslund, K. E., Foa, E. B., & Linehan, M. M. (2012). Treating PTSD in suicidal and self-injuring women with borderline personality disorder: Development and preliminary evaluation of a dialectical behavior therapy prolonged exposure protocol. *Behaviour Research and Therapy, 50*(6), 381–386. https://doi.org/10.1016/j.brat.2012.02.011

Harned, M. S., Lungu, A., Wilks, C. R., & Linehan, M. M. (2017). Evaluating a multimedia tool for suicide risk assessment and management: The Linehan Suicide Safety Net. *Journal of Clinical Psychology, 73*(3), 308–318. https://doi.org/10.1002/jclp.22331

Hellman, I. D., Morrison, T. L., & Abramowitz, S. I. (1986). The stresses of psychotherapeutic work: A replication and extension. *Journal of Clinical Psychology, 42*(1), 197–205. https://doi.org/10.1002/1097-4679(198601)42:1<197::AID-JCLP2270420134>3.0.CO;2-J

Kliem, S., Kröger, C., & Kosfelder, J. (2010). Dialectical behavior therapy for borderline personality disorder: A meta-analysis using mixed-effects modeling. *Journal of Consulting and Clinical Psychology, 78*(6), 936–951. https://doi.org/10.1037/a0021015

Koerner, K. (2012). *Doing dialectical behavior therapy: A practical guide.* Guilford Press.

Koerner, K., & Linehan, M. M. (1997). Case formulation in dialectical behavior therapy for borderline personality disorder. In T. D. Eells (Ed.), *Handbook of psychotherapy case formulation* (pp. 340–367). Guilford Press.

Koons, C. R. (2011). The role of the team in managing telephone consultation in dialectical behavior therapy: Three case examples. *Cognitive and Behavioral Practice, 18*(2), 168–177. https://doi.org/10.1016/j.cbpra.2009.10.008

Linehan, M. M. (1993). *Cognitive–behavioral therapy of borderline personality disorder.* Guilford Press.

Linehan, M. M. (2015). *DBTherapy skills training manual* (2nd ed.). Guilford Press.

Linehan, M. M., Cochran, B. N., Mar, C. M., Levensky, E. R., & Comtois, K. A. (2000). Therapeutic burnout among borderline personality disordered clients and their therapists: Development and evaluation of two adaptations of the Maslach Burnout Inventory. *Cognitive and Behavioral Practice, 7*(3), 329–337. https://doi.org/10.1016/S1077-7229(00)80091-7

Linehan, M. M., Comtois, K. A., Brown, M. Z., Heard, H. L., & Wagner, A. (2006). Suicide Attempt Self-Injury Interview (SASII): Development, reliability, and validity of a scale to assess suicide attempts and intentional self-injury. *Psychological Assessment, 18*(3), 303–312. https://doi.org/10.1037/1040-3590.18.3.303

Linehan, M. M., Comtois, K. A., & Ward-Ciesielski, E. F. (2012). Assessing and managing risk with suicidal individuals. *Cognitive and Behavioral Practice, 19*(2), 218–232. https://doi.org/10.1016/j.cbpra.2010.11.008

Linehan, M. M., Korslund, K. E., Harned, M. S., Gallop, R. J., Lungu, A., Neacsiu, A. D., McDavid, J., Comtois, K. A., & Murray-Gregory, A. M. (2015). Dialectical behavior therapy for high suicide risk in individuals with borderline personality disorder: A randomized clinical trial and component analysis. *JAMA Psychiatry, 72*(5), 475–482. https://doi.org/10.1001/jamapsychiatry.2014.3039

Miller, A. L., Koerner, K., & Kanter, J. (1998). Dialectical behavior therapy: Part II. Clinical application of DBT for patients with multiple problems. *Journal of Practical Psychiatry and Behavioral Health, 4*(2), 84–101. https://journals.lww.com/practicalpsychiatry/Abstract/1998/03000/Dialectical_Behavior_Therapy__Part_II__Clinical.4.aspx

Panos, P. T., Jackson, J. W., Hasan, O., & Panos, A. (2014). Meta-analysis and systematic review assessing the efficacy of dialectical behavior therapy (DBT). *Research on Social Work Practice, 24*(2), 213–223. https://doi.org/10.1177/1049731513503047

Rizvi, S. L., & Ritschel, L. A. (2014). Mastering the art of chain analysis in dialectical behavior therapy. *Cognitive and Behavioral Practice, 21*(3), 335–349. https://doi.org/10.1016/j.cbpra.2013.09.002

Rizvi, S. L., Yu, J., Geisser, S., & Finnegan, D. (2016). The use of "bug-in-the-eye" live supervision for training in dialectical behavior therapy: A case study. *Clinical Case Studies, 15*(3), 243–258. https://doi.org/10.1177/1534650116635272

Sayrs, J. H. R. (2018). Running an effective DBT consultation team: Principles and challenges. In M. Swales (Ed.), *The Oxford handbook of dialectical behaviour therapy.* Oxford University Press. https://doi.org/10.1093/oxfordhb/9780198758723.013.10

Shaw, B. F., Elkin, I., Yamaguchi, J., Olmsted, M., Vallis, T. M., Dobson, K. S., Lowery, A., Sotsky, S. M., Watkins, J. T., & Imber, S. D. (1999). Therapist competence ratings in relation to clinical outcome in cognitive therapy of depression. *Journal of Consulting and Clinical Psychology, 67*(6), 837–846. https://doi.org/10.1037/0022-006X.67.6.837

Waltman, S. H., Hall, B. C., McFarr, L. M., & Creed, T. A. (2018). Clinical case consultation and experiential learning in cognitive behavioral therapy implementation: Brief qualitative investigation. *Journal of Cognitive Psychotherapy, 32*(2), 112–127. https://doi.org/10.1891/0889-8391.32.2.112

Waltz, J., Fruzzetti, A., & Linehan, M. (1998). The role of supervision in dialectical behavior therapy. *The Clinical Supervisor, 17*(1), 101–113. https://doi.org/10.1300/J001v17n01_09

Wingate, L. R., Joiner, T. E., Jr., Walker, R. L., Rudd, M. D., & Jobes, D. A. (2004). Empirically informed approaches to topics in suicide risk assessment. *Behavioral Sciences & the Law, 22*(5), 651–665. https://doi.org/10.1002/bsl.612

6

Functional Analytic Psychotherapy

Supervision and Therapist Self-Development

Mavis Tsai, Robert J. Kohlenberg, Emerson Hardebeck,
Sarah Sullivan-Singh, and Mary Plummer Loudon

Functional analytic psychotherapy (FAP) is a modern behavior therapy, rooted in functional contextualism, that leverages the power of the therapeutic relationship and maximizes therapists' genuineness, empathy, and vulnerability. Each client's unique history—their experiences of joy and anguish, their cultural and generational memories—is closely examined to understand how and for what this person has been reinforced. An FAP therapist enters each session with their particular client's history in mind, tuning in to how this person's daily-life problems occur in the therapy session, and responding to such problems in a tailored way that helps the client move towards a more meaningful life (Holman et al., 2017; Kohlenberg & Tsai, 1991; Tsai et al., 2009; Tsai et al., 2013). A key mechanism of change in FAP is the therapist responding contingently to client problems and improvements as they occur in session. Instead of merely spending the therapy hour talking about problems that occur in the client's outside life, FAP focuses on how these problems are emerging here and now, moment-to-moment, as the client and therapist engage in a real relationship together.

For some therapists, it may be unfamiliar to look for client behaviors during a session that correspond to that client's presenting concerns, but such *clinically relevant behaviors* (CRBs) are more common than one might first imagine. FAP recognizes two different categories of CRBs, referred to as *CRB1s* and *CRB2s*. CRB1s are in-session occurrences of behaviors that are related to problems the client has identified they would like to change; in a successful course of

https://doi.org/10.1037/0000314-007
Training and Supervision in Specialized Cognitive Behavior Therapy: Methods, Settings, and Populations, E. A. Storch, J. S. Abramowitz, and D. McKay (Editors)

FAP, CRB1s will decrease over time. CRB1s can take a nearly infinite number of forms depending on the client's specific history or presentation—for instance, Tsai et al. (2009) explained that CRB1s for a man who reports having no friends might include avoiding eye contact, answering questions by talking at length in an unfocused and tangential manner, having one "crisis" after another, demanding to be taken care of, and getting angry at the therapist for not having all the answers. In contrast, a significant CRB1 for a woman whose primary presenting complaint is that she develops relationships with unattainable men might be developing a crush on her male therapist.

CRB2s are in-session improvements that correspond to a client's goals for therapy. A client will begin to display these behaviors more often over time if treatment is succeeding. At the beginning of therapy, CRB2s are rare by definition; while nearly all clients bring numerous strengths and assets with them into therapy, a behavior is only considered a CRB2 if it is initially outside a client's repertoire. A behavior that a client can engage in with ease may be a CRB1, or if it is not problematic, may simply not be CRB. Moreover, it cannot be overstated that, consistent with the functional contextual theories underlying FAP, CRB1s and CRB2s are idiographically defined. In other words, without knowing a particular client's life history, goals, and case conceptualization, a therapist cannot know whether a certain behavior is a CRB1 or CRB2 for that client. Even a behavior that might appear topographically to be problematic (e.g., yelling at the therapist) might represent an initial step toward a CRB2 for an individual client (e.g., if they have difficulty asserting their needs), and may simply require further gradual shaping to ensure that it is enacted in a form that is likelier to be reinforced in a client's natural environment.

KEY CONCEPTS AND TECHNIQUES FOR TRAINEES TO LEARN

FAP entails implementing five therapeutic rules that orient the focus of treatment to CRBs. Rather than the common rigid connotation of the term "rule," FAP rules are suggestions for therapist behavior that typically lead to positive client change and thus reinforce the therapist. In actual clinical practice, the rules are less clearly distinct from one another than when presented in a textbook for learning purposes, and an FAP therapist is often enacting several rules simultaneously. A primary reason for delineating these rules so concretely is to help therapists harness therapeutic opportunities that they might not otherwise notice.

Rule 1: Watch for CRBs (Be Aware)

This rule has often been said to be the most important one in FAP, as simply following it on its own can result in a significantly more powerful therapy relationship and treatment course. As a therapist becomes more attuned to CRBs taking place in the room, therapy has a way of becoming more immediate, interesting, and meaningful. A therapist's ability to notice CRBs and observe their function will be affected by many variables, including the therapist's own problematic behaviors, which we label "Therapist 1s" or *T1s*. Corresponding improvements in therapist behavior are *T2s*. For example, a therapist who is highly sensitive to criticism may misinterpret a client's effectively assertive delivery of negative feedback as a CRB1, when in fact this behavior was actually a CRB2 for the client. As such, it is critical that FAP therapists continuously practice awareness of how their own learning histories and resultant behaviors may influence their interactions with clients.

Rule 2: Evoke CRBs (Be Courageous)

A necessary condition for FAP treatment to be effective is that the therapy relationship must be similar enough to the rest of the client's life that CRB1s will emerge and eventually be replaced by CRB2s. The degree to which the therapeutic relationship will need to be individually tailored to sufficiently replicate the salient behavioral triggers in a client's life depends on the individual client's history and presenting concerns. Some complaints, such as anxiety, depression, or indecision, are likely to occur directly in the therapy relationship regardless of what paradigm the therapist is using. However, it is also common for clients to express more interpersonal goals for therapy, such as deeply trusting others, taking interpersonal risks, being authentic, or giving and receiving love. In order for such concerns to be not merely talked about but actually experienced and worked with directly in the therapeutic relationship, FAP invites therapists to be completely present, conducting therapy in a manner not typically found in other behavior therapies. In many cases, for the therapy relationship to become evocative enough to give rise to frequent CRB, therapists need to take risks and push their own emotional intimacy boundaries. This entails being courageous enough to genuinely step beyond one's comfort zone, setting the tone for clients to do the same.

"From the very first contact between therapist and client, therapists can begin structuring the therapeutic environment to prepare the client for an intense and evocative therapy that focuses on in-vivo interactions" (Tsai et al., 2009, p. 71). It is often a good idea to offer the FAP rationale, or "FAP rap," as early as possible, informing clients that the therapist will be working with their outside life problems directly as they emerge in therapy because this present-moment focus creates the most impactful change. Often, people believe they are coming to therapy to discuss issues and relationships outside of therapy, so variations of the "FAP rap" should be presented in informed consent documents and early sessions of treatment until the client has a full understanding of why approaching treatment this way may be helpful. It is the therapist's personal invitation to the client to participate in a meaningful interpersonal relationship. For example, a therapist could say, "Unlike therapies that focus on telling you how to do things, research shows that it's really effective to be aware of how your struggles in daily life are actually showing up in therapy.

In other words, I consider our relationship to be a microcosm of your outside relationships. So, I'd like to explore how you interact with me in a way that is similar to how you interact with other people, what problems come up with me that also come up with other people, or what positive behaviors you have with me that you can translate into your relationships with others."

Rule 3: Reinforce CRBs Naturally (Be Therapeutically Loving)

Effective evoking typically results in lots of CRBs, which is where Rule 3, reinforcing CRBs naturally, comes in. To move clients from CRB1s to CRB2s, therapists need to find an expanse of nascent, improved behaviors to authentically reinforce through successive approximations, including CRB2s that might not be reinforced by others in the outside world. The therapist who is aware of the occurrence of CRB2s and sees them as stepping-stones to client goals is likely to respond in a naturally reinforcing manner that will help clients generalize improvements to daily life.

How does a FAP therapist reinforce CRB2s? One way we describe the therapist stance that leads to being naturally reinforcing is to be "therapeutically loving" (Tsai et al., 2013). Our behavioral definition of therapeutic love is a willingness to take steps, within the boundaries of the therapeutic relationship, that will best serve the client's interests. Specifically, we encourage therapists to give clients gifts from their hearts in terms of offering reinforcing self-disclosure in response to CRB2s. We often ask new FAP trainees to ask themselves the following questions to guide their therapeutically loving response when a client emits a CRB2:

> What's alive in you, the therapist, right now? What's hard for you to share with this client about what they have just done? What body sensations, thoughts, memories, images are coming up for you? How are you growing, being inspired or motivated as a result of this interaction with your client?

An example of a powerful, authentic statement in response to a CRB2 might be:

> No matter how hard I tried to connect with my dad as a kid, I never felt let in by him. When you just did [description of the client's CRB2], I felt connected to you and could feel that kid inside me being healed just a bit more. You have no idea how powerful and meaningful that is to me.

What is reinforcing to one client may be punishing to another, however, so the only way we can be certain that our behavior was reinforcing is to observe whether the targeted CRB2 increases in strength (see the discussion of Rule 4).

We tend to focus on authentic positive reinforcement for CRB2s in Rule 3, but sometimes faster progress can be made if therapists simultaneously try to extinguish CRB1s as well. This can be done by ignoring them, by presenting the stimulus again in a different way (e.g., "Are you noticing any sensations in your body?"), by asking about visible signs of possible emotional avoidance (e.g., inappropriate affect, tense body, poor eye contact), by asking about possible avoidance directly (e.g., "What might you be doing to block your feelings right now?"), by prompting and shaping a CRB2 (e.g., "How about if

I name some feelings, and you pick one that seems to fit?") or by addressing previously emitted CRB2s (e.g., "You've been naming your feelings more, which helps me feel really connected. What can I do right now to help you name your feelings?") After a relationship is more solid, therapists can try blocking CRB1s with a kind tone, saying something like, "I feel far away from you when you don't respond."

Rule 4: Be Aware of Your Impact

Rule 4 guides therapists to pay attention to the relationship between changes in the client's target behaviors and the therapist's contingent responding. It bears repeating that, by definition, the only way to know if the client is actually being reinforced for their CRB2s is if they begin to exhibit those very behaviors more frequently or intensely. A common mistake trainees can make is assuming that if they made a strongly worded statement (e.g., an expression of gratitude for what the client did, or an emotional disclosure of how the client impacted them), then they must have reinforced the client. In many cases this may be true; however, because every person has been trained by their unique history to respond to different sorts of stimuli as reinforcing, some individuals will find aversive a therapist response that would be pleasant to another client. Thus, the only way to determine if a response that was intended to be reinforcing was in fact reinforcing is if there is an observed increase in the target behavior afterward—so it is critical for a FAP therapist to be highly attentive to how a client's behavioral repertoire is evolving. Nonetheless, explicitly asking about the client's experience of an intended reinforcer can also offer clues about how a therapist response has been received by the client. For example, the therapist may simply ask, "How was that for you?" or "How did you feel when I said just now that I am inspired by your risk-taking this week?" or "Do you think my response made it more or less likely that you will do what you did again?"

It is important to time these assessment questions strategically. An interaction involving CRB2/Rule 3 may be quite emotional, so attempting right away to "process" it with Rule 4 questions may truncate the natural interaction. Moreover, quickly moving away from the client's CRB2 and the therapist's reaction to it may at times represent a therapist's subtle avoidance of emotional intensity. An approach to Rule 4 that can create more room to lean into the powerful reinforcement and learning opportunities of a Rule 3 interaction is to wait until the next session to engage in much processing of what happened.

Rule 5: Interpret and Generalize

This final rule focuses on therapists making functional analytically informed interpretations and extensions of client behavior. These interpretations can include understanding of learning history that accounts for how problematic behavior was adaptive for clients in the past and how to generalize progress in therapy to daily life. Facilitating generalization is essential; success in FAP has not been achieved unless clients change their behavior in daily life. Thus, provision of homework is also central in Rule 5. Some of the best homework assignments are made when a client has engaged in a CRB2 and the assignment is for the client to take the improved behavior "on the road" and try doing it with significant others.

WHAT PATIENT CHARACTERISTICS MAKE FOR A GOOD TRAINING CASE IN FAP?

In cases where there is another evidence-based practice that more directly targets a client's presenting problem, then that treatment should be applied first. For example, clients who fit the diagnostic criteria for borderline personality disorder should be referred for dialectical behavior therapy. It is important to note, however, that FAP can be integrated into and enhance virtually any form of psychotherapy. Moreover, engaging a client in specific interventions that might appear to be unrelated to typical FAP targets (e.g., exposure and response prevention) can itself function as a potent evoke (e.g., the client might struggle to communicate to the therapist that the exposure protocol is moving too quickly and begin skipping sessions).

In general, however, clients with less specific presenting concerns offer the new FAP therapist a relatively more expansive palette of FAP interventions with which they can paint freely rather than having to manage the complexity of incorporating the colors of another evidence-based practice. In addition, clients presenting with problems and goals specific to relationships are often an especially good fit, as CRBs may be easier to identify and clients may be more immediately interested in exploring the therapy relationship as a means of working on outside goals. By contrast, clients who are not receptive to the FAP rationale regarding why it is important to focus on behaviors occurring in session and the bond between therapist and client may be poor candidates for FAP.

COMMON MISTAKES THAT TRAINEES MAKE AND HOW TO FIX THEM

Organized according to the five rules that comprise FAP, this section discusses the most common mistakes trainees make, as well as corresponding remedies.

Mistakes in Awareness of CRBs (Rule 1)

When watching for CRBs, it is essential for therapists to understand the distinction between the function versus the form of a behavior. That is, client behaviors are grouped based on similar antecedents, consequences, and functions (or the purpose they serve), with specific form or appearance often varying across different clients and across contexts within any one client. Behaviors that look different (i.e., have different forms) can be functionally equivalent. For example, withdrawing into sadness, laughing hysterically, and yelling in anger may all serve the same function (i.e., be functionally equivalent) of distracting the therapist from talking about interpersonal closeness. Likewise, topographically similar behaviors may serve very different functions. For instance, depending on the context, each of the following behaviors could function to facilitate avoidance or engagement and connection: telling a joke, sobbing, always being willing to do homework, disclosing suicidal ideation, sitting in silence, and complimenting the therapist. As therapists learn to notice the shared function among a client's behaviors, they can focus on authentically reinforcing connection and extinguishing/punishing avoidance in the moment rather than being distracted by responding to the topography of a client's behaviors. Completing a case formulation that incorporates the client's salient learning history, values and goals, problematic beliefs, and an inventory of potential CRBs can support the identification of distinct functional classes of behavior that cut across topography.

Mistakes in Being Evocative (Rule 2)

Mistakes in the execution of Rule 2 may assume diverse forms, including offering evokes that are too intense, too passive, too frequent, or not frequent enough. Addressing these issues may involve increasing a supervisee's awareness of the problem (being able to watch recordings of supervisee sessions is helpful) but may well also involve addressing supervisee T1s, such as discomfort and avoidance of delivering negative feedback to clients. For example, supervisees may hesitate to disclose the impact a client is having when they ramble at length or cancel sessions at the last minute. To resolve this avoidance, it is helpful to look at the supervisee's history and consider what makes it so hard for them to be evocative with their clients around this particular issue. In addition, a supervisor might have a supervisee practice the same kind of evocative behavior that is needed with the client in supervision (e.g., the supervisor might ask the supervisee to offer a piece of negative feedback about the supervision process). In this way, supervisors also model effective evoking in supervision by evoking the supervisee T2s.

Mistakes in Reinforcing CRBs (Rule 3)

Numerous mistakes can be made in naturally reinforcing CRBs. We focus on three key ones in this section.

Inadvertently Reinforcing CRB1s or Punishing CRB2s

As discussed earlier, CRB1s and CRB2s are defined by their function, rather than their form, and are idiographic, so the same behavior might be a CRB1 for one client, but a CRB2 for another client with a different history and case conceptualization. In order not to unwittingly punish improvements or reinforce problems, Tsai et al. (2016) instructed therapists to pay attention to

- how each client's behavior, including their CRB1s, emerges from that person's historical and cultural context, including numerous environmental antecedents and consequences they have been exposed to;

- the temptation to pathologize early CRB2s, not understanding them to be growth because their form may be rough, as they are still being shaped (e.g., a client who does not usually express their opinions may seem overly critical of the therapist when they first begin to do so);

- the fact that the same behavior must be interpreted differently across clients, given their different histories and goals (e.g., for a client who is compulsively on time, being late to a session might be a CRB2, but this same behavior could be a CRB1 in a client who is always running late); and

- the ever-changing nature of CRB as clients' repertoires expand over the course of therapy—indeed, behavior that is a CRB2 towards the beginning of therapy may be a CRB1 in the later stages (e.g., asking for the therapist's take on a significant question may be a CRB2 at first for a client who has difficulty relying on others, but if this behavior becomes so entrenched over time that it develops into overreliance on the therapist, then it might be reconceptualized as a CRB1 near the end of therapy and treated as such at that point).

Supervisors need to be in the practice of routinely and repeatedly, across and within clients, asking the question "How is this behavior a CRB1, a CRB2, both, or neither?" and thoughtfully considering the dynamics described earlier with their supervisees.

Not Having the Client's Target Behavior in One's Own Repertoire
In order to be helpful to the numerous clients who present to therapy with various flavors of interpersonal difficulties, an FAP therapist must have access to a broad and flexible repertoire of relational behaviors. Consider a client who struggles to accept love and care, or to open up about their feelings. If this client's therapist is not comfortable with intimacy, then the therapist will probably not act in ways that generate adequate connection with the client, and may also fail to reinforce bids for closeness when the client does emit them. In fact, client behaviors such as asking for more closeness, making personal inquiries about the therapist, or stating how important the therapist is to them might be interpreted indiscriminately as CRB1s by a therapist whose own repertoire of closeness-generating behaviors is underdeveloped. Of course, at times it may be entirely correct to understand such behaviors from clients as CRB1s, but an FAP therapist should have a well-rounded interpersonal repertoire that allows them to accurately discriminate between CRB1s and CRB2s, and to respond accordingly.

Indiscriminate Self-Disclosure

Therapists newer to the strategic use of self-disclosure as both an evoking and reinforcing stimulus may at times err in the direction of self-disclosing in more depth and/or with more frequency than is actually helpful for clients. For example, when a client discloses a significant event, the therapist may be tempted to respond with a similar disclosure that conveys "Something similar happened to me, I know what that is like." In some circumstances, such disclosure may be reinforcing, but in many others it may not be. Hence, supervisors need to model and coach supervisees in both identifying a rationale for self-disclosure and carefully observing the impact of disclosure on the client (Rule 4). In sum, though FAP encourages the use of the therapist's authentic self as a primary tool in the therapy process, autobiographical self-disclosure should only be offered deliberately and thoughtfully. Trainees are encouraged to hone their sensitivity to the effects of their disclosures during supervision, by making personal disclosures to supervisors, who can then advise them about whether or not a particular disclosure seems like it might be helpful to make directly to the client.

Mistakes in Being Aware of One's Impact (Rule 4)

We have observed a pattern in supervision that therapists are often better able to report back on their own in-session behaviors relative to describing the client's in-session behaviors. When asked to describe the important moments in a therapy session, supervisees often report the interventions they performed but may struggle to respond to the subsequent question: "And then what did the client do?" It is natural, especially when learning a new skill, to maintain heightened awareness of one's own behavior, but practicing FAP necessitates supervisees learn to practice a keen awareness of their own behavior, the client's behavior, and the reciprocal impacts being continuously exchanged in the therapy relationship. Rule 4 can be practiced covertly by observing the client's facial expressions, posture, movement, tone, and verbal responses and also explicitly by asking the client: "I just gave you some feedback that might have felt pretty powerful. What's happening for you right now as you take it in?"

One strategy for honing supervisee awareness of their own and the client's behavior is to have supervisees complete a "session bridging form" (adapted from the client session bridging form; Tsai et al., 2009, Appendix D) between supervision sessions that asks them to observe (a) their own problematic and improved behavior in both supervision and client sessions, (b) the impact of the supervisor's behavior on them in the supervision relationship, and (c) the client's CRB1s and CRB2s. The process of completing the supervision bridging questionnaire is a practice of awareness for the supervisee and also provides the supervisor with useful information about both the supervisee's clinical interactions and how the process of supervision is working.

Not Knowing How to Help Clients Generalize (Rule 5)

It is a mistake to expect too much change too quickly; it may take much time and patience for a client to enact change in their outside context. When clients are having difficulty generalizing their gains in therapy, it is important to plan homework very intentionally and with careful consideration of the client's context. Sometimes significant creativity is required to figure out how to engage clients in any homework. In such cases, several strategies that have worked with our clients include sharing a secure, online spreadsheet where client and therapist both track target behaviors (e.g., gratitude lists, meditation time, bids for social connection). This practice can be effective whether clients and therapists are working on the same or different target behaviors but can be especially powerful when working on the same behavior.

Some clients may benefit from checking in by email about target behaviors between sessions, or by checking in about progress on target behaviors at the beginning of each session. Supervisors can coach supervisees in experimenting with these practices with their clients and also can engage supervisees in the practices by setting shared goals for T2s that may be relevant in both client and supervision sessions (e.g., ending sessions on time, leading mindfulness meditations, setting a session agenda).

Another important point is that in comparison to the rich and immediate wealth of reinforcement FAP therapists learn to offer in session to clients, the outside world is rarely as immediately or powerfully reinforcing of new behaviors. Indeed, under some circumstances, a client's social network may balk at behavior changes. After all, a client's problematic behaviors in daily life typically have been long maintained by their social context. For example, a client's spouse may have grown accustomed to the client taking on the coordinating role for the couple's social activities and may not take kindly to the client's request that the spouse assume a more active role in that coordination. In cases such as this, supervisors must prepare trainees to offer an attuned response to the disappointment, reinforce the act of having taken the risk, build hope that future risks can lead to different outcomes, and gently debrief what happened and how the client may wish to revise their planning of future risks.

ETHICAL ISSUES IN TREATMENT APPLICATION

FAP seeks to cultivate a deep and profound therapeutic experience in which strong attachments often develop between therapist and client. The functional contextual emphasis in FAP encourages therapists to think flexibly about the structure of therapy and orient toward practices that most workably support clients' goals rather than adhering to a particular set of standard procedures. This flexibility affords room for creativity and tailoring treatment to suit the client's needs. The combination of flexibility in procedures and a potentially intense therapeutic bond, however, also requires that FAP therapists be extremely thoughtful, careful, and cautious in cultivating an exquisite awareness of both their own reactions to the client, the client's reactions to them, and the maintenance of professional boundaries. FAP supervisors must both model this kind of professional and yet deeply emotional relationship with their supervisees and also ensure that boundaries are a routine topic in supervision. The following sections delineate areas of potential ethical concern and how they relate specifically to FAP.

Exploitation

The intense and emotional nature of the therapeutic relationships that can be created in FAP makes it especially critical for supervisors and supervisees to always ask themselves what is best for their client. Holding this question in awareness reduces the chance that clients will be exploited or harmed. Particular pitfalls to remain wary of include unhealthy dependence on the therapist, sexual involvement, or interminable treatment where both parties are gratified by a relationship that is more like friendship than therapy. It is worth noting that another benefit of the open and vulnerable supervision environment fostered by FAP is that it often encourages supervisees to be especially authentic with their supervisors, sharing fears and uncertainties so they can be attended to before serious issues arise.

Cultural Biases

Because we are all embedded in a particular cultural context that contains certain values and expectations, FAP therapists defining CRB must balance the pull of our own culture with that of the client's. Developing awareness of our own cultural biases and blind spots is critical to avoid reinforcing what may seem like a CRB2 given our own cultural assumptions, but is actually a CRB1 from the client's context, or vice versa. For example, one therapist may have the expectation in his own culture that men ought to be impassive; from that lens, this therapist might unconsciously punish emotional disclosure from a male client, even if this behavior is actually a CRB2 for that client.

Acknowledging the importance of culture cannot be overstated; FAP therapists must be deeply attuned to a client's culture and/or subculture and seek consultation when necessary to learn about a client's culture. The need for multiculturally sensitive interventions is increasingly urgent. Therapists need to be more prepared to address cultural issues surrounding racism, discrimination, and White privilege in order to better serve marginalized populations. FAP enables clinicians to gain awareness of their own cultural assumptions and biases and to expand their multicultural competence as they register their clients' responses to their culturally influenced perspective (Miller et al., 2015).

Being Controlled by Reinforcers That Do Not Benefit Clients

From an FAP perspective, an important ethical consideration is to ensure that the therapist is aware of how what takes place in therapy is or is not beneficial to their client, and that the therapist is primarily reinforced by what is beneficial to their client, rather than what isn't. As an example, consider a client for whom it is a common CRB1 to make overzealous expressions of gratitude and praise towards the therapist. It's easy to imagine how a therapist might recognize this behavior as a CRB1 and would not feel reinforced by it (e.g., they might feel slightly distanced or disappointed when their client acted this way). However, it's just as easy to imagine a therapist who does experience reinforcement from this sort of client behavior, and whose appreciative responses then reinforce and maintain the client's problem. The potential for ethical issues of this nature to arise underscores the importance of practicing Rule 1. Supervisors need to observe what is reinforcing to supervisees in both the supervision and client relationships and, together with the supervisee, consider if there are any problematic sources of reinforcement in operation in either context.

THE BIGGEST CHALLENGE IN FAP SUPERVISION: IN VIVO WORK

Consistent with supervision across all theoretical orientations, FAP supervision attempts to help the supervisee develop their intellectual knowledge about clinical work and case conceptualization, using methods such as modeling of interventions, assigned homework (e.g., readings), setting goals, and offering feedback on recordings or other assessments of performance. A more challenging endeavor in FAP supervision is to create "emotional knowing" for trainees with in vivo work that directly shapes the effectiveness of their behavior related to noticing, evoking, and contingently responding to CRBs. These therapist behaviors are contingency-shaped and, unlike improvements in the FAP knowledge base, improvements in contingency-shaped behavior can occur outside of awareness. This sort of knowledge is described in everyday language as "deep," "emotional," and "intuitive" (Skinner, 1974). One supervisee aptly described the contrast between intellectual knowing versus emotional knowing through supervision:

> Many other supervisors tried to teach me to be emotionally present with my clients. But I am finding that going there is something I do heart-first. To do this task, I needed more than hearing it in supervision, reading it in an article, or watching it on a video. I needed to experience it myself, in-vivo, within the supervisory relationship. That, for me, is the core of FAP and FAP supervision that is transforming me and my work. (Tsai et al., 2009, p. 169)

Thus, in FAP supervision, trainees learn competent therapist behaviors by directly experiencing an intense and supportive interpersonal relationship with their supervisor. The idea that intellectual learning alone is insufficient to help trainees develop competence is well-established, and prior work has noted that in vivo learning in supervision can be an especially effective tool (Safran & Muran, 2001). Other research supporting this kind of approach has found that exploring parallel process in supervision leads to better client outcomes (Tracey et al., 2012), and that trainees who build a stronger alliance with supervisors using self-disclosure come to have a stronger alliance with their clients (DePue et al., 2016; Knox et al., 2011; Park et al., 2019).

When appropriate, by focusing on in vivo work that is relevant to the supervisee's growth as a therapist, supervisors can fuel the learning of FAP by creating a genuine relationship which parallels the therapist–client relationship and in which supervisees feel safe and cared about. This process unfolds through three related methods: (a) contextual modeling, (b) evoking and naturally reinforcing supervisee target behaviors, and (c) parallel process work. Notably, the genuine relationship between supervisor and supervisee is paramount in all three of these techniques.

Contextual Modeling

In typical modeling that happens in other models of supervision, the supervisee is merely observing the supervisor roleplay an intervention. In contrast, a supervisor who is using contextual modeling will implement FAP rules based on what is happening at the moment within the supervision relationship, involving both participants in a more active learning process. A tool that helps with contextual modeling is FAP Questions for Supervisors (Tsai et al., 2009, p. 175), a table of questions that assess awareness of supervisee toward client (e.g., "What feelings/thoughts do your client bring up in you?"), supervisee toward supervisor (e.g., "What feelings/thoughts do I bring up in you?"), and supervisor toward supervisee (e.g., "What feelings/thoughts does my supervisee bring up in me?").

Evoke and Naturally Reinforce Supervisee Target Behaviors

Another activity that is related to contextual modeling is using FAP rules to evoke and naturally reinforce supervisee target behaviors that are related to their growth targets as therapists, including their awareness, courage, and therapeutic love. FAP supervisors and supervisees should together determine what the supervisees' T1s and T2s are, and the supervisor should be sensitive to these as they occur in the supervisory relationship. Because supervision is not therapy, supervisors may choose to disclose in more detail than they would with a client, their own therapist, or even outside-life T1s and T2s, and may be open to the supervisee about being explicitly reinforcing of the supervisor's improvements as well. Typical targets in supervision include decreasing avoidance and increasing courage by taking emotional risks, experiencing or disclosing vulnerable emotions, developing comfort with silence, engaging in productive conflict, challenging someone who is suffering to take necessary action, or engaging in other interpersonal repertoires that are difficult for the trainee.

By responding to supervisee T1s and T2s, FAP supervisors also provide a model to the supervisee of the process of implementing the five FAP rules. For example, being therapeutically loving is an important aspect of Rule 3, equated with being naturally reinforcing and with being reinforced by your supervisees' improvements and successes. Being therapeutically loving is a broad class of therapy behaviors that supervisors can model contextually, and such training is likely to be relevant to supervisees' therapeutic work (Tsai et al., 2009). The supervisory relationship can become emotionally intimate and profound as supervisors demonstrate therapeutic love; ideally, supervisees' experience of this process facilitates their engagement in it with clients.

Thus, FAP supervisors are genuine and open-hearted in seeing, evoking, and authentically reinforcing their supervisees' improvements, target behaviors, and best qualities. A FAP supervisee said to their supervisor: "You mirror back to me the best of who I am, and you see the best of who I am capable of becoming." Like FAP, the intensity of FAP supervision will vary depending on the needs and repertoires of the supervisee, and supervisee progress will be shaped over time.

Focus on Parallel Process

The psychoanalytic idea of *parallel process* is a useful one for FAP supervisors to understand. Like the psychoanalytic traditions, FAP encourages supervisors to take advantage of in vivo learning opportunities when emotional or interpersonal dynamics of the therapy relationship arise within the supervisory relationship. For instance, consider a client who presents as stuck, helpless, and unsure of what to do. Perhaps a diligent supervisee is experiencing little success with this client despite significant effort, leaving the supervisee feeling stuck, helpless, and uncertain. An FAP supervisor who is attuned to this parallel process can use it to create a rich in vivo experience for growth and development. To the degree that the supervisor can use contextual modeling and natural reinforcement to help the supervisee in this case, the trainee will have experienced what it is like to become unstuck from the inside-out and can hold this experience as a guide as they continue to treat their client.

In sum, FAP supervisors can invite their supervisees to develop advanced skills of empathy, intimacy, vulnerability, and presence, especially when supervisors can rise to the occasion of stepping outside their own comfort zones and working directly with what arises in the supervision relationship. A challenge of working this way is that topics can tread quite close to the territory of personal therapy, but FAP supervision remains distinct from therapy because it aims to help the supervisee develop as a therapist and professional; in other words, the personal is explored in supervision to the extent that it is helpful for the therapist's clinical development, but no further.

CONCLUSION

As experiential as it is didactic, FAP supervision focuses not only on the establishment of core competencies in implementing the five rules, but also recognizes that the self-development of the therapist is inextricably linked to therapeutic competence. The experience of FAP supervision is about moving intentionally toward interpersonal connection, and toward seeing the supervisee as a whole person who does not just play the role of a therapist when they step into a therapy room. FAP supervisors are committed to tolerating emotional discomfort, to taking risks without knowing what may happen next, because they value both the professional and the personal growth of their supervisees. The connection between the whole self of the supervisor and the whole self of the trainee, the knowledge of salient parts of one another's personal histories, allows for a profound trust that enriches therapist development. In order for supervisees to become truly willing to visit the most uncomfortable parts of their client's experience, it is immeasurably helpful for their learning experience in supervision to include personally tolerating the combination of unpleasantness and tenderness that can coincide with being fully seen. They come to trust that the alliance they form with clients can serve as a reliable foundation upon which both client and therapist can experiment with new behaviors. As supervisees grow their flexibility about risk-taking and authenticity in the therapeutic relationship, their clients tend to be more willing to take risks and truly change their lives as well.

FAP supervision is a privilege for both the supervisor and supervisee, where they are privy to each other's joys and struggles in life and in clinical work. Most profoundly, supervisor and supervisee often find that over time the foundation of closeness, trust, mutual risk-taking, authenticity, acceptance, and compassion ultimately enhances the supervisee not only as a clinician but also as a powerful human being who can bring change to their communities and to the world.

REFERENCES

DePue, M. K., Lambie, G. W., Liu, R., & Gonzalez, J. (2016). Investigating supervisory relationships and therapeutic alliances using structural equation modeling. *Counselor Education and Supervision, 55*(4), 263–277. https://doi.org/10.1002/ceas.12053

Holman, G., Kanter, J., Tsai, M., & Kohlenberg, R. J. (2017). *Functional analytic psychotherapy made simple: A practical guide to therapeutic relationships.* New Harbinger Publications.

Knox, S., Edwards, L. M., Hess, S. A., & Hill, C. E. (2011). Supervisor self-disclosure: Supervisees' experiences and perspectives. *Psychotherapy, 48*(4), 336–341. https://doi.org/10.1037/a0022067

Kohlenberg, R., & Tsai, M. (1991). *Functional analytic psychotherapy: Creating intense and curative therapeutic relationships.* Plenum Press. https://doi.org/10.1007/978-0-387-70855-3

Miller, A., Williams, M. T., Wetterneck, C. T., Kanter, J., & Tsai, M. (2015). Using functional analytic psychotherapy to improve awareness and connection in racially diverse client–therapist dyads. *Behavior Therapist, 38*(6), 150–156.

Park, E. H., Ha, G., Lee, S., Lee, Y. Y., & Lee, S. M. (2019). Relationship between the supervisory working alliance and outcomes: A meta-analysis. *Journal of Counseling and Development, 97*(4), 437–446. https://doi.org/10.1002/jcad.12292

Safran, J. D., & Muran, J. C. (2001). A relational approach to training and supervision in cognitive psychotherapy. *Journal of Cognitive Psychotherapy, 15*(1), 3–15. https://doi.org/10.1891/0889-8391.15.1.3

Skinner, B. F. (1974). *About behaviorism*. Alfred A. Knopf.

Tracey, T. J., Bludworth, J., & Glidden-Tracey, C. E. (2012). Are there parallel processes in psychotherapy supervision? An empirical examination. *Psychotherapy, 49*(3), 330–343. https://doi.org/10.1037/a0026246

Tsai, M., Callaghan, G. M., & Kohlenberg, R. J. (2013). The use of awareness, courage, therapeutic love, and behavioral interpretation in functional analytic psychotherapy. *Psychotherapy, 50*(3), 366–370. https://doi.org/10.1037/a0031942

Tsai, M., Kohlenberg, R. J., Kanter, J., Kohlenberg, B., Follette, W. C., & Callaghan, G. M. (Eds.). (2009). *A guide to functional analytic psychotherapy: Awareness, courage, love and behaviorism in the therapeutic relationship*. Springer. https://doi.org/10.1007/978-0-387-09787-9

Tsai, M., Mandell, T., Maitland, D., Kanter, J., & Kohlenberg, R. J. (2016). Reducing inadvertent clinical errors: Guidelines from functional analytic psychotherapy. *Psychotherapy, 53*(3), 331–335. https://doi.org/10.1037/pst0000065

7

Supervising the Delivery of Comprehensive Behavior Intervention for Tics

Christopher A. Flessner, Theresa R. Gladstone, and Emily P. Wilton

Tic disorders (e.g., Tourette's disorder, chronic tic disorder, other specified tic disorder) occur in as many as 6.6% of children and adolescents (Khalifa & von Knorring, 2003). While tics often decline in severity through adolescence, a small percentage of patients will exhibit severe symptoms into adulthood (Bloch & Leckman, 2009; Groth et al., 2017). Specific tics can vary widely within and across individuals according to complexity (simple or complex) and type (vocal or motor; Wolicki et al., 2019). The comprehensive behavioral intervention for tics (CBIT) is the first line of psychosocial intervention for tic disorders (Woods et al., 2008).

CBIT was developed utilizing the neurobehavioral model of Tourette's disorder, which posits that, although tic disorders have a neurological basis, tics are also subject to environmental influences (Woods et al., 2007). CBIT can be utilized alone or in conjunction with psychopharmacological interventions (McGuire et al., 2014; Piacentini et al., 2010). Overall, CBIT has demonstrated efficacy across both adults and children (McGuire et al., 2014) and has been shown to be more effective in symptom reduction as compared with supportive therapy (Piacentini et al., 2010; Wilhelm et al., 2012); thus, CBIT is an important intervention for trainees to gain experience in implementing.

CBIT integrates components of psychoeducation, habit reversal training (HRT; Piacentini & Chang, 2006), and broader principles of behavior therapy (Capriotti et al., 2015; Conelea & Woods, 2008a; Piacentini et al., 2010) within its multisession approach to treatment. For example, contextual factors may

https://doi.org/10.1037/0000314-008
Training and Supervision in Specialized Cognitive Behavior Therapy: Methods, Settings, and Populations, E. A. Storch, J. S. Abramowitz, and D. McKay (Editors)

serve as antecedents to (e.g., taking a test, waiting in line, playing video games) or consequences of tic expression (e.g., someone telling the child to stop grunting, someone laughing at the child, the child being removed from the situation after a tic; Capriotti et al., 2015; Conelea & Woods, 2008b); thus, functional assessment and the application of function-based strategies form an important component of CBIT. Throughout CBIT sessions, patients are provided with psychoeducation related to tic disorders and a rationale for treatment. A functional assessment of each of the patient's tics is conducted and a tic hierarchy created to identify the relative impairment associated with each tic. Working in a stepwise fashion (i.e., beginning with the most bothersome tic), HRT (i.e., awareness training, competing response training, social support) is implemented for a different tic at each session. It should be noted, however, that the social support component of HRT and behavioral reward programs are generally not considered "essential" for work with most adults. It is with this overview of CBIT in mind that we proceed to discussing, first, core concepts for trainees to understand prior to implementing this intervention.

KEY CONCEPTS FOR TRAINEES TO LEARN

Several key concepts exist that are important for trainees to understand to effect optimal behavior change using CBIT. Some of these concepts are unique to CBIT (e.g., premonitory sensations). Others are common to a host of behaviorally oriented interventions (e.g., psychoeducation, behavioral principles) but must be adapted appropriately for a tic disorder population. What follows is a brief overview of these core concepts that, in our opinion, all trainees should grasp prior to implementing specific, intervention-related techniques with patients.

Premonitory Sensations/Urges

Premonitory sensations (hereinafter referred to as *premonitory urges*) are a somewhat unique experience specific to tic disorders. These urges represent internal signals that some have likened to the feeling prior to a sneeze or having an itch that needs to be scratched. While premonitory urges do not always occur prior to a tic, approximately 77% to 93% of those with a tic disorder have experienced a premonitory urge (Leckman et al., 1993). It also appears that stronger urges are associated with greater tic severity (Kyriazi et al., 2019; Reese et al., 2014) as well as increased internalizing symptoms (Rozenman et al., 2015). HRT is thought to interrupt the negative reinforcement cycle of premonitory urges and tic expression (Piacentini et al., 2010). As such, incorporating a discussion of premonitory urges throughout treatment is critical and should be assessed and described for each tic. With an accurate description of a patient's premonitory urge(s), clinicians can use this information throughout the course of awareness training and when implementing a competing response to increase the potential efficacy of the intervention (see the Habit Reversal Training section later in this chapter).

Psychoeducation

Psychoeducation is not unique to CBIT; however, the application of this concept must be adapted accordingly in working with a tic disorder population. It is incumbent upon supervisors and their trainees to seek the most up-to-date information about tic disorders. I (Flessner) have found that book chapters devoted to tic disorders in many edited texts are an excellent resource for obtaining information of this sort. Broadly speaking, important components of psychoeducation, as applied via CBIT, include diagnostic criteria for various tic disorders, common tics, prevalence rates, common comorbidities, premonitory urges, as well as a basic understanding of the neurological basis and contextual factors that may influence tic expression (American Psychiatric Association, 2013; Bloch & Leckman, 2009; Conelea & Woods, 2008b; Gloor & Walitza, 2016). Developing an understanding of tic-related background information will allow trainees to convey accurate information to patients, correct misconceptions, and normalize the patient's experience. In our view, however, a solid grounding in basic, behavioral principles is of even greater importance for trainees to adequately implement CBIT and its embedded techniques.

Understanding Behavioral Principles

Developing an understanding of behavioral principles is critical to successful treatment implementation. Previous research has identified antecedents (e.g., social interactions, fatigue, school) and consequences (e.g., attention, escape; Capriotti et al., 2015; Conelea & Woods, 2008b) associated with increased tic expression. As such, trainees must understand a myriad of behavioral principles and concepts, including establishing operations, reinforcement, stimulus control, and punishment. Trainees must be able to identify establishing operations (e.g., sleep deprivation, fatigue) that may influence tic presentation and understand how to modify the patient's environment such that all factors that may increase tic expression (i.e., stimulus control) are minimized. For example, within the context of CBIT, how does tic expression vary at a child's school or place of work as opposed to their home? A foundational concept within CBIT is the understanding that tics may vary across situations or environments and that fluctuation in tic presentation and frequency is a normal occurrence within the context of tic disorders (i.e., psychoeducation). Without said knowledge, implementing CBIT's primary therapeutic techniques—establishing a tic hierarchy, conducting a functional assessment, and implementing HRT—will be exceedingly difficult.

KEY TECHNIQUES FOR TRAINEES TO LEARN

A variety of techniques and strategies are important for the proper implementation of CBIT. A brief overview of some of these follows.

Tic Hierarchy Development

A tic hierarchy is established before conducting either a functional assessment or HRT and is an important progress monitoring tool embedded within CBIT. In creating the tic hierarchy, clinicians begin by developing an operational definition of each tic a patient has described via their initial intake assessment. This assists the clinician in understanding the nature of the tic and will also be useful later as part of implementing HRT (see the Awareness Training section later in this chapter). Somewhat akin to an exposure hierarchy in cognitive behavior therapy for anxiety disorders, tics are ranked from 0 to 10 based on the impairment or distress associated with each; however, trainees will want to inquire as to the broader distress that said tic creates (e.g., "How much does this tic bother you?"). That is, the 0-to-10 scale is used for determining which tic is most distressing (i.e., tic rated the highest) and should be the first target of intervention. In this vein (i.e., starting with the most distressing tic) a tic symptom hierarchy is markedly different than would be the case in the use of an anxiety hierarchy. When working with a young child, it is preferable for clinicians to obtain both parent and child accounts of associated distress. Creating a tic hierarchy is a critical technique for trainees to learn, given its importance in subsequent aspects of treatment (i.e., guiding which tic is addressed session by session) and ascertaining the relative efficacy of CBIT week by week. It has been our experience that this is also a skill most trainees are able to master very early in their professional training.

Functional Assessment

Given previous research suggesting that tics are susceptible to contextual factors (Conelea & Woods, 2008b), conducting a functional assessment and recommending environmental modifications are critical to treatment. With few exceptions (e.g., eye blinking, eye darting; see the ideal training cases section later), the tic rated as most distressing via the tic hierarchy will be the first target of treatment for trainees. A strength of CBIT is that the intervention makes conducting a functional assessment relatively straightforward via a variety of handouts and assessment tools; however, an understanding of core behavioral principles is required to conduct a functional assessment and implement function-based strategies well. As part of the functional assessment, trainees must be able to assess the antecedents and consequences associated with each tic examined. Trainees will then use this information to provide recommendations to the patient and their family members. For example, if a child's tic appears to increase while watching television, this contextual factor may be functioning to reinforce the tics. Recommended environmental modifications will target this hypothesis (e.g., practice therapy-relevant exercises while watching TV).

It is important for trainees to realize that patients and their families often exhibit difficulty recognizing contextual factors surrounding the occurrence of tics or may be unaware of changes in tic expression across environments. For example, it is not uncommon for patients to report, "My tics are bad all of the time." As such, trainees must not only understand how to conduct a functional assessment but also be able to explain concepts to patients and provide examples or ask additional questions to probe further should the patient require these prompts. Supervisors will need to work with trainees as to how best to communicate the information needed most effectively.

Habit Reversal Training

In our opinion, HRT is the most important component of CBIT for trainees to understand. A detailed description of HRT is beyond the scope of this chapter; however, two primary components exist—awareness training and competing response training—and are described, with some tips for supervisors (McGuire et al., 2014).

Awareness Training

As part of awareness training, trainees seek to increase a patient's awareness of the targeted tic as well as the premonitory urge that may precede it. The trainee will ask the patient to describe sensations surrounding the tic in great detail. In some instances, the trainee may ask the patient to demonstrate the tic to gain an enhanced understanding of the movements involved while exhibiting the tic. The trainee should inquire about aspects of the tic that they notice and which the patient may not have mentioned. Trainees will ask their patients to consider any behaviors or "warning signs" that may serve as a signal that the tic is going to occur (i.e., premonitory urge). After a detailed description is obtained, several idiosyncratic exercises are undertaken to reaffirm the patient's ability to identify and label their tic.

Successful implementation of awareness training is necessary to ensure that patients can anticipate the occurrence of a tic and later implement a competing response (see the Competing Response Training section later). From the supervisor's or trainee's perspective, it is important to understand that patients present with varying degrees of insight. The difficulty trainees have in implementing awareness training is likely to be negatively correlated with their patient's level of insight (i.e., greater insight means less difficulty implementing awareness training). Supervisors are well-advised to formulate novel approaches to equip the beginning (or experienced) trainee in delivering this component to HRT. For example, I (Flessner) have often equated awareness training to a high school English assignment I was once given. The assignment was to (in as much detail as needed) write down and explain the steps necessary to make a peanut butter and jelly sandwich. After completing said assignment, I quickly realized that I had missed important steps (e.g., unless one possesses superpowers, it is difficult to make a peanut butter and jelly sandwich without first opening the lid to either condiment). In the same way, patients and beginning trainees may gloss over seemingly meaningless or commonplace facets to a tic (e.g., arm moves back and to the left as part of an arm-jerking tic). An understanding of this fact and differing ways in which to implement this therapeutic technique is likely to exert a significant impact on the efficacy of the second, primary component of HRT—competing response training.

Competing Response Training

Following awareness training, a competing response is selected and implemented contingent on the occurrence of a tic or the observation of a patient's warning signs. In selecting a competing response, the patient should be confident in their ability to implement the competing response and maintain it for 60 seconds or until the urge to tic subsides—whichever is longer. Additionally, a competing response should be socially inconspicuous and able to be easily implemented across environments. After the trainee and patient decide on a competing response together, the trainee engages in several additional exercises designed to ensure the patient understands when and how to implement their competing response.

Trainees must possess an understanding of both the theory underlying the competing response portion of HRT and how to implement it in practice. Therefore, trainees must be prepared to "think on their feet" within session to develop competing responses appropriate for the patient's tic. Trainees are likely to benefit from brainstorming multiple possible competing responses for a specific tic with their supervisor prior to session. Supervisors may wish to share resources that are available to guide new and experienced trainees in the development of appropriate competing responses (Carr, 1995; Piacentini et al., 2010). Additionally, trainees should be able to problem solve barriers, provide corrective feedback, and praise proper implementation of a competing response—all of which are important facets that the supervisor may wish to practice with their supervisee.

CHARACTERISTICS OF IDEAL AND POOR TRAINING CASES

Research is equivocal on patient-level characteristics that predict treatment success or failure using CBIT (Nissen et al., 2019; Sukhodolsky et al., 2017). Even so, we highlight some characteristics that, in our opinion, may make either a desirable or poor training case for someone new to the field.

Some evidence suggests that treatment using CBIT may be just as successful among patients with and without comorbidities (Conelea et al., 2018; Sukhodolsky et al., 2017); however, we believe that a client with few (or mild) comorbidities is likely to make a superior training case. Simply put, fewer comorbidities are likely to result in the need for fewer modifications to a "typical" CBIT case. A client with co-occurring disorders may require the clinician to make decisions as to which concerns to address first as part of treatment planning or even within session. In our view, not all comorbidities are created equal. Several comorbidities, in particular, might be best avoided as part of a training case.

Moderate to severe symptoms of inattention and/or hyperactivity (i.e., attention-deficit/hyperactivity disorder [ADHD]) may require clinicians to evaluate the burden of these symptoms and ensure proper treatment for ADHD, aside from tics (Pringsheim et al., 2019). Studies have corroborated the connection between ADHD and functional difficulties in children with Tourette's disorder (Hoekstra et al., 2004; Sukhodolsky et al., 2003). Children with co-occurring ADHD may be more likely to exhibit disruptive behavior (Sukhodolsky et al., 2003), which may make individual sessions and key aspects of CBIT more challenging for the training clinician to administer. That is, CBIT requires building awareness of the patient's tic(s). A patient with symptoms of ADHD may exhibit marked difficulty focusing on this particular component to HRT. They may become distracted or impulsive, not implementing the competing response well, and needing redirection regularly. Clearly, the management of these symptoms are an important skill for all trainees to develop. If the purpose, however, of a CBIT training case is to develop proficiency in delivering this particular, evidence-based intervention, we believe that choosing a more straightforward case with fewer, milder symptoms of ADHD is preferred.

Obsessive–compulsive disorder (OCD) is a second, commonly co-occurring disorder that should be considered carefully when screening a CBIT training case. While OCD is common in people with Tourette's disorder, administering CBIT with a client who has co-occurring OCD or "gray area" tic-related OCD symptoms may be especially challenging. The first decision to be made is if OCD or the tic disorder should be treated first. As cognitive behavior therapy (CBT) is considered the first line of treatment for OCD (Öst et al., 2015), OCD and tic disorders are unlikely to be addressed simultaneously (Pringsheim et al., 2019). Certainly, one can make the argument that the "true" differences between exposure-based CBT and HRT are less clear than might be implied at first glance. In fact, there have been at least two studies to employ exposure plus response prevention for the treatment of tics (van de Griendt et al., 2013; Verdellen et al., 2004). Despite this and other philosophical debates around this issue, it is generally agreed upon that OCD and tic-related OCD symptoms can be especially difficult to differentiate, particularly among children. It is for all of these reasons, that we strongly recommend a beginning training case exhibit minimal to no OCD-related symptoms.

Shifting our focus away from co-occurring presenting concerns, we recommend that a motivated patient leads to an easier training case. This fact is probably not too surprising to most; however, it is important to consider within the context of CBIT. Put simply, CBIT requires effort, persistence, and consistency from the patient within and between sessions, perhaps more so than is commonplace within other evidence-based treatments. The therapist introduces and practices techniques with the patient and works with them to problem solve deterrents throughout treatment. Much of the work constituted in CBIT occurs at home. Monitoring tics multiple times during the week, pre-defining two to three segments each week to practice HRT, attending to the patient's tics, and performing competing responses are far from convenient between-session tasks, particularly for patients exhibiting more frequent or impairing tics. For example, implementing a 60-second competing response for a tic that occurs multiple times during a 20-minute period may be exhausting and require far more vigilance than a tic occurring only multiple times during a 12-hour period. For youths, this may be especially true if the between-session task(s) detract from a preferred activity. If the client is not motivated to practice at home, CBIT is unlikely to be successful. In our view, lack of motivation is quite different from simply being "busy." Neither may make for an ideal training case; however, a busy patient who is also very motivated (e.g., completes portions of homework, arrives to session on time, remains engaged, etc.) is preferred. Low motivation will likely lead to lack of progress in treatment, difficulty enforcing adherence, and, ultimately, challenge the trainee in domains not explicitly related to gaining proficiency in CBIT.

A final, but important, consideration in identifying an ideal training case pertains to the type of tics exhibited as well as some basic, demographic characterstics. First, a caveat: Assuming each of the ideal training case scenarios described in the preceding paragraphs has been met, concerning oneself with the type of tic a patient presents with is likely of little concern. Most cases though will not meet each of the criterion listed earlier. Generally speaking, we recommend trainees practice administering CBIT within the following context—in order of increasing difficulty: (a) simple motor tics (most); (b) simple vocal tics; (c) complex vocal tics; (d) complex motor tics (most); and (e) simple and complex eye movement. Stated simply, tics involving eye movements can be exceptionally difficult for some patients to address. It has been my (Flessner's) experience, both via previous training and supervisory experiences, that patients tend to struggle with competing responses for tics involving the eyes. It may be best for this class of tics to be addressed after the trainee and patient have established some success with other tics. From a severity perspective, moderately severe tics are likely to be ideal for a training case. As a trainee, it is often easiest for a tic to occur frequently enough during session for the therapist to observe and troubleshoot, but not so much that it takes over and training becomes exhausting to the client. Finally, adults and older children tend to be easier to start with as training cases. This is especially true because, as patients mature cognitively, they are more likely to present with premonitory urges which can, in turn, make facets of HRT easier to implement for the beginning clinician.

COMMON MISTAKES AND HOW TO FIX THEM

Trainees may make a variety of mistakes when first starting out with CBIT. Motivation is a key component of treatment. When working with youths, spending time engaging the patient in creating a reward program that successfully motivates them is crucial. Two common mistakes that trainees make are not spending sufficient time ensuring that (a) the reward or incentive is actually motivating for the patient and (b) the family is implementing the reward program as desired. Therefore, if for example, the therapist finds that competing response practice is minimal at home, they should reassess the effectiveness of the reward program. They may reassess with the family how motivating the reward is, as well as review the family's implementation of the reward system in specific scenarios to understand and alter its execution.

Another common mistake is failing to actively engage the patient early on in treatment. For example, it is important that the patient has some autonomy over aspects of treatment. Choosing the competing response is one such area that the client can be heavily involved. Often trainees may assume there is only one correct competing response for each tic; however, this is not the case. As long as the competing response matches the criteria described in the Habit Reversal Training section earlier, it can be utilized. The patient is the one who will have to implement this behavior. Making sure to engage them in the decision and help them understand why one competing response may be superior to another can help them to take ownership of the treatment.

Finally, choosing the best tic to start HRT with can be an especially challenging task for a trainee. Although our previous description (see the tic symptom hierarchy section) may seem straightforward, in many cases selection is more nuanced. The selection of which tic to target is made on a case-by-case basis, akin to the selection of the first exposure task in CBT for anxiety. It is critical to include the patient (and parent, if applicable) in the decision. The therapist ought to consider both the highest tic on the hierarchy (i.e., tic the client finds most annoying/distressing) and the tic for which implementing a competing response may be easiest (e.g., simple motor tic). Supervisors and trainees new to working with this population are advised to engage in a simple experiential exercise to help "break the tie" if several options exist. Practice the competing response necessary for the tic and choose the tic that the supervisor and trainee deem easiest to treat.

Resolving Trainee Misconceptions About CBIT and HRT

In addition to common mistakes trainees make, there are also several misconceptions about CBIT/HRT that new therapists may possess and are important to dismantle. This is especially important so that the trainee can elaborate and provide psychoeducation if the patient (or their family) have similar misconceptions. First, suppressing tics does not make the tics worse. This misconception, often referred to as the *rebound effect*, is particularly common, in my (Flessner's) experience, among parents and uninformed healthcare professionals. The notion behind the rebound effect is that the act of suppressing a tic leads to the patient needing to "let them out" later (e.g., the tics seem better at school/work and then occur more frequently at home). Studies have consistently refuted this effect, failing to demonstrate an increase in tics following suppression (Himle & Woods, 2005; Himle et al., 2007). Additionally, in a randomized controlled trial, results demonstrate that tic worsening did not occur at a greater rate in CBIT as compared with psychoeducation alone (Piacentini et al., 2010). A more likely explanation for the apparent rebound effect is the natural waxing and waning course of tics. It is also likely that patients actively attempt to suppress tics at school/work and are less likely to do so within the relative "safety" of their home.

A second misconception pertains to the "whack-a-mole" phenomenon. That is, targeting one tic results in a new tic emerging or other tics worsening. Available empirical evidence suggests that this is not the case (Woods et al., 2003, 2010). In fact, Woods et al. (2003) found that nontargeted tics actually decreased via the use of HRT. Finally, some believe that the practice of suppressing (i.e., utilizing a competing response) a tic will result in a detriment to one's ability to focus on other important tasks (e.g., schoolwork). Initially, this may be the case for some patients; however, while accuracy on other cognitive tasks may decrease at the outset of attempts to implement a competing response, with continued practice suppression becomes more automatic (Conelea & Woods, 2008a; Woods et al., 2010).

ETHICAL CONCERNS

When starting CBIT as a trainee, a number of ethical issues are likely to arise that the trainee may wish to discuss with their supervisor. First, competency must be contemplated. CBIT, although grounded in behavioral principles well known to many, is a specific treatment that requires practice and supervision before competency is attained. Trainees should only be supervised by therapists experienced with implementing the therapy. Second, tics frequently co-occur with other conditions. Deciding when and how to treat these co-occurring conditions is a conceptual and ethical concern to which clinicians must attend. Third, it is not uncommon for tics to bother a parent (or spouse) more so than the patient. As such, the trainee and supervisor must carefully consider whether this is the appropriate time to pursue CBIT. In my role as a clinical supervisor, I (Flessner) often caution my supervisees to think about whether (a) pursuing treatment at this time is in the best interest of the child, and (b) the patient may develop a skewed perspective on the efficacy of CBIT. The latter may influence their decision to pursue CBIT or related forms of therapy in the future.

COMMON OBSTACLES IN SUPERVISION

It is important for trainees to study the theory behind CBT, learn the practical skills required for its implementation, and practice the corresponding therapeutic techniques. For example, if a trainee has not yet taken a more advanced class in learning and condition, supervising the implementation of HRT and function-based facets to CBIT may be especially challenging. CBIT requires a good degree of effort, on the part of the patient, to implement. Strong rapport can facilitate the necessary buy-in to increase between-session task compliance. Trainees exhibiting an inability to build rapport with their patient may require their supervisor to spend additional time with foundational therapy skills. Alternatively, the trainee may need to hone these skills with other patients prior to beginning CBIT.

CONCLUSION

CBIT is efficacious in the treatment of tics in youths and adults. CBIT requires knowledge of key behavioral concepts and theory as well as HRT. Competent supervision is key to aiding the trainee in catching common mistakes and scaffolding competent implementation. Assigning trainees more ideal training cases (e.g., motivated client/family, fewer co-occurring problems) and monitoring common trainee mistakes may be especially important to allow for growth and successful training in the implementation of this evidence-based treatment.

REFERENCES

American Psychiatric Association. (2013). *Diagnostic and statistical manual of mental disorders* (5th ed.). https://doi.org/10.1176/appi.books.9780890425596

Bloch, M. H., & Leckman, J. F. (2009). Clinical course of Tourette syndrome. *Journal of Psychosomatic Research, 67*(6), 497–501. https://doi.org/10.1016/j.jpsychores.2009.09.002

Capriotti, M. R., Piacentini, J. C., Himle, M. B., Ricketts, E. J., Espil, F. M., Lee, H. J., Turkel, J. E., & Woods, D. W. (2015). Assessing environmental consequences of ticcing in youth with chronic tic disorders: The Tic Accommodation and Reactions Scale. *Children's Health Care, 44*(3), 205–220. https://doi.org/10.1080/02739615.2014.948164

Carr, J. E. (1995). Competing responses for the treatment of Tourette syndrome and tic disorders. *Behaviour Research and Therapy, 33*(4), 455–456. https://doi.org/10.1016/0005-7967(94)00066-S

Conelea, C. A., Wellen, B., Woods, D. W., Greene, D. J., Black, K. J., Specht, M., Himle, M. B., Lee, H. J., & Capriotti, M. (2018). Patterns and predictors of tic suppressibility in youth with tic disorders. *Frontiers in Psychiatry, 9*, 188. https://doi.org/10.3389/fpsyt.2018.00188

Conelea, C. A., & Woods, D. W. (2008a). Examining the impact of distraction on tic suppression in children and adolescents with Tourette syndrome. *Behaviour Research and Therapy, 46*(11), 1193–1200. https://doi.org/10.1016/j.brat.2008.07.005

Conelea, C. A., & Woods, D. W. (2008b). The influence of contextual factors on tic expression in Tourette's syndrome: A review. *Journal of Psychosomatic Research, 65*(5), 487–496. https://doi.org/10.1016/j.jpsychores.2008.04.010

Gloor, F. T., & Walitza, S. (2016). Tic disorders and Tourette syndrome: Current concepts of etiology and treatment in children and adolescents. *Neuropediatrics, 47*(02), 84–96. https://doi.org/10.1055/s-0035-1570492

Groth, C., Mol Debes, N., Rask, C. U., Lange, T., & Skov, L. (2017). Course of Tourette syndrome and comorbidities in a large prospective clinical study. *Journal of the American Academy of Child & Adolescent Psychiatry, 56*(4), 304–312. https://doi.org/10.1016/j.jaac.2017.01.010

Himle, M. B., & Woods, D. W. (2005). An experimental evaluation of tic suppression and the tic rebound effect. *Behaviour Research and Therapy, 43*(11), 1443–1451. https://doi.org/10.1016/j.brat.2004.11.002

Himle, M. B., Woods, D. W., Conelea, C. A., Bauer, C. C., & Rice, K. A. (2007). Investigating the effects of tic suppression on premonitory urge ratings in children and adolescents with Tourette's syndrome. *Behaviour Research and Therapy, 45*(12), 2964–2976. https://doi.org/10.1016/j.brat.2007.08.007

Hoekstra, P. J., Steenhuis, M. P., Troost, P. W., Korf, J., Kallenberg, C. G., & Minderaa, R. B. (2004). Relative contribution of attention-deficit hyperactivity disorder, obsessive–compulsive disorder, and tic severity to social and behavioral problems in tic disorders. *Journal of Developmental and Behavioral Pediatrics, 25*(4), 272–279. https://doi.org/10.1097/00004703-200408000-00007

Khalifa, N., & von Knorring, A. L. (2003). Prevalence of tic disorders and Tourette syndrome in a Swedish school population. *Developmental Medicine and Child Neurology, 45*(5), 315–319. https://doi.org/10.1111/j.1469-8749.2003.tb00402.x

Kyriazi, M., Kalyva, E., Vargiami, E., Krikonis, K., & Zafeiriou, D. (2019). Premonitory urges and their link with tic severity in children and adolescents with tic disorders. *Frontiers in Psychiatry, 10*, 569. https://doi.org/10.3389/fpsyt.2019.00569

Leckman, J. F., Walker, D. E., & Cohen, D. J. (1993). Premonitory urges in Tourette's syndrome. *The American Journal of Psychiatry, 150*(1), 98–102. https://doi.org/10.1176/ajp.150.1.98

McGuire, J. F., Piacentini, J., Brennan, E. A., Lewin, A. B., Murphy, T. K., Small, B. J., & Storch, E. A. (2014). A meta-analysis of behavior therapy for Tourette Syndrome. *Journal of Psychiatric Research, 50*, 106–112. https://doi.org/10.1016/j.jpsychires.2013.12.009

Nissen, J. B., Parner, E. T., & Thomsen, P. H. (2019). Predictors of therapeutic treatment outcome in adolescent chronic tic disorders. *BJPsych Open, 5*(5), e74. https://doi.org/10.1192/bjo.2019.56

Öst, L. G., Havnen, A., Hansen, B., & Kvale, G. (2015). Cognitive behavioral treatments of obsessive–compulsive disorder. A systematic review and meta-analysis of studies published 1993–2014. *Clinical Psychology Review, 40*, 156–169. https://doi.org/10.1016/j.cpr.2015.06.003

Piacentini, J., Woods, D. W., Scahill, L., Wilhelm, S., Peterson, A. L., Chang, S., Ginsburg, G. S., Deckersbach, T., Dziura, J., Levi-Pearl, S., & Walkup, J. T. (2010). Behavior therapy for children with Tourette disorder: A randomized controlled trial. *Journal of the American Medical Association, 303*(19), 1929–1937. https://doi.org/10.1001/jama.2010.607

Piacentini, J. C., & Chang, S. W. (2006). Behavioral treatments for tic suppression: Habit reversal training. *Advances in Neurology, 99*, 227–233.

Pringsheim, T., Okun, M. S., Müller-Vahl, K., Martino, D., Jankovic, J., Cavanna, A. E., Woods, D. W., Robinson, M., Jarvie, E., Roessner, V., Oskoui, M., Holler-Managan, Y., & Piacentini, J. (2019). Practice guideline recommendations summary: Treatment of tics in people with Tourette syndrome and chronic tic disorders. *Neurology, 92*(19), 896–906. https://doi.org/10.1212/WNL.0000000000007466

Reese, H. E., Scahill, L., Peterson, A. L., Crowe, K., Woods, D. W., Piacentini, J., Walkup, J. T., & Wilhelm, S. (2014). The premonitory urge to tic: Measurement, characteristics, and correlates in older adolescents and adults. *Behavior Therapy*, *45*(2), 177–186. https://doi.org/10.1016/j.beth.2013.09.002

Rozenman, M., Johnson, O. E., Chang, S. W., Woods, D. W., Walkup, J. T., Wilhelm, S., Peterson, A., Scahill, L., & Piacentini, J. (2015). Relationships between premonitory urge and anxiety in youth with chronic tic disorders. *Children's Health Care*, *44*(3), 235–248. https://doi.org/10.1080/02739615.2014.986328

Sukhodolsky, D. G., Scahill, L., Zhang, H., Peterson, B. S., King, R. A., Lombroso, P. J., Katsovich, L., Findley, D., & Leckman, J. F. (2003). Disruptive behavior in children with Tourette's syndrome: Association with ADHD comorbidity, tic severity, and functional impairment. *Journal of the American Academy of Child & Adolescent Psychiatry*, *42*(1), 98–105. https://doi.org/10.1097/00004583-200301000-00016

Sukhodolsky, D. G., Woods, D. W., Piacentini, J., Wilhelm, S., Peterson, A. L., Katsovich, L., Dziura, J., Walkup, J. T., & Scahill, L. (2017). Moderators and predictors of response to behavior therapy for tics in Tourette syndrome. *Neurology*, *88*(11), 1029–1036. https://doi.org/10.1212/WNL.0000000000003710

van de Griendt, J. M. T. M., Verdellen, C. W. J., van Dijk, M. K., & Verbraak, M. J. P. M. (2013). Behavioural treatment of tics: Habit reversal and exposure with response prevention. *Neuroscience and Biobehavioral Reviews*, *37*(6), 1172–1177. https://doi.org/10.1016/j.neubiorev.2012.10.007

Verdellen, C. W., Keijsers, G. P., Cath, D. C., & Hoogduin, C. A. (2004). Exposure with response prevention versus habit reversal in Tourette's syndrome: A controlled study. *Behaviour Research and Therapy*, *42*(5), 501–511. https://doi.org/10.1016/S0005-7967(03)00154-2

Wilhelm, S., Peterson, A. L., Piacentini, J., Woods, D. W., Deckersbach, T., Sukhodolsky, D. G., Chang, S., Liu, H., Dziura, J., Walkup, J. T., & Scahill, L. (2012). Randomized trial of behavior therapy for adults with Tourette syndrome. *Archives of General Psychiatry*, *69*(8), 795–803. https://doi.org/10.1001/archgenpsychiatry.2011.1528

Wolicki, S. B., Bitsko, R. H., Danielson, M. L., Holbrook, J. R., Zablotsky, B., Walkup, J. T., Woods, D. W., & Mink, J. W. (2019). Children with Tourette syndrome in the United States: Parent-reported diagnosis, co-occurring disorders, severity, and influence of activities on tics. *Journal of Developmental and Behavioral Pediatrics*, *40*(6), 407–414. https://doi.org/10.1097/DBP.0000000000000667

Woods, D. W., Conelea, C. A., & Himle, M. B. (2010). Behavior therapy for Tourette's disorder: Utilization in a community sample and an emerging area of practice for psychologists. *Professional Psychology: Research and Practice*, *41*(6), 518–525. https://doi.org/10.1037/a0021709

Woods, D. W., Piacentini, J., Chang, S., Deckersbach, T., Ginsburg, G., Peterson, A., Scahill, L. D., Walkup, J. T., & Wilhelm, S. (2008). *Managing Tourette syndrome: A behavioral intervention for children and adults therapist guide*. Oxford University Press.

Woods, D. W., Piacentini, J., & Walkup, J. T. (Eds.). (2007). *Treating Tourette syndrome and tic disorders: A guide for practitioners*. Guilford Press.

Woods, D. W., Twohig, M. P., Flessner, C. A., & Roloff, T. J. (2003). Treatment of vocal tics in children with Tourette syndrome: Investigating the efficacy of habit reversal. *Journal of Applied Behavior Analysis*, *36*(1), 109–112. https://doi.org/10.1901/jaba.2003.36-109

8

Supervision in Behavioral Activation

Stacey B. Daughters, Catherine E. Paquette, and Elizabeth D. Reese

Behavioral activation (BA) is a reinforcement-based treatment best known for its established effectiveness in the treatment of depression (Mazzucchelli et al., 2009). The premise of BA is that depression is the result of a loss or lack of response-contingent positive reinforcement stemming from a combination of avoidance behavior, the inability to derive enjoyment from naturally rewarding reinforcers, and decreased engagement in rewarding activities (Ferster, 1973; Lewinsohn, 1974). Drawing on a functional analysis framework, low mood and/or anhedonia leads to withdrawal from value-based, enjoyable activities, and this inactivation exacerbates depressive symptoms and decreases the likelihood that the individual will engage in rewarding activities in the future. BA disrupts this cycle by helping the client reengage in value-based activities that make life enjoyable and meaningful.

Two of the most widely used treatment manuals for BA are the *Brief Behavioral Activation Treatment for Depression* (Hopko et al., 2003; Lejuez et al., 2011) and *Depression in Context: Strategies for Guided Action* (Martell et al., 2001). Strengths inherent in the BA approach account for its exponential growth. It is more feasible and accessible than full cognitive behavior therapy, while proving just as effective (Ekers et al., 2008). This is evidenced in its successful provision by support workers with little formal training in psychotherapy (Ekers et al., 2011) and its feasibility and effectiveness in a small group format (Simmonds-Buckley et al., 2019). BA has also proven effective cross-culturally, given the focus on client-driven value-based activities (Chen et al., 2021; Collado et al., 2016; Magidson et al., 2015).

https://doi.org/10.1037/0000314-009
Training and Supervision in Specialized Cognitive Behavior Therapy: Methods, Settings, and Populations, E. A. Storch, J. S. Abramowitz, and D. McKay (Editors)

The benefits of BA, coupled with similar reinforcement-based deficits found in other psychological disorders and symptoms, have led to the successful expansion of BA as an effective treatment for substance use disorder (SUD; Daughters et al., 2018), posttraumatic stress disorder (Etherton & Farley, 2020), and anxiety disorders (Stein et al., 2020). In this chapter, we discuss the supervision of BA principles with transdiagnostic applicability, primarily drawing on examples in the treatment of depression and SUD.

KEY CONCEPTS FOR TRAINEES TO LEARN

BA sessions have a strong emphasis on knowledge and application of the treatment model (see Figure 8.1), namely, the cycle of difficult feelings and sensations, urges, and avoidance/maladaptive behaviors (e.g., isolation, substance use), and how this cycle is experienced by the client. Clients learn that the goal of treatment is to break this cycle by engaging in value-based approach behaviors. The premise of the treatment model is that as an individual becomes

FIGURE 8.1. Behavioral Activation Treatment Model

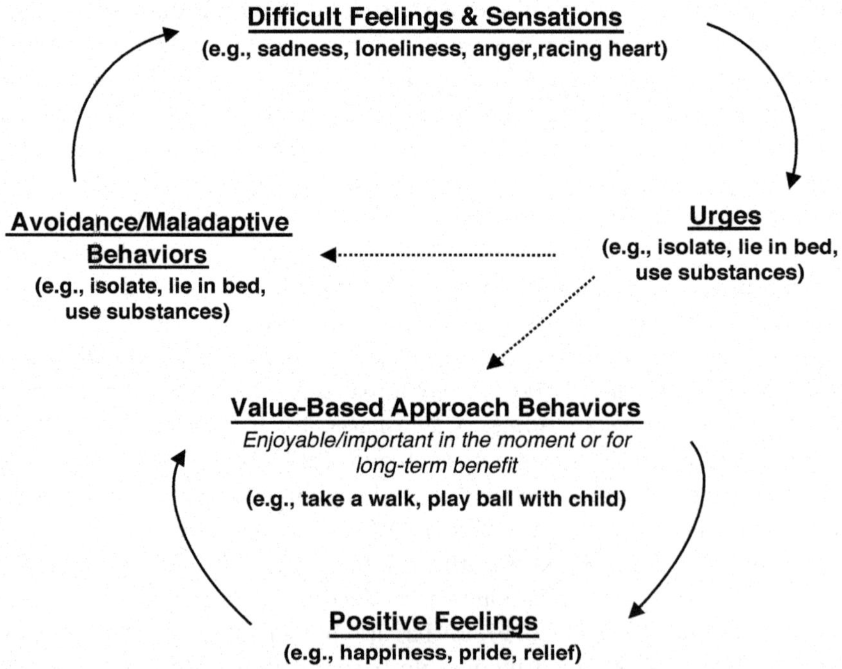

Difficult Feelings & Sensations
(e.g., sadness, loneliness, anger, racing heart)

Urges
(e.g., isolate, lie in bed, use substances)

Avoidance/Maladaptive Behaviors
(e.g., isolate, lie in bed, use substances)

Value-Based Approach Behaviors
Enjoyable/important in the moment or for long-term benefit
(e.g., take a walk, play ball with child)

Positive Feelings
(e.g., happiness, pride, relief)

Note. The goal of BA is to shift client behavior from the upper negative cycle to the lower positive cycle. The client begins to plan value-based activities as well as choose these options more often in response to urges for avoidance/maladaptive behavior. With repeated engagement in value-based activities the client will soon experience fewer avoidance urges and more urges to engage in value-based approach behavior.

more active and regularly engages in activities that generate a sense of enjoyment and/or accomplishment, they are less likely to have the urge to engage in avoidant or maladaptive behaviors in response to difficult emotions. Over time, these new stimulus-response associations will increase urges to engage in value-based approach behavior. At the beginning of treatment, clients monitor and rate their daily activities on enjoyment and importance to identify patterns of inactivation and opportunities to increase engagement in activities that provide pleasure and mastery. Next, they identify possible value-based activities within a variety of life areas (e.g., education/work, hobbies/recreation, relationships). Therapists help clients identify specific and measurable activities that align with their values, with an emphasis on balancing activities that are enjoyable and important ("In order to be a caring friend [value], I will call my friend and ask how she's doing [activity]"). During earlier sessions, clients focus on monitoring their current activities and creating activity hierarchies. In later sessions, the focus shifts to planning and implementing these activities, problem solving challenges to adherence, and posttreatment planning.

BA is rooted in *reinforcement theory*, which posits that a person's behavior is a function of its consequences and that the key to changing behavior is to institute consequences that make desired behaviors more likely to occur (reinforcement) and undesired behaviors less likely to occur (punishment). To be an effective BA practitioner, it is critical for therapists to have a strong grasp on reinforcement theory and the ability to conceptualize how it can be applied to client behavior throughout treatment.

BA relies heavily on *positive reinforcement*—the addition of a desirable consequence—to increase the frequency of naturally rewarding behaviors (e.g., those that promote pleasure and mastery) that are typically diminished in depression and SUD. Positive mood is one of the primary reinforcers leveraged, and to capitalize on the potential of positive mood the therapist must understand specific issues with reinforcement that characterize depression and SUD. This includes *anhedonia*, or a reduced ability to experience pleasure, targeted in BA by linking desired behaviors to specific values held by the individual and rating the anticipated enjoyment and importance of planned activities. Problematic *avoidance* is also targeted, as individuals with low mood demonstrate patterns of avoidance of aversive situations. Behaviors consistent with avoidance (e.g., isolating, substance use) result in decreased opportunities for positive reinforcement and are important to extinguish. The use of activity monitoring in BA helps to identify patterns of avoidance and, through functional analysis, helps clients see how avoidant behaviors maintain symptoms of low mood. Success occurs through repeated positive reinforcement over time, and therapists have an important role in helping to reinforce activation—especially when positive mood is still developing. This includes both verbal and nonverbal strategies, such as leaning in and demonstrating enthusiasm when clients report activation, as well as praising desired behaviors rather than praising the client.

KEY TECHNIQUES FOR TRAINEES TO LEARN

The effective delivery of BA requires mastery of several techniques. The following section reviews key procedures and strategies for introducing the theoretical model, daily monitoring, life areas and values assessment, activity selection, and eliciting support.

Introducing the Theoretical Model to Clients

The theoretical model for BA (Figure 8.1) is a functional analysis of the relationship between feelings (i.e., emotions), urges, and behaviors, and is referred to as the *treatment model* or *treatment rationale*. It is important for the therapist to have a thorough understanding of this model and the ability to flexibly apply it in treatment. Key techniques for training include providing a clear description of the model, helping clients understand their own experiences within the model, and applying principles of the model during the administration of treatment.

It is useful to begin training by learning to introduce the theoretical model. This typically involves talking through the model step by step while creating a visual illustration (e.g., on a whiteboard, client workbook) in which client examples are integrated. The therapist should be prepared to define each term in the model, for example, explaining that difficult feelings are "emotions that might feel uncomfortable or that lead to negative consequences—such as anger, sadness, and frustration" and clarifying that "an urge is something you want to do in the moment, while the behavior is what you actually do." It is also helpful to practice differentiating between feelings, thoughts, and behaviors. For example, if a client offers a thought instead of a feeling, the therapist may ask, "What emotion were you feeling? How did it feel in your body when you had that thought?"

After brainstorming difficult feelings or sensations recently experienced by the client, the therapist helps identify urges that often accompany these feelings and the behaviors that typically follow. Clients often report behaving in line with their urges; however, it can be helpful to elicit examples in which an urge was followed by a different behavior in order to emphasize the difference between urges and behaviors and to prime clients to recognize this as a decision point. By linking maladaptive behaviors back to difficult feelings, the therapist helps clients understand how feelings, urges, and behaviors functionally relate and can create a "negative cycle." Stimulating discussion about how to break the cycle helps to establish the rationale for behavior change. The therapist can practice describing the rationale for targeting behavior while also acknowledging that behavior change is not easy, and that the purpose of the treatment is to learn tools and strategies to help break this cycle by engaging in value-based behavior. When eliciting examples of possible behaviors with which clients can break the cycle, it is important to include both enjoyable and important (i.e., goal-oriented) behaviors; these are sometimes described as activities that promote *pleasure* and *mastery*. When exploring emotional consequences of BA, it is important to highlight the reinforcing effect of value-based behavior, so that clients understand that the positive emotions typically experienced after enjoyable and important activities will make them more likely to continue engaging in such behavior, creating a "positive cycle."

After the trainee has mastered the introduction of the theoretical model, they can practice flexibly applying the model to a variety of examples that could arise during treatment. Early in training this may include relatively straight-forward applications, such as role-playing responding to a client who says they drank alcohol to cope with loneliness and that they felt relaxed afterward (in this case, the therapist could help the client differentiate between immediate consequences vs. longer term emotional consequences [e.g., increased loneli-ness]). Later in training, they may practice drawing on the theoretical model to troubleshoot more challenging situations, such as responding to a client who is emotionally dysregulated (see the common challenges in training and super-vision section later in this chapter). Indeed, most troubleshooting with trainees can be accomplished in the context of the theoretical model.

Daily Monitoring

Monitoring of daily activities is a key component early in treatment that helps identify opportunities to increase environmental reward. Key tasks for thera-pists include providing a rationale and instructions for activity monitoring and helping clients identify patterns of inactivation using the monitoring forms. It may be necessary to practice offering a clear and concise rationale, such as, "Before you try to change your behavior, it is important to have a sense of what you are already doing on a daily basis." It is also helpful to provide clear instructions, including (a) keeping a detailed record of activities throughout the day (even activities that seem unimportant, such as sleeping or watch-ing television), (b) rating each activity on importance and enjoyment, and (c) noting which aspects of the activities were or were not enjoyable. It is important to describe enjoyment and importance as separate, independent dimensions (e.g., "Enjoyment is how fun or pleasurable the activity was, while importance refers to whether it fulfills some goal you have") and to elicit examples of activities that are high on one dimension but low on the other (e.g., watching TV may be high on enjoyment but low on importance, while completing a job application may be important but not very enjoyable). When reviewing monitoring homework, the therapist may practice Socratic ques-tioning to help clients identify areas to target in treatment, such as asking, "What did you learn about yourself as a result of completing the exercise? Are you engaging in many activities that you want to do? Which activities were more enjoyable than others? Why?"

Life Areas, Values, and Activities Assessment

Due to decreased activation seen in both depression and SUDs, clients may have limited repertoires of activities that promote pleasure and mastery.

The life areas, values, and activities (LAVA) assessment involves identifying possible value-based activities in a variety of life areas. Important techniques for the trainee to learn include facilitating discussion of a breadth of life areas, differentiating between values and activities, and helping clients identify activities that are specific and achievable. When eliciting client values, the therapist may start by asking, "What is important to you in this life area?" It is helpful to clearly differentiate values from activities, such as by saying,

> A value is what is important to you within each of these life areas—it is an ideal, quality, or strong belief in a certain way of living. In other words, what are you striving for in each life area? What are the qualities of that life area that are important to you? An activity, on the other hand, is something specific you can do consistent with your values.

The trainee should also practice helping clients refine the activities in their LAVA assessment to make each activity observable, measurable, and in small, discrete pieces.

Activity Selection and Ranking

Starting with activities that are easy to accomplish helps ensure early success with activity planning and completion, thus increasing the likelihood of receiving positive reinforcement and in turn promoting client self-efficacy. To do this, therapists will guide clients in selecting and ranking a sample of activities identified during their LAVA assessment (e.g., 10–15 activities) from easiest to accomplish to hardest to accomplish. When planning activities, clients start by planning the easiest activities and gradually work toward the more difficult ones.

Activity Planning

Successful planning and completion of value-based activities is the core of BA. Techniques for trainees to learn include explaining the rationale for planning activities ahead of time and applying the theoretical model when planning, debriefing, and troubleshooting homework. Planning is essential for increasing activation and is often a significant change in clients' routines. Thus, it is important for therapists to be able to provide a strong and clear rationale for planning ahead. For example, saying,

> Planning activities ahead of time is important, because if you wake up and see activities already planned for the day, it makes it more likely that you will do them. Also, this way, the decision to schedule an activity is not dependent on your current mood.

The therapist may need to emphasize the importance of knowing the value behind each activity, and to planning activities across a variety of life areas. An additional skill involves preemptively problem solving potential obstacles to planning ahead (e.g., asking what could get in the way of scheduling activities each day).

It is helpful for trainees to practice flexibly applying the theoretical model when planning and debriefing activity planning homework. Training role plays might include debriefing homework by placing each completed activity into a treatment model diagram and identifying the antecedents and consequences of the activity using the diagram. Relying on the theoretical model is especially helpful when troubleshooting challenges with activity planning. When clients report not completing homework, the therapist can conduct a functional analysis using the treatment model diagram to examine any difficult feelings, urges, and maladaptive behaviors that interfered with completing activities, and to identify specific value-based activities that could be used to cope with those urges in the future. For example, a client may report feeling depressed and fatigued, having the urge to withdraw, and then spending the day in bed rather than following through on their planned activity of going for a run. In this case, the therapist could practice helping the client understand how these fit into the negative cycle and lead to more feelings of depression. They would then help the client identify specific positive coping behaviors to be used next time they feel the urge to withdraw (e.g., "When I feel the urge to withdraw, I will go for a walk around the block"). The trainee will gain mastery with the theoretical model by using it to examine the consequences of a variety of both maladaptive and value-based behaviors.

Eliciting Support

Social isolation is a risk factor for both mood and substance use disorders (Chou et al., 2011), and increasing social support is an important target within BA. Eliciting support can be emphasized throughout BA treatment; for example, when facilitating the LAVA assessment, the therapist may suggest asking friends, family, or others in the therapy group for ideas of value-based activities. Toward the end of BA treatment, identifying one or more "support person(s)" is a helpful part of posttreatment planning. Trainees should practice helping clients identify individuals who can be supportive of their treatment goals and guiding them in identifying specific ways in which they want to be supported. For example, a client dealing with depression may request that their partner go for one walk each day with them to help support their value of staying active. Some clients may have difficulty identifying support people; after helping the client think through options (even including other clients in the group or treatment setting), the therapist may suggest behaviors related to finding and developing new supportive relationships (e.g., reaching out to a new acquaintance).

RECOMMENDATIONS FOR TRAINING CASES

Following learning of core BA principles, training cases can provide beginning clinicians with the opportunity to integrate theoretical foundations of BA into clinical practice. BA was originally developed to treat psychological conditions such as depression, where the primary diagnostic features can be conceptualized as originating from low rates of positive reinforcement (Dimidjian et al., 2011).

Thus, we recommend that trainees practice first administering BA to a client whose clinical presentation aligns with this conceptualization (e.g., major depressive disorder [MDD] with primary anhedonia) and is not further complicated by comorbid psychological disorders. A "beginner" training case of this nature ideally allows the trainee to practice providing core BA content in a straightforward manner, helps to solidify comfort with BA content, and builds confidence in the clinical application of this material without additional, clinically relevant symptoms distracting from core content.

While a beginner training case provides a foundational training opportunity for clinicians learning BA, it is common for individuals seeking mental health services to meet diagnostic criteria for multiple psychological disorders (Kessler et al., 2005). Thus, it is advantageous for clinicians intending to utilize BA as part of their therapeutic repertoire to also practice applying BA with clients who present with psychological conditions often comorbid with MDD (e.g., SUD and anxiety-related disorders; Hasin et al., 2018). We designate these "advanced" training cases, as they require the therapist to adapt core content of BA to additional presenting concerns or simultaneously attend to symptoms impacting an individual's willingness or ability to engage in BA treatment.

Consider the example of a client with comorbid MDD and panic disorder. In this instance, opportunities for engagement with positively reinforcing stimuli, particularly from the external environment, is limited not only by depression symptoms (e.g., anhedonia) but additionally by a fear of experiencing panic-like symptoms during activity engagement. This fear compounds motivation for avoidance behavior, contributing to missed positive reinforcement opportunities (and potentially reinforcing depression symptoms). This can negatively impact the course of treatment, as a client with this presentation may be less willing to engage in particular aspects of BA treatment (e.g., may plan activities but fail to complete them) or willing only to engage in select activities that do not elicit distress.

In such a case, the therapist may be tasked with balancing an emphasis on BA core principles while targeting avoidance behavior. In this example, we recommend using the BA treatment model to highlight the relationship between difficult feelings and sensations associated with panic disorder (e.g., fear, heart racing), subsequent behaviors engaged in by the client (e.g., avoidance, isolation), and both short and long-term consequences of these behaviors (e.g., experience of additional difficult emotions such as loneliness and sadness, decreased access to future positive reinforcement opportunities, and ultimate continuation of psychological symptoms related to both depression and panic). In addition, the therapist may also find it helpful to incorporate anxiety symptom ratings alongside enjoyment and importance ratings during activity monitoring.

There are multiple ways to adapt BA to accommodate comorbidities, such as the one described in the previous example. However, the clinical skill needed to do so requires solid, foundational experience with BA, conceptualization of comorbid symptoms within the BA framework, and an overall flexible approach to treatment. Thus, supervised training cases are an ideal step in clinical training. We additionally recommend relevant readings that discuss adaptation of BA to various psychological presentations to facilitate further knowledge accumulation and training for clinicians treating such "advanced" clinical cases (Daughters et al., 2016; Hopko et al., 2006).

COMMON MISTAKES TRAINEES MAKE AND HOW TO FIX THEM

Clinicians new to BA often face challenges common across clinical populations and treatment settings. Here we highlight these challenges using clinical examples and offer potential solutions.

Introducing Activity Planning Too Quickly

When a client is unable to demonstrate understanding of the treatment model, particularly by explaining how their own feelings, urges, and behaviors perpetuate the maintenance of clinical symptoms (e.g., depression), they may not fully adopt the principle that engagement in enjoyable and important behaviors is linked to an increase in future, positive feelings and behavior change. Similarly, client difficulty conceptualizing or identifying core values risks future subsequent generation and planning of activities that are not truly aligned with client values. Without the foundational understanding of the treatment model and LAVA concepts, clients may see little benefit in engaging in theory-driven aspects of treatment including value-based activity planning. Techniques therapists can use to assess conceptual understanding of BA concepts include asking the client to complete each of the following in-session and unassisted: (a) complete the treatment model diagram (Figure 8.1) using a personal example from the past week, and (b) identify a new value and associated hierarchy of activities.

Client Difficulty Completing Planned Activities

Client inability to complete scheduled activities becomes problematic and antithetical to BA success, as it perpetuates a negative reinforcement cycle of negative emotions (e.g., frustration), avoidance of activity planning, decreased motivation for treatment, and the continued maintenance and/or exacerbation of depressive symptoms. The strategy that is most helpful for increasing activity completion is the identification of activities that are specific, measurable, and attainable. In other words, ask the client to determine what exactly they will do (specificity), answer questions regarding the activity such as when, where, how long, and how much (measurability), and break the activity down into small, achievable steps (attainability). Consider the example of a client who schedules the activity "working out." The therapist can help the client revise this activity to include more specific information about what is deemed "working out" (e.g., lifting weights, jogging, taking an exercise class), and include measurable qualities about where (e.g., at a specific gym, park, or room in their home), when (e.g., on Tuesday at 3:00 p.m.) and for how long (e.g., 30 minutes). Drawing on the daily monitoring stage of treatment can be particularly helpful to the therapist when assessing the attainability of planned activities. For example, the activity of "jog 3 miles" may not be attainable for a client who has only recorded physical activity that includes walking for 20 minutes a few times a week. Therapists can help their client break activities into smaller, more immediately feasible parts (e.g., jog for 1 minute, walk for 5 minutes), the success of which will increase feelings of enjoyment, mastery, and positive reinforcement for future activity engagement.

Encouraging Quantity Over Quality

Early therapists often fall into the trap of enthusiastically assisting their client in the overscheduling of activities. Consider the following scenario: A therapist helps her client generate and schedule five values-related activities per day for at home practice. The therapist leaves the session feeling confident in her provision of treatment due to the client's expressed enthusiasm to complete activities for the upcoming week. During the next week's homework review, the client reports completing two activities on the first day and no other activities that week. The client states that they feel more depressed than ever and disappointed in themself for failing to follow through on their home practice.

This is a classic scenario of an activity schedule that is unattainable, thereby perpetuating the negative cycle of the treatment model. This behavior is particularly common among clients prone to all-or-nothing thinking patterns. A technique that helps prevent this scenario is to begin by scheduling one or two value-based activities per day. Early client success will be followed by increases in motivation for future activity planning, opening the door to incrementally increasing daily planned activities. For clients resistant to starting with only one or two activities per day, it can be helpful to identify life areas and values that align with activities the client is already completing successfully (e.g., going to work, attending treatment sessions). Including these activities in the client's daily plan can provide a boost of positive reinforcement when checking them off after completion.

Ignoring Difficulties With Homework Compliance

Homework completion is a critical component of BA success. Yet some trainees find it challenging to address homework compliance issues. Consider a client who does not complete any scheduled activities over the previous week. There may be a multitude of reasons for this. Perhaps the scheduled activities were not aligned with client values, the planned activities were too difficult, the client scheduled too many activities, or the client felt that they did not have enough support from others. Attending to homework compliance issues early in treatment and allotting adequate time in session for problem solving is critical for the identification of barriers to treatment success. It can be particularly helpful to utilize the treatment model when troubleshooting homework completion. For example, the therapist can help the client identify difficult emotions (e.g., guilt), urges (e.g., "I felt like giving up on therapy"), and behaviors (e.g., "I avoided doing the rest of my homework for the week") and draw connections back to the maintenance of psychological symptoms (e.g., depression). This method has the added benefit of reinforcing core treatment concepts.

Emotion Regulation and Crisis Management

It is not uncommon for a client to present to a session emotionally aroused and highly motivated to share the details of a recent life event. Consider the following scenario: A client presents to treatment in visible distress, pacing back and forth, and reveals to the therapist that they just had an argument over the phone with their child. The therapist attempts to begin session by reviewing homework, but the client continues to perseverate. The therapist provides validation to the client and attempts to redirect the client to reviewing homework. The client clenches their fists together, stating how angry they are with their child, and then proceeds to describe the financial strain of saving money for the child's tuition. The therapist, unsure of what to do, listens to the client describe the situation, while noting that the client is becoming more and more visibly agitated as the session continues. The session ends without any review of home practice nor introduction of novel BA content.

It is easy for acute client distress to become the session focus for early trainees, at the cost of BA provision. One method of addressing client distress in the moment while adhering to the BA framework is to use in-session affect (e.g., anger) as an example of a difficult emotion in the treatment model. By identifying urges (e.g., lashing out) and behaviors (e.g., continuing to think or talk about the event) associated with current affect, the therapist can aid the client in identifying the cycle of behavior playing out in session, highlighting consequences of perseverative behavior (e.g., maintaining distress, sacrificing focus on treatment). This method additionally allows the client the opportunity to change behavior (i.e., engage in a value-based approach behavior) in the moment in order to break this negative cycle and return to treatment content. The therapist can facilitate this transition into the positive cycle in session by leading the client in a mindfulness practice or grounding exercise, thereby providing an opportunity to reduce emotional intensity while illustrating real-time engagement in an activity that can then be linked to the client's personal values later in the session.

Cultural Competence

Although client-generated values, activities, and pacing means BA tends to be inherently culturally sensitive, often a lack of awareness of a client's cultural background can interfere with treatment progress. Consider the following scenario: A client who is a Chinese woman with MDD is initially highly engaged in treatment. The White male therapist is encouraged by the client's ability to grasp the treatment model; apply it to her own cycle of mood, urges, and avoidant behavior; and complete daily monitoring. Yet progress suddenly stalls when the client is asked to generate personal values and activities. She indicates she "doesn't know" and seems to look to the therapist for answers. He does not want to do the work for his client, assumes she needs more time, and therefore suggests that she work on the LAVA worksheet during home practice. The next week the client arrives for treatment without any new values or activities. The client continues to demonstrate difficulty generating values. Fearing a lack of progress, the therapist provides suggested values, which she adopts, and they are able to complete the session agenda.

This scenario demonstrates the importance of cultural awareness, as well as a new therapist feeling pressure to maintain progress and thus doing the work for the client. Cultural beliefs can drive a client's expectation of client–therapist roles. In this instance, it was revealed in a future session that the client holds cultural beliefs regarding deference to males and authority figures. It is recommended that new trainees develop cultural competence (Comas-Díaz, 2012; see also Chapter 18, this volume, for more information on multiculturalism in CBT supervision). One approach that can be used to enhance these skills is to role-play conversations surrounding client cultural beliefs and expectations throughout different phases of treatment.

Time Management

BA manuals contain predefined content for each session, often with accompanying checklists and time recommendations. Yet, time management often becomes a challenge for new therapists who do not yet have the experience to estimate the duration of each treatment module or example. This becomes increasingly challenging when faced with obstacles mentioned previously, such as crisis management, poor homework compliance, or client difficulty comprehending the treatment model. It can be especially helpful for trainees to role-play sticking to the recommended time allotted to each module within a session, generate transition phrases to use when their client is resistant to move on from a specific module, and to have session checklists on-hand during the treatment session.

ETHICAL CONSIDERATIONS

While much emphasis has been placed on flexibility in the application of the BA treatment model, it is important for trainees to recognize when a client is presenting with psychological symptoms and conditions for which BA is not an empirically supported treatment or for which BA provision requires specialized training. For example, if a trainee observes psychotic symptoms in a client presenting with MDD, a thorough assessment, consultation, and possible referral is recommended. Similarly, if a therapist who has only received training in BA for major depression learns during the course of therapy that their client meets criteria for SUD, it is recommended that the therapist obtain training in BA for SUD prior to attempting to treat substance use within a BA framework.

Therapist assumptions about client background, views, and expectations can impact BA treatment progress. Here we discuss the importance of the therapist remaining open and curious about each clients' education level, literacy, financial security, and cultural beliefs. Generating, planning, and tracking value-based activities is academic in nature, and thus it is important for clinicians to be aware of any assumptions regarding their clients' literacy and educational background. Challenges with this framework may be observed in clients with limited exposure to creating lists, hierarchies, and abstract thinking. It may be helpful for therapists to establish baseline functioning in these domains by probing with questions such as, "Tell me about times you have thought about your values," or "Tell me about any experience you have had writing down future plans." If literacy is a concern, therapists can use alternative strategies such as stickers in place of written monitoring (Magidson et al., 2015). Client financial constraints may be a barrier to treatment progress, and therapists are encouraged to support clients' identification of low-cost activities.

SUPERVISION OBSTACLES

A BA supervisor will often be faced with providing guidance to therapists who experience challenges. Recommended supervision techniques include trainee role plays, supervisor modeling of the timing and structure of treatment modules, review of audio and video recordings, and group supervision, which can increase trainee exposure to challenging scenarios and problem-solving approaches. It can also be challenging to supervise a BA trainee who has a history of approaching treatment from a nonbehavioral theoretical orientation. For example, a seasoned cognitive therapist new to BA may be resistant to ignoring thoughts in the context of the treatment model. Similarly, a psychodynamic therapist may find that BA does not attend enough to client processing or existing belief systems. In these instances, it may be helpful to acknowledge the role of cognitions or past experiences in the context of the BA model. For example, rumination or all-or-nothing thinking can be categorized as an avoidant or maladaptive behavior. In regard to client processing, it may help to discuss the "outside-in" philosophy behind BA, namely, that new experiences can help change a clients' belief system rather than the "inside-out" philosophy that it is first important to address client beliefs. While there may be some resistance, the successful adoption of BA can be aided by a supervisors' openness, flexibility, and ability to discuss these alternative philosophies within the context of the BA model.

CONCLUSION

BA has experienced exponential growth over the past 2 decades, from its established effectiveness as a treatment for depression among adults to its transdiagnostic application across multiple age groups and cultures. As highlighted in this chapter, this growth is in direct response to the accessibility and feasibility of applying BA. That said, BA is not simply the increase in activity engagement or pleasant events. Its successful implementation requires adequate supervision and training to ensure new trainees can conceptualize and apply the BA treatment model and value based activity planning and completion.

REFERENCES

Chen, Y. Anand, D., Li, H., Xu, P., & Daughters, S. B. (2021). Feasibility, acceptability and future adaptation of the Chinese translated behavioural activation (C-BA) treatment for depression: A pilot study. *International Journal of Psychology, 56*(2), 238–248. https://doi.org/10.1002/ijop.12704

Chou, K. L., Liang, K., & Sareen, J. (2011). The association between social isolation and *DSM-IV* mood, anxiety, and substance use disorders: Wave 2 of the National Epidemiologic Survey on Alcohol and Related Conditions. *The Journal of Clinical Psychiatry, 72*(11), 1468–1476. https://doi.org/10.4088/JCP.10m06019gry

Collado, A., Calderón, M., MacPherson, L., & Lejuez, C. (2016). The efficacy of behavioral activation treatment among depressed Spanish-speaking Latinos. *Journal of Consulting and Clinical Psychology, 84*(7), 651–657. https://doi.org/10.1037/ccp0000103

Comas-Díaz, L. (2012). *Multicultural care: A clinician's guide to cultural competence.* American Psychological Association.

Daughters, M., Magidson, J. F., Lejuez, C. W., & Chen, Y. (2016). LETS Act: A behavioral activation treatment for substance use and depression. *Advances in Dual Diagnosis, 9*(2/3). Online publication. https://doi.org/10.1108/ADD-02-2016-0006

Daughters, S. B., Magidson, J. F., Anand, D., Seitz-Brown, C. J., Chen, Y., & Baker, S. (2018). The effect of a behavioral activation treatment for substance use on post-treatment abstinence: A randomized controlled trial. *Addiction, 113*(3), 535–544. https://doi.org/10.1111/add.14049

Dimidjian, S., Barrera, M., Jr., Martell, C., Muñoz, R. F., & Lewinsohn, P. M. (2011). The origins and current status of behavioral activation treatments for depression. *Annual Review of Clinical Psychology, 7*(1), 1–38. https://doi.org/10.1146/annurev-clinpsy-032210-104535

Ekers, D., Godfrey, C., Gilbody, S., Parrott, S., Richards, D. A., Hammond, D., & Hayes, A. (2011). Cost utility of behavioural activation delivered by the non-specialist. *The British Journal of Psychiatry, 199*(6), 510–511. https://doi.org/10.1192/bjp.bp.110.090266

Ekers, D., Richards, D., & Gilbody, S. (2008). A meta-analysis of randomized trials of behavioural treatment of depression. *Psychological Medicine, 38*(5), 611–623. https://doi.org/10.1017/S0033291707001614

Etherton, J. L., & Farley, R. (2020). Behavioral activation for PTSD: A meta-analysis. *Psychological Trauma: Theory, Research, Practice, and Policy.* Advance online publication. https://doi.org/10.1037/tra0000566

Ferster, C. B. (1973). A functional analysis of depression. *American Psychologist, 28*(10), 857–870. https://doi.org/10.1037/h0035605

Hasin, D. S., Sarvet, A. L., Meyers, J. L., Saha, T. D., Ruan, W. J., Stohl, M., & Grant, B. F. (2018). Epidemiology of adult *DSM-5* major depressive disorder and its specifiers in the United States. *JAMA Psychiatry, 75*(4), 336–346. https://doi.org/10.1001/jamapsychiatry.2017.4602

Hopko, D. R., Lejuez, C. W., Ruggiero, K. J., & Eifert, G. H. (2003). Contemporary behavioral activation treatments for depression: Procedures, principles, and progress. *Clinical Psychology Review, 23*(5), 699–717. https://doi.org/10.1016/S0272-7358(03)00070-9

Hopko, R., Robertson, S. M. C., & Lejuez, C. W. (2006). Behavioral activation for anxiety disorders. *The Behavior Analyst Today, 7*(2), 212–232. https://doi.org/10.1037/h0100084

Kessler, R. C., Demler, O., Frank, R. G., Olfson, M., Pincus, H. A., Walters, E. E., Wang, P., Wells, K. B., & Zaslavsky, A. M. (2005). Prevalence and treatment of mental disorders, 1990 to 2003. *The New England Journal of Medicine, 352*(24), 2515–2523. https://doi.org/10.1056/NEJMsa043266

Lejuez, C. W., Hopko, D. R., Acierno, R., Daughters, S. B., & Pagoto, S. L. (2011). Ten year revision of the brief behavioral activation treatment for depression: Revised treatment manual. *Behavior Modification, 35*(2), 111–161. https://doi.org/10.1177/0145445510390929

Lewinsohn, P. M. (1974). A behavioral approach to depression. In R. J. Friedman & M. M. Katz (Eds.), *The psychology of depression: Contemporary theory and research* (pp. 157–174). John Wiley & Sons.

Magidson, J. F., Lejuez, C. W., Kamal, T., Blevins, E. J., Murray, L. K., Bass, J. K., Bolton, P., & Pagoto, S. (2015). Adaptation of community health worker-delivered behavioral activation for torture survivors in Kurdistan, Iraq. *Global Mental Health (Cambridge, England), 2*, E24. https://doi.org/10.1017/gmh.2015.22

Martell, M. E., Addis, M. E., & Jacobson, N. S. (2001). *Depression in context: Strategies for guided action.* W. W. Norton.

Mazzucchelli, K., Kane, R., & Rees, C. (2009). Behavioral activation treatments for depression in adults: A meta-analysis and review. *Clinical Psychology: Science and Practice, 16*(4), 383–411. https://doi.org/10.1111/j.1468-2850.2009.01178.x

Simmonds-Buckley, M., Kellett, S., & Waller, G. (2019). Acceptability and efficacy of group behavioral activation for depression among adults: A meta-analysis. *Behavior Therapy, 50*(5), 864–885. https://doi.org/10.1016/j.beth.2019.01.003

Stein, A., Carl, E., Cuijpers, P., Karyotaki, E., & Smits, J. (2020). Looking beyond depression: A meta-analysis of the effect of behavioral activation on depression, anxiety, and activation. *Psychological Medicine, 51*(9), 1491–1504. https://doi.org/10.1017/s0033291720000239

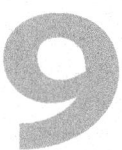

Supervising Child Behavior Management

Deborah J. Jones, Rex Forehand, Nicholas Long, and Robert J. McMahon

Collectively, disruptive behavior disorders (DBDs; i.e., oppositional defiant disorder, conduct disorder), which co-occur often with attention-deficit/ hyperactivity disorder (ADHD), affect over a million youth worldwide (Merikangas et al., 2009, 2010; Polanczyk et al., 2015). Untreated DBDs predict later antisocial behavior, substance use, underachievement, employment instability, and chronic illness (e.g., Fergusson et al., 2005; Odgers et al., 2007; Piquero et al., 2009). Early identification and intervention can save millions of dollars per high-risk child; yet, too few youth receive evidence-based treatment (e.g., Cohen & Piquero, 2009; Deković et al., 2011; Farahmand et al., 2011). Therefore, opportunities to train and supervise therapists in the evidence-based treatment for early-onset (3–8 years old) DBDs (i.e., behavioral parent training [BPT]), are essential.

The origins of BPT date back to the 1960s with the emergence of data to support the utility of therapists teaching parents to use behavioral strategies to modify child behavior (Kotchick et al., 2004; Long et al., 2017). The evolution of this triadic approach (i.e., therapist, parent, child; Tharp & Wetzel, 1969) was subsequently influenced by Patterson's (1982) work demonstrating that punitive and increasingly coercive (e.g., nagging, threatening, yelling) parenting increased (rather than decreased) child noncompliance. Concurrent with Patterson's work, Hanf developed a two-phase BPT program that focused on reducing this coercive cycle via skill modeling, role plays, and practice (Kaehler et al., 2016; Long et al., 2017; Reitman & McMahon, 2013). Hanf's trainees and

https://doi.org/10.1037/0000314-010
Training and Supervision in Specialized Cognitive Behavior Therapy: Methods, Settings, and Populations, E. A. Storch, J. S. Abramowitz, and D. McKay (Editors)

colleagues went on to develop a family of evidence-based BPT programs that share her framework: Webster-Stratton's *Incredible Years* (2011), Cunningham's *Community Parent Education Program* (2013), McMahon and Forehand's *Helping the Noncompliant Child* (2003), Barkley's *Defiant Child* (2013), and Eyberg and Funderburk's *Parent–Child Interaction Therapy* (2011). BPT, which is now considered the standard of care for early-onset DBDs (Kaminski & Claussen, 2017; McMahon & Frick, 2019), has also shown effects for comorbid symptomatology in children (e.g., internalizing problems) and parents (e.g., depression), and its effects on behavior are largely consistent across demographics, including race/ethnicity, with few exceptions (e.g., less effective for low-income families given engagement challenges discussed later; see Gonzalez & Jones, 2016; Kaehler et al., 2016; Long et al., 2017). This chapter focuses on Helping the Noncompliant Child (HNC; Forehand & McMahon, 1981; McMahon & Forehand, 2003) as an example.

KEY CONCEPTS FOR TRAINEES TO LEARN

HNC, which was developed for families of young (3–8 years old) children with high levels of noncompliance and other problem behavior (e.g., aggression, oppositionality), is a therapist-delivered, two-phase program with weekly sessions. Phase I, *Differential Attention*, focuses on increasing parent–child relationship quality and, in turn, the child's "okay" behavior (i.e., behavior parents want to see or see more of, e.g., using an "inside voice," sharing, and compliance). Parents are taught a series of skills that progress from *Attends* (e.g., "You are using your inside voice") to *Rewards* (e.g., "Good job using your inside voice!") to planned *Ignoring* (e.g., no looking, talking, or touching when the child yells instead of using their inside voice). Skills are taught in the context of the *Child's Game* (i.e., child-directed play), which parents are instructed to practice daily (10–15 minutes), and also to use the skills throughout the day.

In Phase II, *Compliance Training*, parents are taught the *clear instruction sequence*, which includes guidance on how to give an effective instruction (e.g., "Put on your shoes" instead of "Will you put on your shoes?" or "Let's put on your shoes"). Essentially, ensuring parents are giving effective or clear instructions both decreases the likelihood of child noncompliance (e.g., Parent: "Will you put on your shoes?" Child: "No!") and increases the likelihood that both the therapist and the parent feel confident that a child's failure to comply is not a function of misunderstanding (e.g., "But you asked if I wanted to, and I say 'no'!"). If the child complies within 5 seconds to the clear instruction, the parent is taught to use their Phase I Attends and Rewards skills (e.g., "You are picking up your shoe. You put on your right shoe, you put on your left shoe. Thank you for putting on your shoes!"). Alternatively, if the child does not comply within 5 seconds, parents are taught to give one *Warning* (e.g., "If you do not put on your shoes, you will go to Time Out"). If the child complies to the Warning, parents are taught to use Attends and Rewards in the same way they would if the child had complied without the Warning. If the child, however, does not comply to the Warning within 5 seconds, the parent is taught to use *Time Out* (e.g., "Because you did not put on your shoes, you have to go to Time Out"). Once the Time Out is completed (i.e., 3 minutes with the child being quiet and still the last 15 seconds), parents are taught to repeat the original clear instruction (e.g., "Put on your shoes") and the sequence continues until compliance is achieved. A *standing rule* (i.e., an automatic Time Out) is also taught as an option for safety-related behaviors (e.g., aggression).

During Phase II, the clear instruction sequence and standing rules are taught in the context of the *Parent's Game* or a parent-directed activity (e.g., clean up). However, parents are told that they should continue to engage in the Child's Game at home daily, which allows ongoing practice of Phase I skills in the context of child-directed, appropriate play. Parents are also instructed to use the skills outside of the session in order to continue the generalization of skills to the home and other settings, which is critical for behavior change. HNC is a mastery-based program for which parents must demonstrate that skill use meets behavioral criteria before progressing from one skill to the next, to move from Phase I to II, and to complete the program (see McMahon & Forehand, 2003, for more detail).

KEY TECHNIQUES FOR TRAINEES TO LEARN

HNC skills are taught in the context of the aforementioned triadic model that includes the therapist, parent, and child in the room together for the entirety of the session. This offers repeated opportunities for planned modeling, role-plays, and use of the skills, as well as in vivo opportunities that arise within and across sessions based on the child's level of problem behavior. The therapist uses *Setting Instructions* to orient the child to how the session will proceed, including what is expected in terms of the child's behavior. For example, a therapist may say,

> Your mom and I will be talking on our side of the room. While we are talking, you will stay on this side of the room with these toys. If you interrupt us, your mom and I will ignore you. That means that we will not look at you, talk to you, or touch you while we are talking. We will take a break in a few minutes and come back over to play with you.

HNC is a very active treatment with sessions characterized by the therapist and parent(s) moving back and forth between their side and the child's side of the room. Setting Instructions are given with each transition to cue the child that positive attention will pause and the "no look, talk, or touch" rules will go back into place. With particularly young children and/or children with more inhibitory control issues who may benefit from physical cues, we have also used colored tape on the floor to demarcate therapist/parent and child "sides" of the room.

HNC skills are taught using a variety of techniques: modeling and role plays, practice with the child (with and without coaching/mastery coding), and therapist discussion with the parent about the use of skills at home. Therapists first briefly describe and provide a rationale for each new skill to the parent. For example,

> The next skill is Rewards. Rewards can be an unlabeled verbal reward (e.g., "good job!"), a labeled verbal reward (e.g., "Good job using your inside voice!"), or positive physical attention (e.g., pat on back, high five). We use rewards because we want to give positive attention to your child's okay behavior—behaviors you want to see more often. Labeled verbal rewards are best, as they let your child know exactly what you like about their behavior. Rewards will work best if you use them initially every time and as soon as possible after the behavior occurs.

The therapist then role-plays the new skill with the therapist pretending to be the parent and the parent pretending to be the child (then vice versa). These role plays can be done on the parent and/or child side of the room and the choice may depend in part on the child's personality, presenting issues and/or behavior in session. For example, if the therapist and parent want an opportunity for in vivo use of the skills, they may do these role plays on their side, which provides an opportunity to practice planned Ignoring if the child comes to their side and tries to engage (as well as Attends and Rewards when the child returns to the other side of the room). Alternatively, if a therapist and parent are looking for more opportunities to give positive attention to a child, for example one who is younger and may need more practice in order to understand the Setting Instructions, they may do the role-plays on the child's side of the room and include the child in those. Either way, therapists and parents briefly discuss those role plays and, if needed, problem solve; then they move to the parent practicing the skills with the child. This occurs first with the therapist providing active coaching to the parent regarding their skill use (e.g., "Really nice job with that labeled verbal Reward. How could you use the combination of Attends, Rewards, and Ignoring right now in response to your child's whining?"). Then, the therapist tells the parent to continue their skill use but phases out coaching for a brief period (e.g., 5 minutes) of observation when behaviors are coded to see if mastery criteria are reached.

After observation/coding, the therapist and parent again give the Setting Instructions and then return to their side of the room to discuss, debrief, and talk about how to generalize the skill to the home and/or other settings. Continued Child's Game and skill use are assigned for daily home practice. Ideally, therapists also schedule a brief midweek call with parents to discuss, cheerlead, and/or problem solve skills use at home, which then can be used to inform the subsequent session.

CHARACTERISTICS OF IDEAL TRAINING CASES

When considering a family's "fit" with the treatment model, a key consideration is a parent's understanding that HNC is an active process that requires their engagement (e.g., weekly sessions, daily home practice, midweek call) in order to see change in their child's behavior. If parents are committed to treatment, HNC takes an average of eight to 12 sessions for families to meet mastery criteria with the program skills and experience clinically significant change in their child's behavior. This investment of time, energy, and resources is particularly difficult for lower income families for whom engagement is more difficult, which weakens outcomes (for reviews, see Chacko et al., 2016; Gardner et al., 2009; Leijten et al., 2013; Lundahl et al., 2006; Reyno & McGrath, 2006; Shaw & Taraban, 2017). Therefore, more financially stable families may make better initial training cases.

Another consideration as it relates to the selection of training cases is maltreatment history. BPT has been used with and may be helpful for families with maltreatment histories (for reviews, see Long et al., 2017; Lundahl et al., 2006); however, given the higher risk nature of such cases, as well as the fact that behavior can get worse in the context of Ignoring before it gets better (i.e., extinction burst), families without current or past maltreatment are likely more optimal training cases for novice therapists. Similarly, BPT in general and HNC in particular are not necessarily contraindicated for parents with comorbid psychopathology, such as depression, which does often co-occur with children's problem behavior. Some data suggest maternal depression may improve as a function of BPT (for a review, see Gonzalez & Jones, 2016); however, careful assessment and management of depression may also be necessary given reliance on the parent as the mechanism of change. Therefore, parents without depression or other current psychopathology likely provide better initial training cases.

In terms of child comorbidities, BPT in general, including HNC, has been shown to reduce children's internalizing symptoms, which often co-occur with DBDs (Rothenberg et al., 2020; for a review, see Gonzalez & Jones, 2016). BPT has also been used with other disorders, such as autism, although with more varying effects (for reviews, see Chorpita et al., 2011; Kaehler et al., 2016; Long et al., 2017); therefore, better initial training cases may be those in which children present with DBDs alone or comorbidity limited to internalizing symptoms alone. Finally, various physical impairments that prevent and/or interfere with children being responsive to the skills and/or make it difficult or impossible for parents to use the skills (e.g., vision or hearing impairments) may also require more modifications to the treatment, which may be less optimal for a beginning-level therapist.

COMMON MISTAKES AND HOW TO CORRECT THEM

HNC provides a guide for the implementation of BPT with families of young children with high levels of noncompliance and other problem behaviors. It is through our collective clinical experience using the manual with many families over the years that we have identified common challenges in the delivery of BPT. In this section, we highlight common challenges and provide recommendations for avoiding those challenges or adjusting accordingly based on the presenting needs and context of the child and family.

Adhering Strictly to Technique Without Flexibility

As described earlier, HNC is an evidence-based treatment with a prescribed format; set of skills; and techniques used to teach, model, and practice those skills. As such, one potential pitfall is for trainees to become "technicians" of the treatment, rather than having a comprehensive understanding of the behavioral and social theories underlying the treatment and associated techniques. It is critical for the therapist to not only understand child management principles but to believe they will be effective in changing behavior. If one becomes "only a technician," then it will be difficult to explain the rationale behind the skills to parents, which is especially critical early in the process when skills are taught in isolation and seemingly out of context (e.g., Attends without Rewards or Ignoring). This can feel arbitrary and less than helpful to parents feeling high levels of distress and frustration related to their child's problem behavior. In addition, therapists with a poor understanding of social learning theory underlying the program's format and skills are more prone to avoid parent questions about the treatment process or particular skills, or have more difficulty responding to such questions effectively, which is critical to parent commitment to and engagement in HNC. Finally, reliance on technique alone without a good understanding of behavioral theory makes it much more difficult for therapists to respond and adjust in session based on the nature of the child's presenting issues and the parent's response to those presenting issues. This takes us to the next point about flexible use of treatment.

As with all evidence-based interventions, HNC must be flexible and based on the presenting needs and context of the child and family. One common example of this follows from the aforementioned discussion of the Setting Instructions. It is common for children, particularly those with early-onset DBDs, to test the limits of the Setting Instructions (e.g., crossing to the therapist and parent's side of the room, crawling under their chairs, turning on and off the lights). While the session may be focusing on the initial skill of Attends, the therapist can use this in vivo noncompliance as an opportunity to introduce and model Ignoring in response to the problem behavior (e.g., child on their side of room) and positive attention (i.e., Attends) as the child returns to the child side of the room. With this example, we have learned that some children can turn this into a way to continue to get attention by immediately returning to the parent side of the room as soon as the Setting Instructions are reissued (e.g., hovering over the tape separating the two sides of the room, dipping their shoes over the line onto the therapist and parent side, hopping back and forth). So, supervisors and therapists and, in turn, therapists and parents will need to tailor how best to use the skills (including using them out of order), in order to make sure they are decreasing rather than increasing the problem behavior (e.g., wait until the child is back on the child side of the room and playing with the toys for a particular period of time before giving positive attention).

Another scenario that may require flexible use of the HNC model is when a child presents early on with high levels of safety-related problem behaviors in the session (e.g., hitting, throwing toys, running out of the session). In such cases, therapists may need to determine if and how much response they are getting using the Phase I skills (Attends and Rewards) with the desirable alternatives of these not-okay behaviors (e.g., gentle hands, keeping the toys on the floor or table, sitting at the table or on the floor with the toys). If therapists and parents are using these skills appropriately, and at sufficiently high rates, yet the child continues to engage in high levels of safety-related behaviors, implementing Phase II skills earlier in treatment may be occasionally indicated (i.e., Clear Instruction, Warning, Time Out or Standing Rule). Alternatively, rigid adherence to the Phase I and II structure could potentially lead to both the therapist and parent feeling ineffective, worsen rather than improve the child's behavior, and decrease the likelihood that the parent continues to invest time and resources in services.

Flexible use of HNC has its limits as well, as evidenced by another potential pitfall for trainees, which is to spend most, if not all, of the session talking with the parent rather than going back and forth between the parent and child sides of the room practicing skills. Having a child with a behavioral issue is stressful and, as we said earlier, can co-occur with parent depression. Parents of children with behavior disorders are also more likely to have co-occurring relationship conflict. Therefore, it is easy for trainees to lose focus on the child's behavior and instead spend the session talking about the parent's stress, which can lead to worse treatment process and outcome (Chorpita et al., 2014; Guan et al., 2019). Instead, trainees need to learn to balance listening to and validating parents with maintaining a focus on the presenting issue (i.e., the child's behavior), which is better served by the parent learning specific skills and practicing the skills in session. This is the only way child misbehavior will eventually change at home; that is, parents have to learn the skills in the clinic and then, with the therapist's assistance, generalize them to the home.

Talking Too Much About Skills Rather Than Practicing Them

Trainees can also run the risk of talking too much about the skills and parent skill use, rather than using the session to practice, coach, and observe. HNC therapists-in-training may be more vulnerable to this pitfall when working with parents who are particularly analytic and want to spend significant time dissecting in detail the parent–child interactions. Similarly, this may occur with socially anxious parents for whom learning new skills and being observed and coded using those skills repeatedly increases their anxiety. Both types of parents may not want to spend the session practicing and being observed. Socially anxious parents in particular may also increase the likelihood of another potential pitfall for trainees, which is to limit providing active, directive, and constructive coaching feedback for fear of hurting the parent's feelings or increasing their anxiety. We recognize this is challenging but remind beginning-level therapists that not providing constructive feedback decreases the likelihood that the parent's skill use (i.e., the mechanism of change in treatment) and, in turn, the child's behavior, will improve. Thus, again, we recommend that therapists focus the session on modeling, role playing, and practice, as this is what will bolster parents' competence and skill use.

Not Sufficiently Encouraging Parents to Complete Homework

Another common pitfall of beginning therapists is to tell parents that "it's okay" that they did not do their daily home practice. While failing to do homework occasionally is expected, frequent or ongoing failure to complete homework is problematic, as it decreases the likelihood that families will benefit from treatment. So, again, we encourage therapists to support and validate parents (e.g., "It really does sound like it has been an incredibly stressful week") and remind parents that progress is contingent upon in- and out-of-session practice ("Let's talk about how to build in practice to your day in spite of all that is going on"). One strategy we have suggested to trainees in such situations is for them to empathize with parents that adding one more thing to their day or week is going to be stressful in the short term, but that using the parenting skills at home is a way to decrease stress in the long term, as they begin to feel more positive about their relationship with their child and their ability to effectively manage the child's behavior.

Not Spending Enough Time Mastering a Difficult Skill

A final point regarding potential pitfalls concerns the mastery criteria. Again, HNC is a mastery-based program for which parents must meet criteria on one skill to proceed to the next, to move from Phase I to II, and to complete the program. The reliance on mastery criteria means that families move through the program at their own pace, with some families requiring more sessions to master one or more skills than other families, which can feel frustrating for both the therapist and the parent. For example, Attends provides parents with a strategy to maintain sustained positive attention to the child's okay behavior (e.g., "You are picking up your shoe. You put on your right shoe. You put on your left shoe"). Without the context of the other skills, however, Attends can feel arbitrary or, as some parents say, "weird" or "awkward" and, thus, may not necessarily feel intrinsically or immediately motivating or rewarding. While it would be easy with such complaints for a beginning therapist to move on from Attends before the parent meets mastery criteria, we instead want them to emphasize that Attends is a foundational skill—a building block—that may require multiple sessions of practice until the parent meets criteria. Indeed, what many parents realize when therapists take this approach is that most children come to enjoy Attends (i.e., their parent's sustained positive attention). This occurs particularly when parents use a positive, excited tone of voice, smiles, and also lean in to convey their interest. In turn, the use of Attends can (and often does) become intrinsically motivating for parents once they are comfortable with using attending regularly, as they start to see their children smile, enjoy, and even ask for their parents to attend. We have even observed some children start to attend to their own behavior when they are not receiving enough attention in session—a good reminder that is time for the therapist and parent to stop talking and go to the child's side of the room!

ETHICAL ISSUES

As with any evidence-based intervention, supervisors must help trainees navigate potential ethical issues that arise in the course of treatment. One issue was already noted, which stems from parent's expectations about the focus and course of treatment. If parents expect treatment to focus on the child alone and/or to focus initially on the not-okay behavior, then therapists must help them to understand the rationale for the treatment plan (i.e., the parent as a mechanism of change; start with increasing okay behavior then decreasing not-okay behavior). To extend this point, parents may have thoughts and feelings about particular skills. These reactions tend to focus on: (a) Attends and Rewards (i.e., parents who think they should not have to give their child positive attention for what they should or are supposed to do); (b) Ignoring (i.e., parents who find it uncomfortable/distressing or believe that it is neglectful to withhold attention); and (c) Time Out (i.e., parents who either think it is neglectful to withhold attention from a child or who think Time Out is not punitive enough).

It is possible that some parents will decide that HNC in general or the skills in particular are a poor fit for their family. In this case a referral to a therapist with a different approach is warranted. However, in many cases, psycho-education can help a parent see the value of learning child management strategies. For example, with Attends and Rewards we talk about how it is normal for young children to not yet have intrinsic motivation for many prosocial behaviors and that they develop that motivation by what is pleasing to and reinforced by adults. Another helpful approach is to talk to parents about adults also being more likely to do things and do them more frequently when someone notices, tells them "good job," and, in the case of employment, pays them to do it! With Ignoring, we (a) highlight to parents that it is planned (i.e., parents identify which child behaviors [e.g., yelling] they are going to target in advance to ignore); (b) tell the child that when those behaviors occur the parent will not look, talk, or touch (i.e., Ignore); and (c) when the child does the opposite of those behaviors (e.g., using an inside voice), the parent gives positive attention (i.e., Attends, Rewards).

For Time Out, the strategies depend on parents' particular questions and concerns. For some parents, the concern is that Time Out is not punitive enough. These parents may prefer, for example, spanking. In this case, we use a variety of nonjudgmental strategies, such as talking with parents about feeling bad when they have to spank, as well as that spanking does not seem to be working with this child (i.e., they are seeking help). Building upon this conversation, we ask parents if they are willing to try an alternative to spanking that is brief and does not lead to feeling sad or guilty about physically disciplining their child. We highlight that Time Out is new and different and, therefore, may feel more challenging in the short term, but that it is more likely to decrease or eliminate the behavior in the long term without the unintended side effects of spanking. Indeed, most parents we have worked with are willing to try Time Out and, once they are coached to do it correctly, see the benefit fairly quickly. On the other hand, some parents express concerns that Time Out is too punitive, is isolating, and that it has long-lasting negative effects on children's attachment and sense of security. This has been at least in part fueled by some negative press on Time Out in the media, which unfortunately is not based on data. In fact, data clearly show that Time Out, when used as intended and correctly (i.e., brief, removal of positive attention as a consequence for noncompliance), is associated with better short- and long-term outcomes for children, including those most vulnerable (e.g., children with maltreatment and trauma histories; for reviews, see Dadds & Tully, 2019; Quetsch et al., 2015).

SUPERVISION CHALLENGES

We believe that supervising new HNC therapists is incredibly rewarding; however, there are some challenges as well. We have addressed some of these earlier, as they relate to the common challenges faced by all new therapists (e.g., teaching skills as a technician rather than understanding the theory or principle behind the skills; talking with parents rather than practicing with the child). One strategy to address some of these in-session challenges is to use a checklist that reminds new therapists about what to cover and how to cover it during the session. The HNC manual (McMahon & Forehand, 2003) provides session outlines that supervisors and therapists in training can use. These can also be tailored or made more specific based on the therapist's level of comfort and training, as well as based on any topics discussed in supervision. For example, we have built in more frequent reminders for therapists and parents to pause ongoing discussion in order to give the child positive attention. There is a lot to accomplish in each session, which involves a balance of brief talking and more action-oriented learning of skills, and often against a backdrop of high levels of not-okay behavior (e.g., yelling, throwing toys, turning off lights). As a result, it is easy for beginning-level therapists to lose track of their place in session, lose track of time, and/or, as noted earlier, fall into the trap of a parent-focused talk therapy session. To address this, supervision may also address estimated time frames for each item on the checklist to aid with session management.

Supervisors can also help beginning therapists with time and session management by, if possible, watching sessions either live or by video. We have many examples of therapists telling us a session was "terrible" only to watch it and realize that the child's behavior was challenging, but the therapist used the session effectively to model and engage the parent in skill use to manage that behavior. Alternatively, we have also heard from therapists that a session went "well" only to watch a video that revealed a session full of traditional "talk therapy" with the parent as the client and little or no attention to the child. In turn, beginning-level therapists can benefit greatly from supervisors providing more informed feedback about session management, adherence to the treatment, and effective teaching of skills. This allows the trainee to learn and adjust accordingly in the subsequent session. Of course, we recognize that this may be a challenge, if not impossible, in some clinical settings and recommend audio recordings of the session, if that is more feasible, particularly for new therapists.

If more than one therapist is starting HNC training, we find group supervision that includes therapists watching (or listening to) one another's sessions to be highly beneficial, for both addressing challenges and sharing successes. This provides modeling of session format, how different therapists explain and use the skills in session, and a broader exposure to the range of families and presenting issues for which HNC is effective. Group supervision also encourages new therapists to think more deeply about cases as a function of both the group's input on their session(s) and constructive feedback they provide to their peers.

It is ideal for therapist training and quality of service provision if supervisors can continue to provide individual and/or group supervision to new therapists over multiple cases. Therapists will employ the same format, principles, and skills with each family, but sessions will also look and feel different based on if and how the therapists are tailoring the treatment plan to the individual family's unique context and presenting issues. For example, HNC sessions with the family of a child presenting with clinically significant oppositional behavior is going to look and feel different than with the family of a child presenting with high levels of aggression and property destruction. So, supervision that continues through the course of treatment for individual families, as well as across multiple families, is ideal to ensure that therapists continue to balance adherence to the treatment while also adapting and adjusting based on what is happening in session with a particular family.

Beyond a focus on what is happening in session and the best ways to provide new therapists with feedback, a serious challenge faced by all BPT therapists is poor family engagement (with subsequent increased risk of dropout). BPT (including HNC) is time-intensive (eight–12 weekly sessions, daily home practice, and midweek calls) and can also be resource-intensive as well (e.g., child care for nonparticipating siblings). Perhaps not surprisingly, then, attrition rates hover at 50%, with the highest rates of dropout occurring for the lowest income families (for reviews, see Chacko et al., 2016; Gardner et al., 2009; Lundahl et al., 2006; Reyno & McGrath, 2006; Shaw & Taraban, 2017). Families rescheduling, not showing up for sessions, and/or discontinuing services prematurely can feel discouraging for all therapists, but particularly new therapists.

In terms of how to use supervision to address poor engagement and associated therapist frustration, we have found that therapists able to make clear connections between what is happening in the therapy room and at home (e.g., skill use, Child's Game), identifying and cheerleading parents' progress and successes, and problem solving challenges can be helpful for maintaining or boosting parental motivation and commitment. That said, stressors may arise that make it difficult for families to continue, or parents may feel like they have achieved enough benefit (e.g., after Phase I) so that the pros of discontinuing outweigh the cons of completing services (i.e., Phase II). In this case, supervisors can work with therapists to encourage them to talk with parents in final sessions or phone calls regarding how to use the skills they have learned to maintain any gains.

A final supervision challenge is related more broadly to theory and, as such, may be most relevant for more experienced therapists who are seeking training and supervision in HNC. As discussed earlier, BPT has its roots in behavioral theory, and HNC relies heavily on the principles of social learning theory (e.g., role plays, modeling) and behavior modification (e.g., differential attention). The reliance on behavioral theory and techniques, however, may be unfamiliar and even uncomfortable to some more-experienced therapists, depending on the theoretical orientation in which they were originally trained, as well as their experience. Therefore, a primer in behavioral theory may be necessary for buy-in among even experienced therapists in order to ensure they fully understand the rationale for the treatment and, in turn, feel comfortable explaining it to parents in session. Additionally, we believe there are opportunities for talking with therapists about what theoretical orientations and approaches to treatment they are more familiar with in order to determine whether the approaches can enhance and/or complement one another. For example, a therapist more comfortable with cognitive theory and therapy may find the reliance on behavioral strategies alone frustrating given their lack of experience with young children and the limits of their cognitive development. Brief cognitive work with the parent, however, may be appropriate. For example, helping a parent to identify thoughts about their child's behavior that make it difficult to use Ignoring (e.g., "I should be able to control my child's behavior," "My child should not whine," "My child is trying to upset me") may facilitate parents' skill use and, thus, allow them to progress in the program.

CONCLUSION

HNC is one example of evidence-based BPT, which is the standard of care for early-onset DBDs (Kaminski & Claussen, 2017; McMahon & Frick, 2019). Yet, too many families have difficulty accessing evidence-based BPT, and those who do too often receive medication management in spite of its significantly more limited effect in this age range relative to therapy (see Comer et al., 2013, 2014, for reviews). This remains the case in spite of BPT's potential to also reduce child internalizing and parent depressive symptoms, thereby affording the potential for an efficacious and cost-effective treatment model (Gonzalez & Jones, 2016). Expanding the reach and impact of BPT programs like HNC, however, depends on therapists experienced in child behavior management offering high-quality training and supervision opportunities. As we have described here, there are many subtleties to effective BPT intervention for child DBDs, which cannot be learned from relying on a treatment manual alone.

REFERENCES

Barkley, R. A. (2013). *Defiant children: A clinician's manual for assessment and parent training* (3rd ed). Guilford Press.

Chacko, A., Jensen, S. A., Lowry, L. S., Cornwell, M., Chimklis, A., Chan, E., Lee, D., & Pulgarin, B. (2016). Engagement in behavioral parent training: Review of the literature and implications for practice. *Clinical Child and Family Psychology Review, 19*(3), 204–215. https://doi.org/10.1007/s10567-016-0205-2

Chorpita, B. F., Daleiden, E. L., Ebesutani, C., Young, J., Becker, K. D., Nakamura, B. J., Phillips, L., Ward, A., Lynch, R., Trent, L., Smith, R. L., Okamura, K., & Starace, N. (2011). Evidence-based treatments for children and adolescents: An updated review of indicators of efficacy and effectiveness. *Clinical Psychology: Science and Practice, 18*(2), 154–172. https://doi.org/10.1111/j.1468-2850.2011.01247.x

Chorpita, B. F., Korathu-Larson, P., Knowles, L. M., & Guan, K. (2014). Emergent life events and their impact on service delivery: Should we expect the unexpected? *Professional Psychology: Research and Practice, 45*(5), 387–393. https://doi.org/10.1037/a0037746

Cohen, M. A., & Piquero, A. R. (2009). New evidence on the monetary value of saving a high-risk youth. *Journal of Quantitative Criminology, 25*(1), 25–49. https://doi.org/10.1007/s10940-008-9057-3

Comer, J. S., Chow, C., Chan, P. T., Cooper-Vince, C., & Wilson, L. A. (2013). Psychosocial treatment efficacy for disruptive behavior problems in very young children: A meta-analytic examination. *Journal of the American Academy of Child & Adolescent Psychiatry, 52*(1), 26–36. https://doi.org/10.1016/j.jaac.2012.10.001

Comer, J. S., Elkins, R. M., Chan, P. T., & Jones, D. J. (2014). New methods of service delivery for children's mental health care. In C. A. Alfano & D. C. Beidel (Eds.), *Comprehensive evidence-based interventions for children and adolescents* (pp. 55–72). John Wiley & Sons.

Cunningham, C. (2013). *The community parent education program: A group-based, family-systems-oriented workshop for parents of children with disruptive behavior disorders.* Taylor & Francis.

Dadds, M. R., & Tully, L. A. (2019). What is it to discipline a child: What should it be? A reanalysis of time-out from the perspective of child mental health, attachment, and trauma. *American Psychologist, 74*(7), 794–808. https://doi.org/10.1037/amp0000449

Deković, M., Slagt, M. I., Asscher, J. J., Boendermaker, L., Eichelsheim, V. I., & Prinzie, P. (2011). Effects of early prevention programs on adult criminal offending: A meta-analysis. *Clinical Psychology Review, 31*(4), 532–544. https://doi.org/10.1016/j.cpr.2010.12.003

Eyberg, S. M., & Funderburk, B. W. (2011). *Parent–child interaction therapy protocol.* PCIT International.

Farahmand, F. K., Grant, K. E., Polo, A. J., Duffy, S. N., & DuBois, D. L. (2011). School-based mental health and behavioral programs for low-income, urban youth: A systematic and meta-analytic review. *Clinical Psychology: Science and Practice, 18*(4), 372–390. https://doi.org/10.1111/j.1468-2850.2011.01265.x

Fergusson, D. M., Horwood, L. J., & Ridder, E. M. (2005). Show me the child at seven: The consequences of conduct problems in childhood for psychosocial functioning in adulthood. *Journal of Child Psychology and Psychiatry, 46*(8), 837–849. https://doi.org/10.1111/j.1469-7610.2004.00387.x

Forehand, R. L., & McMahon, R. J. (1981). *Helping the noncompliant child: A clinician's guide to parent training.* Guilford Press.

Gardner, F., Connell, A., Trentacosta, C. J., Shaw, D. S., Dishion, T. J., & Wilson, M. N. (2009). Moderators of outcome in a brief family-centered intervention for preventing early problem behavior. *Journal of Consulting and Clinical Psychology, 77*(3), 543–553. https://doi.org/10.1037/a0015622

Gonzalez, M. A., & Jones, D. J. (2016). Cascading effects of BPT for child internalizing problems and caregiver depression. *Clinical Psychology Review, 50*, 11–21. https://doi.org/10.1016/j.cpr.2016.09.007

Guan, K., Park, A. L., & Chorpita, B. F. (2019). Emergent life events during youth evidence-based treatment: Impact on future provider adherence and clinical progress. *Journal of Clinical Child & Adolescent Psychology, 48*(Suppl. 1), S202–S214. https://doi.org/10.1080/15374416.2017.1295382

Kaehler, L. A., Jacobs, M., & Jones, D. J. (2016). Distilling common history and practice elements to inform dissemination: Hanf-Model BPT programs as an example. *Clinical Child and Family Psychology Review, 19*(3), 236–258. https://doi.org/10.1007/s10567-016-0210-5

Kaminski, J. W., & Claussen, A. H. (2017). Evidence base update for psychosocial treatments for disruptive behaviors in children. *Journal of Clinical Child and Adolescent Psychology, 46*(4), 477–499. https://doi.org/10.1080/15374416.2017.1310044

Kotchick, B. A., Shaffer, A., Dorsey, S., & Forehand, R. L. (2004). Parenting antisocial children and adolescents. In M. Hoghughi & N. Long (Eds.), *Handbook of parenting: Theory and research for practice* (pp. 256–275). Sage Publications.

Leijten, P., Raaijmakers, M. A., de Castro, B. O., & Matthys, W. (2013). Does socio-economic status matter? A meta-analysis on parent training effectiveness for disruptive child behavior. *Journal of Clinical Child and Adolescent Psychology, 42*(3), 384–392. https://doi.org/10.1080/15374416.2013.769169

Long, N., Edwards, M. C., & Bellando, J. (2017). Parent training interventions. In J. L. Matson (Ed.), *Handbook of childhood psychopathology and developmental disabilities treatments* (pp. 63–86). Springer.

Lundahl, B., Risser, H. J., & Lovejoy, M. C. (2006). A meta-analysis of parent training: Moderators and follow-up effects. *Clinical Psychology Review, 26*(1), 86–104. https://doi.org/10.1016/j.cpr.2005.07.004

McMahon, R. J., & Forehand, R. L. (2003). *Helping the noncompliant child: Family-based treatment for oppositional behavior* (2nd ed.). Guilford Press.

McMahon, R. J., & Frick, P. J. (2019). Conduct and oppositional disorders. In M. J. Prinstein, E. A. Youngstrom, E. J. Mash, & R. A. Barkley (Eds.), *Treatment of disorders in childhood and adolescence* (4th ed., pp. 102–172). Guilford Press.

Merikangas, K. R., He, J. P., Brody, D., Fisher, P. W., Bourdon, K., & Koretz, D. S. (2010). Prevalence and treatment of mental disorders among US children in the 2001–2004 NHANES. *Pediatrics, 125*(1), 75–81. https://doi.org/10.1542/peds.2008-2598

Merikangas, K. R., Nakamura, E. F., & Kessler, R. C. (2009). Epidemiology of mental disorders in children and adolescents. *Dialogues in Clinical Neuroscience, 11*(1), 7–20. https://doi.org/10.31887/DCNS.2009.11.1/krmerikangas

Odgers, C. L., Caspi, A., Broadbent, J. M., Dickson, N., Hancox, R. J., Harrington, H., Poulton, R., Sears, M. R., Thomson, W. M., & Moffitt, T. E. (2007). Prediction of differential adult health burden by conduct problem subtypes in males. *Archives of General Psychiatry, 64*(4), 476–484. https://doi.org/10.1001/archpsyc.64.4.476

Patterson, G. R. (1982). *Coercive family process.* Castalia.

Piquero, A. R., Farrington, D. P., Welsh, B. C., Tremblay, R., & Jennings, W. G. (2009). Effects of early family/parent training programs on antisocial behavior and delinquency. *Journal of Experimental Criminology, 5*(2), 83–120. https://doi.org/10.1007/s11292-009-9072-x

Polanczyk, G. V., Salum, G. A., Sugaya, L. S., Caye, A., & Rohde, L. A. (2015). Annual research review: A meta-analysis of the worldwide prevalence of mental disorders in children and adolescents. *Journal of Child Psychology and Psychiatry, 56*(3), 345–365. https://doi.org/10.1111/jcpp.12381

Quetsch, L. B., Wallace, N. M., Herschell, A. D., & McNeil, C. B. (2015). Weighing in on the time-out controversy: An empirical perspective. *Clinical Psychologist, 68*(2), 4–19. https://incredibleyears.com/wp-content/uploads/Weighing-in-on-Time-Out-Borduin-et-al.pdf

Reitman, D., & McMahon, R. J. (2013). Constance "Connie" Hanf (1917–2002): The mentor and the model. *Cognitive and Behavioral Practice, 20*(1), 106–116. https://doi.org/10.1016/j.cbpra.2012.02.005

Reyno, S. M., & McGrath, P. J. (2006). Predictors of parent training efficacy for child externalizing behavior problems—A meta-analytic review. *Journal of Clinical Child Psychology and Psychiatry, 47*(1), 99–111. https://doi.org/10.1111/j.1469-7610.2005.01544.x

Rothenberg, W. A., Anton, M. T., Gonzalez, M., Lafko Breslend, N., Forehand, R., Khavjou, O., & Jones, D. J. (2020). BPT for early-onset behavior disorders: Examining the link between treatment components and trajectories of child internalizing symptoms. *Behavior Modification, 44*(2), 159–185. https://doi.org/10.1177/0145445518801344

Shaw, D. S., & Taraban, L. E. (2017). New directions and challenges in preventing conduct problems in early childhood. *Child Development Perspectives, 11*(2), 85–89. https://doi.org/10.1111/cdep.12212

Tharp, R. G., & Wetzel, R. J. (1969). *Behavior modification in the natural environment.* Academic Press.

Webster-Stratton, C. (2011). *The Incredible Years parents, teachers, and children's training series: Program content, methods, research and dissemination 1980–2011.* Incredible Years.

II

SPECIAL SETTINGS
AND POPULATIONS

10

Supervising the Delivery of Cognitive Behavioral Therapy in Community Clinics

Alison Salloum and Brian E. Bunnell

Supervision is critical for the effective implementation of cognitive behavioral therapy (CBT) and evidence-based practices (EBPs) in community clinics. Multicomponent training approaches (e.g., manuals, workshops, consultation, live or recorded observation, supervisor trainings, booster trainings, supervised completion of cases) and workshops with active follow-up (e.g., observation, feedback, consultation, coaching) are effective in helping community clinicians increase skills and competence. Training must be accompanied by a trained supervisor who provides feedback on the implementation of the treatment with real clients in community settings (Herschell et al., 2010). While there are numerous CBT techniques to use with clients in community settings, this chapter prioritizes three main factors related to the supervision of delivery of CBT in community settings in order to assist supervisors in providing supervision during implementation of these CBT components. These factors are (a) assessment (e.g., case conceptualization), (b) a specific CBT technique (e.g., exposure; see also Chapter 1, this volume, for more information about exposure therapy), and (c) the CBT process (e.g., structure-related skills).

While supervision in community settings may involve group and individual supervision and may include informal and/or "in real time" supervision, designated time for clinical supervision must be protected. In a study with 56 supervisors and 207 clinicians from 25 community mental health clinics, Dorsey et al. (2017) found that approximately 20% of supervision time was spent on nonclinical issues, and about 20% of clinicians indicated that they

https://doi.org/10.1037/0000314-011

Training and Supervision in Specialized Cognitive Behavior Therapy: Methods, Settings, and Populations, E. A. Storch, J. S. Abramowitz, and D. McKay (Editors)

received supervision every other week or less frequently. The authors suggested that agencies consider nonclinical supervisors to address administrative issues as well as EBP peer support groups to provide additional support. Supervisors and clinicians need to discuss clinician needs and prioritize these functions during the supervision of CBT. For example, Dorsey et al. (2017) found that both supervisors and clinicians rated case conceptualization/formulation and therapy intervention/approaches as their top choice for more time in supervision. Supervisors were more likely to rate more time to focus on issues of therapeutic alliance; clinicians were more likely to rate wanting more time to focus on crisis and case management issues. In terms of nonclinical functions, approximately one third of both supervisors and clinicians rated needing more time allocated in supervision for the supervisory relationship and process. Findings support the need for community supervisors and clinicians to clarify and prioritize the functions of supervision such that key concepts and techniques in the delivery of CBT can be addressed. These findings also support the chapter authors' experiences, where we found case conceptualization, exposure, and structure-related skills (e.g., managing crises and time, staying CBT-focused) to be major challenges associated with supervision. These three topics serve as the basis for the rest of this chapter.

KEY CONCEPTS AND TECHNIQUES FOR TRAINEES TO LEARN

This section focuses on key concepts and techniques for supervisors working with trainees on case conceptualization, exposure, and structure-related skills. Case conceptualization provides an important time for supervisors to work with trainees to use theory to develop a comprehensive understanding of clients' presenting problems and strengths, and to provide trainees with practical assessment methods to guide and monitor treatment. Similarly, supervisors can use theory to help trainees consider multiple strategies to establish exposures. When teaching how to implement structure-related skills, supervisors can model many of these skills during supervisory meetings.

Case Conceptualization

Clients presenting for treatment at community clinics often have co-occurring psychological conditions as well as environmental stressors and challenges (e.g., financial strain, limited transportation, housing conditions/instability). Thus, assessment and case conceptualization are critical to planning and tailoring CBT. CBT case conceptualization can provide a comprehensive understanding of both etiology and maintenance of the client's problems within a theoretical framework that explains the client's psychopathology and elucidates clients' strengths, which helps prioritize treatment strategies (Easden & Kazantzis, 2018). It is a collaborative process between the clinician and client, as well as between the clinician and supervisor. During the case conceptualization process, supervisors can help clinicians (a) select assessment tools to identify symptom severity and monitor treatment progress, (b) understand clients' top concerns and track progress on improving these issues, (c) elicit clients' strengths and understanding of the influence of culture, and (d) better understand clients' maladaptive or unhelpful thoughts.

Exposure Therapy

Exposure therapy is a key technique for community clinicians to learn as it is a key component of many CBT protocols for anxiety and fear-based problems, which are common in such settings. Community clinicians may have negative beliefs about exposure therapy, such as that clients will have difficulty tolerating exposure, that those with comorbid and complex issues will not benefit, and that exposure is associated with high rates of dropout (Deacon et al., 2013). In addition to these beliefs, clinicians' own anxiety about implementing exposure may result in suboptimal use of exposure or avoidance of the technique altogether (Meyer et al., 2014). Effective training in exposure therapy can help to lessen clinicians' negative beliefs and anxiety, and help facilitate its appropriate use (Deacon et al., 2013; Reid et al., 2018). Many community therapists are open to using exposure-based CBT; however, ongoing supervision and organizational support (e.g., assessment of cases that could benefit from exposure-based CBT, incentives for improved patient outcomes, "champions" who value the treatment or who are skilled in exposure-based treatment, training and ongoing supervision) are needed to help community clinicians become comfortable and skilled in its implementation (Wolitzky-Taylor et al., 2018).

Teaching and reinforcing the theories and research that guide exposure-based treatment, such as emotional processing theory and inhibitory learning theory, are also important to helping clinicians learn how and when to implement exposures (Abramowitz, 2013). Although more research is needed on the mechanisms of exposure therapy and how to optimize its use, consideration of these models can help supervisors and clinicians consider different strategies and approaches to exposures. Inhibitory learning theory, for example, posits that the relationship between a conditioned stimulus and unconditioned stimulus does not dissipate, but that new learning, associations, and meaning can occur within different contexts and over time through exposures (Craske et al., 2008). Craske et al. (2014) discussed eight approaches to consider for optimizing exposures that supervisors can help their supervisees practice.

1. *Expectancy violation:* Design the exposure as a behavioral test where what the client expects to happen does not occur. This strategy entails having the client articulate what they are worried about or expect will happen when engaging in the feared/avoidant situation, so that they learn that this association does not always occur and that they can have a different experience.

2. *Deepened extinction:* Engage the client in isolated exposures to separate stimuli that elicit a similar fear response. Then combine those cues in the same exposure.

3. *Occasional reinforced extinction:* In some cases, allow the expected negative outcome to occur (e.g., social rejection), or the expectancy of the negative outcome to not be articulated at the beginning of the exposure and a negative (safe) outcome to occur, enabling an inhibitory learning approach to "extend beyond behavioral testing" (Craske et al., 2014, p.13).

4. *Removal of safety signals:* Remove "safety behaviors" and "safety signals," although preventing the use of safety behaviors/signals may need to be gradual.

5. *Variability:* After the client has completed an "easy," or low anxiety-producing exposure, consider varying the stimuli (e.g., duration and levels of intensity, order in the hierarchy) to enhance new learning and associations.

6. *Retrieval cues:* Work with the client to develop cues that remind the client what they have learned when faced with the fear stimuli in the future. However, it is recommended that these cues not be used in the beginning of the therapy and may better serve as relapse prevention strategies.

7. *Multiple contexts:* Work with the client to complete exposures in multiple settings and/or times to decrease the likelihood that the fear will be renewed when the stimulus is encountered in a new context.

8. *Reconsolidation:* Exposure to the fear stimuli during the memory reconsolidation time frame may weaken and/or change the memory; although how to incorporate this into practice is not clear at this time as additional research is needed (Craske et al., 2014; Lee et al., 2017).

While this brief presentation of these eight strategies does not include the theory and research that support each strategy, it illustrates ways in which theory and research can be used during supervision to encourage and guide the implementation of exposures.

Structure-Related Skills

While there are numerous CBT strategies that clinicians may use, the within-session structure is important for its delivery. Recently, these "structure-related skills" (e.g., setting an agenda, assigning homework, eliciting feedback from clients, pacing the session) have been shown to be therapist-level treatment fidelity factors for CBT competence (Goldberg et al., 2020). In community settings where there is often a fast-paced work environment with back-to-back therapy sessions, these skills help the clinician and the client stay focused within the session on addressing the treatment plan (e.g., top problems). However, implementing structure-related skills in a collaborative manner takes practice and skill. In a dissemination study with community mental health clinicians learning CBT, 71.4% to 90.5% of clinicians had difficulties with structure-related skills. Promisingly, these skills improved with training, especially agenda setting and pacing (Waltman et al., 2017). As clinicians improve in these areas, clients will also learn the structure of CBT sessions, which will help them to know what to expect and how to better utilize the time. Supervisors can structure the supervision meeting in a way that allows modeling for clinicians on how to implement these structure-related skills.

IDENTIFYING APPROPRIATE TRAINING CASES

This section considers case conceptualization, exposure therapy, and structure-related skills for supervisors when identifying training cases. Given that community clinics often provide services to people with complex presenting problems, even cases that meet some of the suggestions for training cases can be quite complex. Thus, trainees may experience difficulties with implementation of CBT and may need ongoing support from supervisors to help navigate challenges and integrate lessons learned.

Case Conceptualization

While some community clinics offer specialized therapy for specific conditions, many community-based mental health agencies provide an array of services, often requiring clinicians to provide treatment for numerous conditions. Thus, when training and supervising community clinicians on the process of case conceptualization, it is often helpful to start with cases where the clinician has a general understanding of the research and theory related to the client's primary condition(s) or problem(s). It is also helpful to identify clients with strong motivation to change, who are able to engage collaboratively with the clinician in conceptualizing and prioritizing problems, and who are willing to engage in selected treatment strategies. Finally, we recommend using a framework that incorporates understanding the client's thoughts, emotions, and behaviors, and a dynamic, collaborative approach that includes understanding the role of culture in the client's experiences, as well as identifying the client's strengths (Kuyken et al., 2016). As the field moves toward tailored and transdiagnostic treatments, case conceptualization that integrates core mechanisms to be targeted in treatment and understanding of clients' experiences and strengths will be critical to initial treatment planning and ongoing decision making.

Exposure Therapy

Similar to clinicians needing confidence in exposure-based treatment (Reid et al., 2018), it is helpful to identify training cases where the client has confidence in the approach. Thus, if a client has had exposure-based therapy before and did not respond to treatment, the case might not be suitable for initial training in CBT for community clinicians, as the client may doubt the technique and have questions about the clinician. It also may be helpful for initial training cases to be clients who are not severely dysregulated, so that both the clinician and client have capacities to tolerate the distress of the exposure work. Similarly, cases where there are safety concerns (e.g., suicidal ideation, nonsuicidal self-harm) may also be excluded as initial training cases. It is not always possible to select initial training cases for learning and practicing exposure-based therapy; thus, training, ongoing supervision, and practice can help clinicians gain competence and confidence.

Structure-Related Skills

It can be difficult to select a good training case for community clinicians to practice implementing structure-related skills. However, the clinician may assess at intake or during the initial assessment session if the client is able to stay focused on answering the questions or if the client veers off on tangents. It may be easier for community clinicians to practice implementing structure-related skills with clients who remain on task during the assessment phase, although in fairness to clients, they have often not been educated about the structure within CBT sessions during the assessment. Thus, having a combination of clients who stay on task and those who often veer to other topics or tasks allows the clinician to practice. Clients who indicate that they want to do therapy homework, feel confident that they will complete homework, and find homework helpful typically serve as good initial training cases (Cooper et al., 2017; Hayasaka et al., 2015).

COMMON MISTAKES AND HOW TO CORRECT THEM

This section includes practical strategies to address common challenges that occur during case conceptualization (e.g., use of assessment measures, linking case conceptualization to CBT protocols or CBT strategies, inclusion of strengths of the clients, primary concerns, the role of culture and beliefs, and maladaptive thoughts), exposure therapy, and structure-related skills (e.g., implementing an agenda and time management).

Case Conceptualization

Accredited clinics often have to demonstrate that assessment measures and post assessments are completed, but "completed" does not necessarily mean "utilized." The use of technology can assist with having clients rapidly complete assessments and scoring for interpretation, discussion with clients, and guidance of treatment. However, some clinicians may worry that having clients complete assessment measures may inhibit therapeutic alliance and contribute to stigmatization. Clinicians need to be trained to introduce the assessment in a way that provides psychoeducation to the client and can be used to validate their experience, which in turn can help build alliance. For example, the clinician may say,

> We will have a lot of time to talk today, so that I can better understand what you are experiencing, which will help us develop a good plan together to help you.

> We ask all of our clients to complete these assessments that include a wide range of experiences. You might not experience them all and there may be other experiences that are not on these assessments that we will talk about later. We know to ask these kinds of questions because many people have experienced similar problems.

If the client is a child or if there are reading level concerns, the clinician might say, "Completing the assessments may take about 20 minutes. If you would like, I can work with you to complete them, or you can complete them by yourself." When youth are involved, it is helpful and time-efficient to have the caregiver complete the assessments while clinicians are talking with the youth and vice versa. If clinics ask clients to come early to complete the assessments, it is important that the client knows why they are being asked to complete the assessments and how the information will be used.

Diagnoses help clinicians in planning treatment, although some clinicians may not match the principal problem to the best EBP. If there is a primary diagnosis, clinicians may want to consider EBPs for a single diagnosis, although many of EBPs have demonstrated improvements in secondary problems. For example, a youth who has experienced a trauma and has a diagnosis of PTSD will likely also experience improvement in internalizing and externalizing problems when receiving trauma-focused CBT (e.g., Jensen et al., 2014; Webb et al., 2014). Training in EBPs takes time and resources, which often presents challenges within community settings. Therefore, agency supervisors may consider being trained and go on to provide training within the agency on common CBT techniques (e.g., exposure therapy, cognitive therapy, mindfulness, applied behavior analysis, behavioral activation, behavior management; see also Chapters 1–9, this volume, for more information about these and other CBT techniques). It is also prudent to have supervisors and managers conduct an analysis of the most common principal diagnoses for adults and youth, and then receive training in a specific CBT EBP for these conditions. Having all community clinicians trained in a CBT EBP for the most prevalent diagnosis would also allow clinicians to practice the CBT techniques and provide context for collaborative learning, group supervision, and peer support. As the field advances, community clinics may consider training in transdiagnostic treatments, which can be effective in the simultaneous treatment of multiple types of disorders (e.g., depression and anxiety; González-Robles et al., 2018).

Some clinicians may stop assessment once a *DSM* diagnosis has been established, which limits case conceptualization. Thus, supervisors should work with clinicians to gather information, such as the unique strengths of the client, the top concerns of the client that impact their everyday life, and how the client's culture and beliefs manifest in how the client experiences the problem, as well as how these beliefs may hinder or promote healing and maladaptive thoughts. A functional analysis of the problem using cognitive and behavioral principles to understand the relationship between situational factors, cognitive factors (beliefs and assumptions), and emotional or behavioral responses is also critical. Whether the community setting uses an electronic record system or hard copy files, having these factors incorporated within the assessment structure will help to ensure that all of these factors are systematically assessed, which will help the supervisor, clinician, and client better conceptualize the client's experiences and treatment plan. The assessment for case conceptualization and assessment tools will need to take into account the developmental stage of the client. Each setting will need to decide the best approach for guiding the assessment of these factors and including supervisors and clinicians in decision-making about what is included as part of assessment may help with implementation.

The following information provides some ideas to consider when assisting a clinician with assessment and case conceptualization. In terms of assessing strengths, a list of specific assessment tools that assess different domains such as self-efficacy, social support and relationships, resilience, coping, acceptance, and so forth can be found in the book *Tools for Strengths-Based Assessment and Evaluation* (Simmons & Lehmann, 2012). Alternatively, including structured questions that elicit further conversation and can inform treatment may be helpful, such as, "How have you coped thus far with [name the problem using the client's words], and what would you consider some of your strengths or anything about you that can help you during therapy (e.g., support from others, mindfulness practices, and cognitive strategies)?" Community clinics may also consider a systematic approach to elicit from clients what they see as the top concerns/problems to be addressed in therapy. For youth and their caregivers, the Top Problems measure may be used (Weisz et al., 2011).

Most training programs include information on cultural competency or, more recently, on cultural humility (Greene-Moton & Minkler, 2020), but this needs to be intentionally translated into practice in community settings and with clients. Community clinics often serve diverse populations, including those who have been marginalized and experienced discrimination. Thus, a collaborative case conceptualization approach is needed that allows the clinician time to listen to and validate the client's experience. Supervisors and clinicians should incorporate time in supervision to discuss cultural differences and similarities between the clinician and client, and how community practices may better meet the needs of underserved populations. There are also resources related to cultural adaptation of CBT that can be used for clinical training and to guide dialogue in supervision (Hinton & Patel, 2017; Iwamasa & Hays, 2019).

Clinicians may have difficulty identifying maladaptive or unhelpful cognitions with their clients. Sometimes, understanding the client's main problems may help the clinician to assess for common maladaptive thoughts related to the condition. For example, for clients who are seeking therapy due to trauma, inventories assessing maladaptive beliefs following trauma may be helpful, such as the Posttraumatic Maladaptive Belief Scale (Vogt et al., 2012) for adults or the Children's Post-traumatic Cognitions Inventory (McKinnon et al., 2016). Having standardized handouts for all community clinicians that have graphics explaining automatic thoughts, the "cognitive triangle" of how thoughts, feelings, and behaviors are related, as well as a list of common cognitive distortions can help the clinician and client begin to identify unhelpful cognitions.

Supervisors can use the client's worksheets identifying cognitions and the case conceptualization information to help develop broader cognitive themes that may be maintaining the client's problems.

Exposure Therapy

Challenges related to implementing exposures include the clinician's reluctance to implement or engineer exposures that would elicit high client distress, and uncertainties about what exposures to suggest to the client. Assuming the clinician has received adequate training in how to implement exposure therapy, supervisors can try several strategies to help. First, an open discussion about the clinician's beliefs and fears about exposures needs to occur. To help facilitate discussions regarding reservations about exposure, the supervisor may ask the clinician to complete the Therapist Beliefs About Exposure Scale (Deacon et al., 2013), which assesses a number of common cognitions known to be associated with the improper use (or avoidance) of this technique. Second, having clinicians watch or listen to recordings of other therapists working with clients to set up exposures, or shadow the supervisor during exposure sessions, can help demystify the process.

Once the clinician shows buy-in to using exposure properly, it can be helpful to use a handout with the client that explains the rationale for exposures. This approach helps the clinician more clearly explain the purpose and helps with buy-in from the client. Fourth, if supervision is occurring in groups, the supervisor might have all clinicians develop a tentative exposure plan so that they have the opportunity to think through how they might establish exposures with clients from the clinic. Supervisors can set up a shared file with examples of community clients' exposure plans for different conditions so that clinicians develop in-house resources of ideas. Finally, having steps for the clinician to think through before a session where exposures are set up can help them feel more prepared.

Supervisors might use the following steps to help clinicians think through setting up exposures:

1. Create a list from the information collected as part of the assessment of all information endorsed as avoided, feared, or potential fear cues.

2. Create a list from the assessment of impairment that is occurring as a result of avoidance and fear, and what level of motivation the clinician thinks the client has to change.

3. Consider additional information gained during sessions that may apply to Steps 1 and 2.

4. Think about two potential exposures based on Steps 1 through 3 and articulate what the clinician thinks the client fears or worries would happen if the exposure occurred. Have the clinician articulate how the client's expectation would be violated or what new meaning is to be gained.

5. Work with the client to complete a fear hierarchy and, with client input, establish the first exposure—often an easy exposure that allows the client to practice.

6. In supervision, review the inhibitory learning strategies discussed previously and how these methods might apply to the information gathered thus far (e.g., what does the client need to learn through exposure practices?). Also, discuss what the clinician thinks would be the most distressing exposure for the client, or what steps are needed to address impairment. It is often helpful to map out potential exposures.

7. Suggest the clinician continue to work with the client to set up exposures and seek supervision as needed.

Structure-Related Skills

Whether the clinician is following a specific CBT protocol or implementing common CBT strategies to address the client's problems, straying from the agenda and running out of time in the session are often challenges. Clients who have numerous stressors (e.g., financial concerns, relationship problems, and parenting challenges) may want time to vent and share with the clinician their most recent stressor, which often results in clinicians providing supportive counseling. While this may be helpful, without targeted treatment for the mental health problems, the target symptoms will often persist. Thus, the client is left to deal with the stressor with the weight of the symptoms. In such situations, supervisors can help clinicians to learn how to set collaborative agendas that allow for check-ins but also segue into CBT strategies, or save time at the end of the session for the client to discuss these types of stressors.

The supervisor may also help the clinician consider whether the client is bringing the aforementioned stressors to the forefront due to the immediate needs that should be addressed first, or whether this is serving as a way to avoid talking about more difficult mental health issues. If the client agrees to have the session recorded for the supervisor and clinicians to review together, supervision may entail role-playing after recorded segments how the clinician could listen to and validate the experience *and* address the CBT agenda or use CBT strategies to address what the client is experiencing. It can also be helpful for the clinician and client to sketch out how much time they will spend on each topic, so that both can manage the time together, and have the agenda displayed where both the clinician and client can see it during the session. Lastly, of course if the stressor leads to crisis, helping the client with the crisis may take precedence over the agenda. Supervisors can help clinicians learn about community resources that may help clients with stressors and when to engage in or get another professional involved to offer case management and/or advocacy.

ETHICAL ISSUES

Given the diversity of clients receiving community mental health services and the wide range of presenting problems, competence may present as an ethical issue for new clinicians who lack the experience and training needed to help specific clients. Competence may also be an issue for seasoned clinicians who have not kept up with advances in CBT. Thus, it is imperative that supervisors meet consistently with clinicians and have candid discussions about the clinician's competence in providing CBT. Supervisors also need to take inventory of their own competence to provide effective supervision conditions where they may have less training and experience. Supervisors can work to get training and consultation for both the supervisor and clinician to increase competence. Competence goes beyond skills in CBT and understanding of different diagnoses and conditions, and must include how one's (e.g., clinician, supervisor, and client) culture and experiences, including racism and discrimination, influence the assessment and treatment process. Supervisors play a unique role within community agencies, as they not only help clinicians care for clients but also help the clinic to be more responsive to clinicians, clients, and the community it serves.

OBSTACLES IN SUPERVISION

Setting-specific issues related to sustaining EBPs in community-based clinics affect supervisors' and clinicians' delivery of CBT. Financial support, leadership, prioritizing implementation, providing reinforcement, integrating workflow issues, workforce challenges, and client compatibility with the EBP have all been documented as factors that affect sustainability of EBPs. Supervisors play an important role in sustaining EBPs in community settings by training new clinicians, providing ongoing and advanced training for experienced clinicians, conducting weekly supervision, monitoring treatment fidelity and outcomes, and seeking expert consultation when needed (Bond et al., 2014). However, if the clinic culture does not value EBPs, both the supervisor and clinician may not be recognized by leadership for their good clinical care and may be penalized for taking time for consistent weekly supervision, reading additional materials, and focusing on fidelity and outcomes, rather than the primary focus of billable hours. Research suggests that the implementation climate, the degree to which the organization values, supports, and rewards EBP implementation, is a key predictor for both supervisors providing key CBT strategies to clinicians (Dorsey et al., 2017; Lucid et al., 2018) and community clinicians implementing CBT techniques (Beidas et al., 2015). Thus, supervisors must be cognizant of these challenges and barriers, and work with leadership and clinicians to improve the implementation culture and provide a sustainable supportive environment for supervision of CBT.

CONCLUSION

This chapter provides suggestions and strategies for those supervising clinicians in community settings. We have focused on matters of case conceptualization, conducting exposure-based therapy, and structure-related skills. In the context of busy clinic days, often with clients with high acuity and complex problems, structuring clinic processes and offering specific strategies to strengthen CBT approaches are helpful to clinicians. This is especially true when they occur within a supportive, respectful, and strong supervisor–clinician relationship. Supervisors are in a pivotal role to provide clinicians supervision on delivering CBT in community clinics and to help administrators and others foster a climate that values effective treatment and recognizes the need for CBT supervision and training. Thus, supervisors also need colleagues that they can go to for consultation, supervision, support, and ongoing training in CBT, especially since they often play the dual role of helping clinicians and administrators.

REFERENCES

Abramowitz, J. S. (2013). The practice of exposure therapy: Relevance of cognitive-behavioral theory and extinction theory. *Behavior Therapy, 44*(4), 548–558. https://doi.org/10.1016/j.beth.2013.03.003

Beidas, R. S., Marcus, S., Aarons, G. A., Hoagwood, K. E., Schoenwald, S., Evans, A. C., Hurford, M. O., Hadley, T., Barg, F. K., Walsh, L. M., Adams, D. R., & Mandell, D. S. (2015). Predictors of community therapists' use of therapy techniques in a large public mental health system. *JAMA Pediatrics, 169*(4), 374–382. https://doi.org/10.1001/jamapediatrics.2014.3736

Bond, G. R., Drake, R. E., McHugo, G. J., Peterson, A. E., Jones, A. M., & Williams, J. (2014). Long-term sustainability of evidence-based practices in community mental health agencies. *Administration and Policy in Mental Health, 41*(2), 228–236. https://doi.org/10.1007/s10488-012-0461-5

Cooper, A. A., Kline, A. C., Graham, B., Bedard-Gilligan, M., Mello, P. G., Feeny, N. C., & Zoellner, L. A. (2017). Homework "dose," type, and helpfulness as predictors of clinical outcomes in prolonged exposure for PTSD. *Behavior Therapy, 48*(2), 182–194. https://doi.org/10.1016/j.beth.2016.02.013

Craske, M. G., Kircanski, K., Zelikowsky, M., Mystkowski, J., Chowdhury, N., & Baker, A. (2008). Optimizing inhibitory learning during exposure therapy. *Behaviour Research and Therapy, 46*(1), 5–27. https://doi.org/10.1016/j.brat.2007.10.003

Craske, M. G., Treanor, M., Conway, C. C., Zbozinek, T., & Vervliet, B. (2014). Maximizing exposure therapy: An inhibitory learning approach. *Behaviour Research and Therapy, 58*, 10–23. https://doi.org/10.1016/j.brat.2014.04.006

Deacon, B. J., Farrell, N. R., Kemp, J. J., Dixon, L. J., Sy, J. T., Zhang, A. R., & McGrath, P. B. (2013). Assessing therapist reservations About exposure therapy for anxiety disorders: The Therapist Beliefs About Exposure Scale. *Journal of Anxiety Disorders, 27*(8), 772–780. https://doi.org/10.1016/j.janxdis.2013.04.006

Dorsey, S., Pullmann, M. D., Kerns, S. E. U., Jungbluth, N., Meza, R., Thompson, K., & Berliner, L. (2017). The juggling act of supervision in community mental health: Implications for supporting evidence-based treatment. *Administration and Policy in Mental Health, 44*(6), 838–852. https://doi.org/10.1007/s10488-017-0796-z

Easden, M. H., & Kazantzis, N. (2018). Case conceptualization research in cognitive behavior therapy: A state of the science review. *Journal of Clinical Psychology, 74*(3), 356–384. https://doi.org/10.1002/jclp.22516

Goldberg, S. B., Baldwin, S. A., Merced, K., Caperton, D. D., Imel, Z. E., Atkins, D. C., & Creed, T. (2020). The structure of competence: Evaluating the factor structure of the cognitive therapy rating scale. *Behavior Therapy, 51*(1), 113–122. https://doi.org/10.1016/j.beth.2019.05.008

González-Robles, A., Díaz-García, A., Miguel, C., García-Palacios, A., & Botella, C. (2018). Comorbidity and diagnosis distribution in transdiagnostic treatments for emotional disorders: A systematic review of randomized controlled trials. *PLOS ONE, 13*(11), e0207396. https://doi.org/10.1371/journal.pone.0207396

Greene-Moton, E., & Minkler, M. (2020). Cultural competence or cultural humility? Moving beyond the debate. *Health Promotion Practice, 21*(1), 142–145. https://doi.org/10.1177/1524839919884912

Hayasaka, Y., Furukawa, T. A., Sozu, T., Imai, H., Kawakami, N., Horikoshi, M., on behalf of the GENKI Project. (2015). Enthusiasm for homework and improvement of psychological distress in subthreshold depression during behavior therapy: Secondary analysis of data from a randomized controlled trial. *BMC Psychiatry, 15*(1), 302. https://doi.org/10.1186/s12888-015-0687-3

Herschell, A. D., Kolko, D. J., Baumann, B. L., & Davis, A. C. (2010). The role of therapist training in the implementation of psychosocial treatments: A review and critique with recommendations. *Clinical Psychology Review, 30*(4), 448–466. https://doi.org/10.1016/j.cpr.2010.02.005

Hinton, D. E., & Patel, A. (2017). Cultural adaptations of cognitive behavioral therapy. *Psychiatric Clinics of North America, 40*(4), 701–714. https://doi.org/10.1016/j.psc.2017.08.006

Iwamasa, G. Y., & Hays, P. A. (Eds.). (2019). *Culturally responsive cognitive behavior therapy: Practice and supervision* (2nd ed.). American Psychological Association. https://doi.org/10.1037/0000119-000

Jensen, T. K., Holt, T., Ormhaug, S. M., Egeland, K., Granly, L., Hoaas, L. C., Hukkelberg, S. S., Indregard, T., Stormyren, S. D., & Wentzel-Larsen, T. (2014). A randomized effectiveness study comparing trauma-focused cognitive behavioral therapy with therapy as usual for youth. *Journal of Clinical Child and Adolescent Psychology, 43*(3), 356–369. https://doi.org/10.1080/15374416.2013.822307

Kuyken, W., Beshai, S., Dudley, R., Abel, A., Görg, N., Gower, P., McManus, F., & Padesky, C. A. (2016). Assessing competence in collaborative case conceptualization: Development and preliminary psychometric properties of the Collaborative Case Conceptualization Rating Scale (CCC-RS). *Behavioural and Cognitive Psychotherapy, 44*(2), 179–192. https://doi.org/10.1017/S1352465814000691

Lee, J. L. C., Nader, K., & Schiller, D. (2017). An update on memory reconsolidation updating. *Trends in Cognitive Sciences, 21*(7), 531–545. https://doi.org/10.1016/j.tics.2017.04.006

Lucid, L., Meza, R., Pullmann, M. D., Jungbluth, N., Deblinger, E., & Dorsey, S. (2018). Supervision in community mental health: Understanding intensity of EBT focus. *Behavior Therapy, 49*(4), 481–493. https://doi.org/10.1016/j.beth.2017.12.007

McKinnon, A., Smith, P., Bryant, R., Salmon, K., Yule, W., Dalgleish, T., Dixon, C., Nixon, R. D., & Meiser-Stedman, R. (2016). An update on the clinical utility of the Children's Post-Traumatic Cognitions Inventory. *Journal of Traumatic Stress, 29*(3), 253–258. https://doi.org/10.1002/jts.22096

Meyer, J. M., Farrell, N. R., Kemp, J. J., Blakey, S. M., & Deacon, B. J. (2014). Why do clinicians exclude anxious clients from exposure therapy? *Behaviour Research and Therapy, 54*, 49–53. https://doi.org/10.1016/j.brat.2014.01.004

Reid, A. M., Guzick, A. G., Fernandez, A. G., Deacon, B., McNamara, J. P. H., Geffken, G. R., McCarty, R., & Striley, C. W. (2018). Exposure therapy for youth with anxiety: Utilization rates and predictors of implementation in a sample of practicing clinicians from across the United States. *Journal of Anxiety Disorders, 58*, 8–17. https://doi.org/10.1016/j.janxdis.2018.06.002

Simmons, C. A., & Lehmann, P. (2012). *Tools for strengths-based assessment and evaluation.* Springer Publishing.

Vogt, D. S., Shipherd, J. C., & Resick, P. A. (2012). Posttraumatic maladaptive beliefs scale: Evolution of the personal beliefs and reactions scale. *Assessment, 19*(3), 308–317. https://doi.org/10.1177/1073191110376161

Waltman, S., Hall, B. C., McFarr, L. M., Beck, A. T., & Creed, T. A. (2017). In-session stuck points and pitfalls of community clinicians learning CBT: Qualitative investigation. *Cognitive and Behavioral Practice, 24*(2), 256–267. https://doi.org/10.1016/j.cbpra.2016.04.002

Webb, C., Hayes, A., Grasso, D., Laurenceau, J. P., & Deblinger, E. (2014). Trauma-focused cognitive behavioral therapy for youth: Effectiveness in a community setting. *Psychological Trauma: Theory, Research, Practice, and Policy, 6*(5), 555–562. https://doi.org/10.1037/a0037364

Weisz, J. R., Chorpita, B. F., Frye, A., Ng, M. Y., Lau, N., Bearman, S. K., Ugueto, A. M., Langer, D. A., Hoagwood, K. E., & the Research Network on Youth Mental Health. (2011). Youth top problems: Using idiographic, consumer-guided assessment to identify treatment needs and to track change during psychotherapy. *Journal of Consulting and Clinical Psychology, 79*(3), 369–380. https://doi.org/10.1037/a0023307

Wolitzky-Taylor, K., Fenwick, K., Lengnick-Hall, R., Grossman, J., Bearman, S. K., Arch, J., Miranda, J., & Chung, B. (2018). A preliminary exploration of the barriers to delivering (and receiving) exposure-based cognitive behavioral therapy for anxiety disorders in adult community mental health settings. *Community Mental Health Journal, 54*(7), 899–911. https://doi.org/10.1007/s10597-018-0252-x

11

Supervising the Delivery of Cognitive Behavioral Therapy in College Counseling Centers

Michael Rogers and Jonathan Mitchell

The use of cognitive behavioral therapy (CBT) in college counseling centers is widespread, as it is well-aligned with the core features of higher education, leveraging emerging technology, novel methods of communication, and innovative models of care to serve a diverse and ever-changing student population. The varied approaches within a cognitive behavioral frame empower students to actively develop new, more adaptive perspectives and reactions toward themselves and their world. For both traditional (e.g., enrolled in a 4-year, campus-based undergraduate program) and nontraditional (e.g., enrolled in a 2-year or nonresidential program, older-than-typical, or part time) college students, such a pursuit is central to the purpose of higher education. Furthermore, as counseling centers have seen demand increase over the last 5 decades (Cornish et al., 2017; Hodges, 2001), CBT offers brief, concrete, and generalizable interventions that permit these centers to meet that need.

Contemporary clinical models in college counseling are diverse (Brunner et al., 2014; Mitchell et al., 2019); nonetheless, trends exist in the field that align well with CBT. First, short-term or brief models are common (Brunner et al., 2017; Robinson et al., 2020; Shefet, 2018). Empirical and anecdotal evidence suggest that brief treatment (i.e., 10 session or fewer) may be most effective in yielding clinically significant change across a number of presenting concerns (Boswell et al., 2020). CBT may be especially effective in this setting because the pace of the semester schedule lends itself to brief and/or episodic courses of treatment. Second, concrete skill development and solution-building

https://doi.org/10.1037/0000314-012
Training and Supervision in Specialized Cognitive Behavior Therapy: Methods, Settings, and Populations, E. A. Storch, J. S. Abramowitz, and D. McKay (Editors)

tend to characterize first-line interventions for issues related to adjustment, life transition, or somatic complaints and sociocultural stressors (Arch & Craske, 2009; Brunner et al., 2014; McNealy & Lombardero, 2019). Setting realistic goals and working to resolve these acute issues supports both healthy emotional development and academic success. Finally, CBT's numerous empirically supported techniques allow for relatively straightforward dismantling and application of these techniques to specific concerns in a short period of time. Students frequently seek convenient and easily understood strategies for resolving their concerns in the present and in the future. Indeed, the blending of education and intervention in CBT is a particularly compelling concept for college counseling.

KEY CONCEPTS FOR TRAINEES TO UNDERSTAND

Cognitive behavioral approaches help clients to view cognition and behavior as functionally related to the experience of emotion and the environmental context in which thoughts and behaviors occur. An important premise for trainees to impart is that while initial cognitive behavioral responses to environmental demands may be adaptive, their function can become maladaptive over time, leading to the emergence of discrete psychological syndromes. Trainees can teach clients to notice these patterns, identify the reasons they occur (e.g., attentional biases and/or maladaptive core belief systems; Hazlett-Stevens & Craske, 2002), and replace them with viable alternatives. For example, a history of having been bullied in middle school and/or high school may lead an incoming college freshman to develop a core belief that others are dangerous and to be avoided when possible. Avoiding others due to the fear of being hurt could cause the student to miss out on study partners, social connections, internship opportunities, and reduce help-seeking behavior from professors, teaching assistants, and student affairs programs. Assisting your trainee in skillfully applying CBT to challenge this belief and its accompanying behaviors can help change the course of the student's academic performance, college experience, and future career options.

Cognitive Restructuring

Maladaptive cognitive patterns (i.e., cognitive errors) often involve the over- or underextension of expectations or beliefs, typically about the self, the world, or the future. The trainee's primary goal in cognitive restructuring is to help the client explore their thought patterns and to generate initial hypotheses about how unhelpful patterns may be at work in the client's presenting concerns (King et al., 2020). Since college students may be especially prone to cognitive errors in a variety of academic, social, and career preparation settings (Lapsley & Woodbury, 2015), it is important to introduce this concept early in treatment.

Clients often present to counseling centers with the intent to resolve a discrete issue or acute conflict (e.g., social anxiety in residence halls), offering trainees a chance to focus on a clear target for intervention. Trainees help the client identify cognitive contributions to that specific presenting concern and explore the connection to their emotions and behavior. More adaptive beliefs can be considered and adopted once the evidence for the differing beliefs is examined and selectively reinforced. Once this premise is established, trainees and clients may collaboratively question whether similar patterns exist in other domains, thereby extending the impact of the cognitive restructuring in other related areas of life.

Behavior Therapy

There are predictable relationships between a given behavior, the context that often precedes it, and the consequences that typically follow (Drossel et al., 2009). CBT leans heavily on defining and modifying these operant contingencies, particularly ones that are associated with or perpetuate the core features of a disorder. The primary focus of behavioral interventions in CBT involves the differential reinforcement (i.e., extinction and counterconditioning) of both overt and covert behaviors. In practice, behavioral activation and exposure interventions highlight these two processes for depression and anxiety, respectively; both interventions disrupt negative reinforcement of withdrawal and encourage practice of behaviors incompatible with core symptoms.

The secondary focus of these interventions is teaching clients to seek out new learning experiences that enable useful patterns to replace maladaptive ones. It is common for students to find that behavior patterns intended to help them cope actually maintain their distress. One salient example involves college students' tendency to overextend themselves across a range of pursuits. Students frequently report feeling overwhelmed after taking up a variety of tasks, many of which are indeed important but nonetheless demanding. Mood and anxiety symptoms in this instance then prompt broad withdrawal and avoidance behaviors. While effective in offering a measure of initial relief, these behaviors inevitably give way to more anxiety and distress and a greater likelihood the student will further avoid these demands. As in cognitive restructuring, teaching clients to critically examine behavioral responses can help disrupt reflexive action and replace it with deliberate choice, underscoring the degree to which students may influence the course of their presenting concerns.

KEY TECHNIQUES FOR TRAINEES TO MASTER

CBT is deeply rooted in the scientific method and the principles of empiricism. Ongoing observation, hypothesis testing, and data-informed solution building are hallmarks of the approach. Supervisors can aid trainee development by advancing their skill in each of these key techniques. Skill development is central to the supervisor's role in contributing to trainee growth and maintaining client welfare.

Goal Setting and Outcome Measurement

A client's initial goals often involve a broad desire for symptom reduction, well-being enhancement, or some combination of the two. While this desire is reasonable, the process of goal setting must not only clarify discrete changes that will be pursued, but also (a) prioritize changes in the context of the client's current functioning and (b) ensure goals can be measured. Prioritizing goals can contribute to early successes that may be leveraged to pursue larger change. To this end, supervisors may encourage trainees to follow specific goal-setting models (e.g., SMART goals) and integrate goal setting very early in the assessment process to improve clarity and inform case conceptualization (Bailey, 2019). For example, a common desire among college students seeking treatment is to improve their ability to study without distractions caused by anxious worry or self-doubt. Therefore, a well-developed goal may look like (a) learn a technique to redirect attention after such interruptions, (b) practice the technique while studying, and (c) utilize the technique to increase the amount of time spend in productive study.

Selecting a viable method by which to measure outcomes is equally important; whether through a formal assessment instrument or unique metric developed for a specific client, aligning goals, intervention, and measurement increases the likelihood that even small positive changes will be detected and built upon. Using the goal around increasing productive study, a supervisor might suggest an approach in which the client demonstrates the ability to use the technique in session with assistance, use the technique in session without assistance, and use the technique outside of session for increasing periods of time as a way to track progress.

Self-Monitoring

CBT should focus upon tangible, concrete, or otherwise observable features of the client's concerns. For the trainee, these observations serve as guideposts of progress and are essential in delivering the right intervention at the right time. Teaching clients the process of self-monitoring allows them to actively apply the scientific method to their concerns. In turn, the trainee and their supervisor benefit by collecting additional data that may help to direct interventions.

Self-monitoring exercises typically feature a structured record form that prompts the client to describe specific circumstances in which a symptom is present as well as the cognitive behavioral antecedents and consequences associated with that circumstance. Supervisors should remind trainees that they should refrain from overapplying constraints and discourage clients from censoring what they record. Capturing a full spectrum of cognitions is useful in identifying thematic cognitive patterns, and monitoring a wide range of behaviors can highlight linked or associated actions not previously clear to the client.

When the results of self-monitoring are reviewed in session, the clients learn to view circumstances with a more objective, critical eye and identify the helpful or unhelpful functions they serve in the client's life. Supervisors might suggest using a thought record for the trainee's client to use while studying to record the content and frequency in which disruptions occur and estimate the time it takes to use the technique to redirect attention. The content revealed might then be helpful for identifying assumptions and habits that can be checked.

Checking Assumptions and Habits

Throughout the self-monitoring process, trainees should adopt a stance of curiosity and operate from the understanding that the client's established cognitive behavioral responses represent only one way of handling the core symptoms. Supervisors should encourage direct questioning and genuine curiosity about the clients' utility, accuracy, and efficacy to yield a keener awareness of patterns in thought, behavior, and habit, which can help the client explore feasible alternatives.

Checking assumptions and habits generally begins by naming a particular cognitive behavioral pattern identified through the self-monitoring exercises, placing this pattern in context, and prompting the client to expand upon how their reaction unfolded. The trainee then invites the client to brainstorm responses that, by virtue of refuting evidence, contradictory experiences, or incompatible facts, argue against the cognitive behavioral pattern in question. Supervisors should point out to trainees who use this intervention that raising awareness is a necessary but insufficient condition for change. This sequence will often require repeated trials and is most effective when the client is engaged in on-going self-monitoring. Perhaps the self-doubt our trainee's client experiences while studying comes from an assumption that the client is "not smart enough" to complete the homework. This might be refuted with evidence of past completed assignments, positive academic progress, the role of persistence, and identifying cognitive distortions about the level of intelligence required for the task. Developing short "checking" statements the client can believe in may assist the client in more quickly redirecting attention during study sessions when self-doubt is triggered.

In order to experience the full benefit of this technique, trainees should encourage clients to test the effectiveness of these new thoughts and behaviors as a scientist may test hypotheses. Self-monitoring is once again useful in this process as the client observes outcomes that emerge from new patterns. These new data points in turn help to inform how the client's goals are adjusted and evaluated.

CLIENT CHARACTERISTICS IN IDEAL TRAINING CASES

Supervisors should encourage trainees to attend to client characteristics as a way to predict who may benefit from a cognitive behavioral approach. Clients who fit well with CBT are likely to favor data-driven or scientific explanations for events and circumstances around them. Individuals who are persuaded by observation—qualitative or quantitative—tend to respond well because this "real-world" stance minimizes subjective labeling of experiences that can be viewed as biased (McLellan et al., 2019). Additionally, individuals who tend to learn through concrete and experiential means may fair better with CBT. The emphasis on practical skills can offer effective solutions in following a standardized set of criteria (Glenn et al., 2013). Finally, those who are generally more content-oriented (as opposed to process-oriented) will enjoy the emphasis on specific details generated through cognitive restructuring and tend to succeed in building connections between the assigned diagnosis, observed symptoms, and cognitive content (Beutler et al., 2018).

These individual qualities should not be viewed as exclusionary. Indeed, while some client characteristics may be theoretically disadvantageous for training purposes, they may actually present an opportunity to innovatively apply CBT principles for the trainee, with supervisor assistance. For instance, trainees who feel stuck working with a given client because of perceived resistance or other obstacles may be operating under their own assumptions, beliefs, expectations, or faulty behavioral patterns, which can be molded through the process of supervision (Cummings et al., 2015).

COMMON TRAINEE MISTAKES AND HOW TO CORRECT THEM

Perhaps the most important supervisory task is naming and defining the explicit mistakes observed on the part of the trainee. Common trainee mistakes can range from misdiagnosis or inadequate assessment early in treatment to nonadherence to the treatment plan as therapy progresses. Supervisors can normalize the process of making mistakes and emphasize that correcting mistakes can help the trainee build new skills and enhance clinical competence.

CBT can be delivered in a variety of ways and the skillful provision of treatment requires a well-formulated conceptualization that is directly connected to interventions delivered. Kim et al. (2016) described four types of common errors that new clinicians make when providing CBT: (a) forgetting the functional analysis, (b) leaving the patient behind, (c) getting caught up in cognitions, and (d) overrelying on the therapeutic alliance. Understanding the nature of these trainee mistakes in a college counseling setting directly informs the type of supervision intervention(s) that are most helpful to apply.

Forgetting the Functional Analysis

Most trainees in university counseling centers carry a primarily theoretical understanding of CBT. As they apply this understanding, CBT techniques may be utilized without fully grasping the function of a target symptom, thought, or behavior. It is vital for trainees to perform a functional analysis prior to attempting interventions. Doing so allows trainees to individualize their treatment to the particular concerns of the student rather than using a one-size-fits-all approach.

For example, a student's description of sleep difficulties may prompt a trainee to launch into a semiprepared overview of sleep hygiene and its rationale. For some clients, this will be helpful. However, it may be that sleep problems follow the student's deliberate avoidance of getting into bed because, when they do, negative self-talk plagues them while trying to fall asleep. In such a case, other interventions are likely to be necessary before sleep hygiene strategies will be helpful. Supervisors should strive to routinely ask questions that necessitate a trainee performing a functional analysis. Such questions may include: What use has the target behavior served in the past? What use does the target behavior serve now? Why might it be difficult to give up this behavior?

Functional analysis is also critically important in the execution of specific techniques. For many trainees, the use of handouts typifies the cognitive behavioral approach and serves as a foundational technique in delivering interventions. Used skillfully, handouts can be especially beneficial; clients may learn labels for their maladaptive thinking styles, build techniques to catch themselves in these patterns, or feel relief that they aren't alone in their way of thinking. However, handouts used without full understanding of functional context may inhibit the therapeutic process. Trainees whose initial approach is summarized as "I have a handout for that" may end up reducing the complexity of therapy to listening quickly for a problem, referencing a marginally relevant handout, and asking the client to work through it for the next session. Experienced cognitive behavioral therapists are more likely to choose tools based on the functional understanding of the target symptoms, explain these tools within session, and personalize them to the client's circumstance. Supervisors can emphasize the importance of functional analysis prior to implementing interventions and can help trainees distinguish between use of clinical handouts as therapeutic aids rather than self-help literature.

Finally, as many counseling centers operate on a short-term model, trainees may feel pressured to quickly identify and institute solutions to effect change in the time allotted. Often, this pressure leads trainees to overlook the function of cognitive behavioral events. It can be helpful to share examples from the supervisor's own experience that confirms change is more quickly achieved by following a thoughtfully constructed treatment plan with clear therapeutic goals rather than jumping directly into general interventions.

Leaving the Client Behind

Some trainees may rush ahead in intervention delivery and may find themselves a few steps ahead of the client, particularly in terms of readiness for change and treatment buy-in. This can breed frustration on the part of the trainee, as their client may not approach interventions or homework with the same eagerness. While most experienced clinicians identify with this frustration from time to time, trainees may unwittingly contribute to this situation by failing to ensure the client is in agreement with the goals and rationale of a given treatment plan.

Unfortunately, efforts to build goal and task agreement can exacerbate the problem, leaving the client further behind. At times, trainees use overly complicated explanations of what CBT is and how it works, particularly when they are feeling uncertain or uncomfortable. These descriptions may drag on for long periods, during which clients may experience increasing boredom, disengagement, and confusion. Regrettably, these explanations may also give the impression that the trainee applies the same approach regardless of the concern, that the trainee is not interested in hearing the client's unique experience, or that the client is no longer the focus of treatment. This may negatively impact client engagement, which has been linked to positive outcomes in psychotherapy (Holdsworth et al., 2014).

Supervisors can address this mistake with a number of interventions. Audio or video playback can be used to accurately capture the trainee's delivery as well as the client's reaction in order to raise awareness. If the trainee engages in this behavior in supervision when trying to describe their interventions, a supervisor should also identify it in the moment. Once a supervisor and trainee have witnessed the behavior and considered the ways that clients may respond, it is important to reflect on why they may be engaging in that behavior with a particular client or set of clients. For instance, the behavior may occur when the trainee feels insecure about addressing a certain issue or when unfamiliar with a presenting concern. It is also possible that the trainee is trying to establish their credibility with someone who they think may doubt it due to personality, age, relative levels of education, cultural mistrust, and so on. Understanding when and why it occurs can help the supervisor and trainee know where to focus in supervision to address those concerns.

Trainees should be encouraged to adopt a more facilitative style when explaining CBT principles. They can set a goal of seeking a greater amount of interaction and feedback from clients when discussing the CBT approach. One exercise that may be helpful is to ask trainees to experiment with limiting interventions to two to four sentences. Trainees are also encouraged to adapt the examples they use when talking about CBT to the client's presenting issue or some of their interests (e.g., art, science, sports, theater, nature). To check for understanding and encourage interaction, trainees can ask clients to "teach back" the concept in their own words.

Trainees can also leave clients behind by not taking into account their readiness for change. Highly effective approaches such as behavioral activation only work when a client is willing to attempt the plan. Clients, particularly inquisitive clients, such as college students, typically need to understand how engaging in actions that might be hard or unfamiliar (e.g., challenging core beliefs, calling a friend when the client feels the desire to self-isolate) will benefit them. Trainees need to spend the required time to match the target concern with the tasks the client is prepared to undertake. For some clients seeking counseling, this will be accomplished in the first session. For others, this may take multiple sessions or the whole course of treatment. Supervisors can help trainees understand that the pace of therapy cannot go faster than the pace of the client.

Caught Up in Cognitions

In addition to its efficacy (Hofmann et al., 2012), one of the reasons that CBT is so widely used in counseling centers is that it pairs well with the learning environment in colleges and universities. Every day, students are asked to examine what they previously learned, incorporate exposure to new information, and decide what they now believe based on that process. While the new information and perspective are valuable, it's ultimately what the students do with that knowledge that is the most beneficial for them. Just as some trainees may jump to behavioral interventions before clients are ready, other trainees may spend an inordinate amount of time examining a client's thought processes and neglect the behavioral interventions (e.g., exposure, behavioral activation) that are also needed to make the desired changes.

College students experiencing social anxiety, for example, may benefit from understanding the nature of their anxious thoughts and challenging the notion that others are viewing them negatively. However, anxiety reduction occurs as a direct consequence of engaging in social interactions while practicing the skills to cope with distress. Exposure therapy, which is a highly effective part of CBT (Foa & McLean, 2016; see also Chapter 1, this volume), relies on clients approaching the stimuli that they normally seek to avoid, withstanding the rise of anxiety, and recognizing that the feared outcome either didn't occur or was tolerable. For the socially anxious student, simply understanding all the variables that went into a learned response is not likely to be enough to change their level of anxiety in social situations. Supervisors can assist trainees to see that by solely staying with cognitions they may be colluding with the client to avoid discomfort and ultimately limiting the progress they make. Supervisors can help trainees explore any discomfort they may feel utilizing behavioral interventions such as exposure, which sometimes stem from clients reporting a high degree of distress or unwillingness to engage behaviorally.

Overreliance on the Alliance

University counseling centers offer ample opportunities to work with intelligent, motivated, and mostly self-referred clients, who often seek treatment in order to make positive changes in their lives. With such a population, establishing a strong working alliance is especially appealing and welcome. However, newer clinicians may be particularly prone to engaging in behaviors that prioritize rapport while undercutting the client's ability to make progress toward their goals.

For example, trainees may seek to use reassurance of client fears to improve their client's self-esteem rather than hold clients to the difficult work of challenging those thoughts themselves. This leaves the client reliant upon the therapist for affirmation rather than being able to develop the capacity to affirm themselves. Overreliance may also manifest in trainees' hesitation following through on interventions over fear of damaging the relationship. Clients being treated with CBT are often asked to complete homework assignments between appointments, and follow-up on that homework in session is vital. Newer trainees sometimes conclude that "homework doesn't work," while failing to note they may not insist the client complete the tasks that were collaboratively agreed upon.

Making progress on goals in CBT treatments parallels the process of molding CBT skills in supervision. Trainees—in much the same way as clients—may feel both excitement and dread as they approach their next supervision session: excitement for the support, validation, and insight they receive and dread that they will continue to be asked to focus on and make difficult changes in order to achieve their goals.

ETHICAL ISSUES IN TREATMENT APPLICATION

Supervisors contend with a variety of practical and ethical issues, including the need to verify the execution of the trainee's therapeutic work (e.g., confidentiality, informed consent, record keeping) and ensure adherence to general ethical principles in their clinical practice (American Psychological Association, 2017). Perhaps one of the most important ethical issues when providing counseling services to diverse populations is to choose an effective treatment within the scope of the clinician's competence. Extant literature demonstrates that CBT is among the most validated of evidence-based therapeutic treatments (Hofmann et al., 2012). In view of CBT's applicability to a wide range of presenting concerns, as found in the generalist setting of a college counseling center, it is an ethical choice for supervisors and trainees to utilize this theoretical frame when both have a sufficient foundational knowledge and skill. Nonetheless, there are several ethical issues to consider when working from a cognitive behavioral lens.

Maintaining Treatment Fidelity While Adapting to Students' Needs

The empirical support of CBT is most robust when the treatment is delivered with high fidelity to the protocol while allowing for appropriate flexibility and personalization. Given the real world setting of a university counseling center, it can be challenging for trainees to maintain treatment fidelity based on time constraints and the inherent demands of the academic environment. Trainees can struggle at times to attend to all facets of a manualized CBT treatment, depending on what point in the semester a student presents for counseling or how many sessions are available. Many centers use a session limit—a policy aimed at managing clinical demand with available resources—that may also reduce the number of sessions to below the recommended number of sessions in a treatment protocol. Supervisors can assist trainees by helping them to adapt a protocol for time available for treatment.

College students usually have the requirement to be concurrently enrolled in classes, and in order to continue receiving care, they often must maintain their academic standing. As such, in addition to the trainee following a specific treatment protocol within a time frame, they may also experience pressure to minimize negative impact of the relevant mental health issue on the student's academic performance. This pressure may require the trainee and supervisor to further adapt treatment from what is outlined in a CBT protocol. Thankfully, CBT is a highly adaptable approach. To ethically address treatment fidelity, the supervisor must be able to embody creative flexibility and a thorough understanding of CBT principles to help trainees customize CBT treatment protocols to the specific circumstance of the individuals being served and the environments in which they operate.

Developing Multicultural Competence

Like most psychotherapy outcome research, the empirical data validating CBT have been based upon samples with an overrepresentation of White participants (Williams et al., 2016), raising a question about external validity of CBT treatment protocols with ethnically diverse groups of students. Understanding and addressing the need for cultural adaptation within CBT treatment is vital to upholding the ethical principle of beneficence and nonmaleficence. There is a growing body of research examining cultural adaptations of cognitive behavioral therapy for specific populations and the findings are generally positive (Benuto & O'Donohue, 2015; Zigarelli et al., 2016). Such outcomes reflect one of the central tenets of multicultural counseling, which is that if counseling does not take into account cultural variables, it is unlikely to be effective for the client, no matter how technically precise (Sue & Sue, 2012). Therefore, it is ethically essential that supervisors assess and continue to develop multicultural competence in trainees as part of their ability to provide effective CBT.

Without adequate development of multicultural knowledge, skills, and awareness, trainees run the risk of pathologizing client's cultural beliefs. For example, consider a trainee working with an international student who has a cultural belief that direct eye contact with authority figures is disrespectful. A trainee without sufficient multicultural awareness may attempt to cognitively restructure that belief or find refuting evidence, rather than try to assist the client in finding strategies to navigate a new setting that still honors the client's cultural beliefs. Supervisors can help trainees question the assumptions they use in order to determine what is an adaptive versus maladaptive belief and encourage the development of a clinical approach that includes cultural humility (Hook et al., 2016).

Supervisors are encouraged to assist trainees in modifying their provision of CBT by reading and incorporating relevant research that shares possible adaptations for specific populations, such as Latinx (Organista, 2019), African

Americans (Kelly, 2006), Southeast Asians (Hinton & Jalal, 2019), and others. To avoid stereotyping, supervisors and trainees must also be able to assess the degree to which an individual client may or may not hold views that are characteristic of a cultural group to whom they belong. Skillful assessment and adaption of treatment in this way is known as dynamic sizing (Liu, 2007). To use dynamic sizing effectively, a clinician must have the knowledge of potential issues impacting diverse populations, awareness of how their own identities interact with their clients' identities, and the skill to address this directly with clients.

COMMON OBSTACLES IN SUPERVISION AND HOW TO ADDRESS THEM

Obstacles that may that arise between the supervisor and trainee not only impede the process of effective supervision but also impact the change process being pursued in treatment. A serious obstacle occurs when supervisees engage in intentional nondisclosure with their supervisor, thereby limiting the amount of information a supervisor has access to and cutting the supervisee off from a greater level of the supervisor's assistance. Another obstacle is when supervisors rely purely on supervisees to recall all the information from their counseling sessions with college students, likewise limiting their effectiveness. Finally, when supervisees take on cases outside their competence level or the supervisor's ability to effectively supervise, both training and client welfare can suffer.

Open and forthcoming communication is vital in supervision to accurately appraise the trainee's developmental level and clinical competence, to protect the welfare of clients, and to select supervision interventions that best reinforce the trainee's strengths and address growth areas. However, it is fairly common for trainees to deliberately withhold some amount of information from supervisors (Ladany et al., 1996), and there can be benign reasons for nondisclosure, such as time constraints and an accurate assessment that information is minor or unnecessary to share. When supervisees have relevant and important information that they deliberately keep from supervisors, it is more problematic.

Predictors for problematic intentional nondisclosure include negative social judgment (e.g., supervisors being viewed as not moral, not competent, or not friendly), poor supervisor working alliance, and the trainee's anxious or avoidant attachments styles (Cook & Welfare, 2018). Supervisors can counter these factors by focusing on a strong supervisory relationship early on, normalizing and reinforcing the disclosure of mistakes, and deliberately addressing types of information expected to be shared within the supervision contract. Additionally, our ability to model nondefensiveness, use of supervision best practices, and valuing of diversity is our strongest tool in reducing this phenomenon.

Supervision that overly relies upon trainee recall may suffer from distortions of memory, dynamics that the trainee does not observe or recognize, or intentional nondisclosure due to supervisees' embarrassment or fear of negative evaluation. This may prompt the supervisor to invest time in a less helpful area while neglecting a skill deficit or a problematic client–therapist dynamic (Haggerty & Hilsenroth, 2011). One of the best ways to resolve this issue is to utilize video recordings of counseling sessions, either as homework or within session. Some supervisees shy away from watching themselves on video due to discomfort or fear of negative evaluation, and therefore may attempt to fill supervision time with talking more generally. Supervisors should collaboratively set an agenda that includes time for watching the video and gently insist on the practice while explaining the rationale and it's benefits for trainee growth.

Specific formats may assist with ameliorating a trainee's unease. Gonsalvez et al. (2016) described a method in which the supervisor and trainee each write down five observations about a videotaped session and then compare their impressions. This tactic helps to ensure the feedback is less overwhelming and allows supervisees to benefit from when the observations are similar (validation) and where they diverge (unique observations from the supervisor). Additionally, watching video during supervision allows for discussion of alternative interventions and can increase the effectiveness of role plays.

The clinical severity within university counseling centers has been steadily rising over the past few decades (Xiao et al., 2017). At times this leads trainees to pick up clients that are too complex or severe for their current level of competence. Often trainees will still advocate to work with clients outside of their scope of competence based on a desire to gain experience, a desire to maintain rapport developed during initial contact, and/or through a misperception of their competence level. This puts the supervisor in the position of having to turn down the supervisee's request. To avoid or minimize ruptures within the supervision relationship, supervisors are encouraged to discuss the exclusionary criteria of cases early. If a transfer is indicated, reasoning should be discussed with the trainee in relation to client welfare and the potential detrimental impact on the trainee's development. Spending an inordinate amount of time on case management of a client beyond their competence can detract from the trainee's time to engage in self-reflection, conceptualization, and refining of intervention skills.

CONCLUSION

CBT is a first-line evidence-based treatment that fits well with the cognitive complexity that college students typically possess, the learning-focused environment of higher education, and the increasingly short-term nature of university counseling center settings. Trainees benefit from skill development in key components such as goal setting, outcome measurement, encouraging client self-monitoring, and helping clients to check their assumptions and habits.

Skilled supervisors are required to correct the mistakes that early trainees commonly make, assisting them to apply CBT theory and interventions in a nuanced way that accounts for clients' individual experience and environmental factors. There is an ethical imperative to understand both CBT principles and multicultural counseling elements in order to adapt treatment protocols to individuals of culturally diverse backgrounds and the real-world demands of the college and university context. Supervisors also work to ensure that trainees are practicing within their scope of competence in using CBT with cases that match their developmental level. Well-informed supervisors, who create strong relationships in which trainees are encouraged to bring up errors, and who use best practices in supervision, such as video playback, are well-positioned to improve trainee competence and client outcomes.

REFERENCES

American Psychological Association. (2017). *Ethical principles of psychologists and code of conduct* (2002, amended effective June 1, 2010, and January 1, 2017). https://www.apa.org/ethics/code/

Arch, J. J., & Craske, M. G. (2009). First-line treatment: A critical appraisal of cognitive behavioral therapy developments and alternatives. *Psychiatric Clinics of North America, 32*(3), 525–547. https://doi.org/10.1016/j.psc.2009.05.001

Bailey, R. R. (2019). Goal setting and action planning for health behavior change. *American Journal of Lifestyle Medicine, 13*(6), 615–618. https://doi.org/10.1177/1559827617729634

Benuto, L. T., & O'Donohue, W. (2015). Is culturally sensitive cognitive behavioral therapy an empirically supported treatment? The case for Hispanics. *International Journal of Psychology & Psychological Therapy, 15*(3), 405–421.

Beutler, L. E., Kimpara, S., Edwards, C. J., & Miller, K. D. (2018). Fitting psychotherapy to patient coping style: A meta-analysis. *Journal of Clinical Psychology, 74*(11), 1980–1995. https://doi.org/10.1002/jclp.22684

Boswell, J. F., Constantino, M. J., & Goldfried, M. R. (2020). A proposed makeover of psychotherapy training: Contents, methods, and outcomes. *Clinical Psychology: Science and Practice, 27*(3), Article e12340. https://doi.org/10.1111/cpsp.12340

Brunner, J., Wallace, D., Keyes, L. N., & Polychronis, P. D. (2017). The comprehensive counseling center model. *Journal of College Student Psychotherapy, 31*(4), 297–305. https://doi.org/10.1080/87568225.2017.1366167

Brunner, J. L., Wallace, D. L., Reymann, L. S., Sellers, J.-J., & McCabe, A. G. (2014). College counseling today: Contemporary students and how counseling centers meet their needs. *Journal of College Student Psychotherapy, 28*(4), 257–324. https://doi.org/10.1080/87568225.2014.948770

Cook, R. M., & Welfare, L. E. (2018). Examining predictors of counselor-in-training intentional nondisclosure. *Counselor Education and Supervision, 57*(3), 211–226. https://doi.org/10.1002/ceas.12111

Cornish, P. A., Berry, G., Benton, S., Barros-Gomes, P., Johnson, D., Ginsburg, R., Whelan, B., Fawcett, E., & Romano, V. (2017). Meeting the mental health needs of today's college student: Reinventing services through Stepped Care 2.0. *Psychological Services, 14*(4), 428–442. https://doi.org/10.1037/ser0000158

Cummings, J. A., Ballantyne, E. C., & Scallion, L. M. (2015). Essential processes for cognitive behavioral clinical supervision: Agenda setting, problem-solving, and formative feedback. *Psychotherapy, 52*(2), 158–163. https://doi.org/10.1037/a0038712

Drossel, C., Rummel, C., & Fisher, J. E. (2009). Assessment and cognitive behavior therapy: Functional analysis as key process. In W. T. O'Donohue & J. E. Fisher (Eds.), *General principles and empirically supported techniques of cognitive behavior therapy* (pp. 15–41). John Wiley & Sons.

Foa, E. B., & McLean, C. P. (2016). The efficacy of exposure therapy for anxiety-related disorders and its underlying mechanisms: The case of OCD and PTSD. *Annual Review of Clinical Psychology*, *12*(1), 1–28. https://doi.org/10.1146/annurev-clinpsy-021815-093533

Glenn, D., Golinelli, D., Rose, R. D., Roy-Byrne, P., Stein, M. B., Sullivan, G., Bystritksy, A., Sherbourne, C., & Craske, M. G. (2013). Who gets the most out of cognitive behavioral therapy for anxiety disorders? The role of treatment dose and patient engagement. *Journal of Consulting and Clinical Psychology*, *81*(4), 639–649. https://doi.org/10.1037/a0033403

Gonsalvez, C. J., Brockman, R., & Hill, H. R. M. (2016). Video feedback in CBT supervision: Review and illustration of two specific techniques. *The Cognitive Behaviour Therapist*, *9*, E24. https://doi.org/10.1017/S1754470X1500029X

Haggerty, G., & Hilsenroth, M. J. (2011). The use of video in psychotherapy supervision. *British Journal of Psychotherapy*, *27*(2), 193–210. https://doi.org/10.1111/j.1752-0118.2011.01232.x

Hazlett-Stevens, H., & Craske, M. G. (2002). Brief cognitive-behavioral therapy: Definition and scientific foundations. In F. W. Bond & W. Dryden (Eds.), *Handbook of brief cognitive behaviour therapy* (pp. 1–20). John Wiley & Sons. https://doi.org/10.1002/9780470713020.ch1

Hinton, D. E., & Jalal, B. (2019). Dimensions of culturally sensitive CBT: Application to Southeast Asian populations. *American Journal of Orthopsychiatry*, *89*(4), 493–507. https://doi.org/10.1037/ort0000392

Hodges, S. (2001). University counseling centers at the twenty-first century: Looking forward, looking back. *Journal of College Counseling*, *4*(2), 161–173. https://doi.org/10.1002/j.2161-1882.2001.tb00196.x

Hofmann, S. G., Asnaani, A., Vonk, I. J. J., Sawyer, A. T., & Fang, A. (2012). The efficacy of cognitive behavioral therapy: A review of meta-analyses. *Cognitive Therapy and Research*, *36*(5), 427–440. https://doi.org/10.1007/s10608-012-9476-1

Holdsworth, E., Bowen, E., Brown, S., & Howat, D. (2014). Client engagement in psychotherapeutic treatment and associations with client characteristics, therapist characteristics, and treatment factors. *Clinical Psychology Review*, *34*(5), 428–450. https://doi.org/10.1016/j.cpr.2014.06.004

Hook, J. N., Watkins, C. E., Jr., Davis, D. E., Owen, J., van Tongeren, D. R., & Ramos, M. J. (2016). Cultural humility in psychotherapy supervision. *American Journal of Psychotherapy*, *70*(2), 149–166. https://doi.org/10.1176/appi.psychotherapy.2016.70.2.149

Kelly, S. (2006). Cognitive-behavioral therapy with African Americans. In P. A. Hays & G. Y. Iwamasa (Eds.), *Culturally responsive cognitive-behavioral therapy: Assessment, practice, and supervision* (pp. 97–116). American Psychological Association. https://doi.org/10.1037/11433-004

Kim, E. H., Hollon, S. D., & Olatunji, B. O. (2016). Clinical errors in cognitive-behavior therapy. *Psychotherapy*, *53*(3), 325–330. https://doi.org/10.1037/pst0000074

King, B. R., Boswell, J. F., Schwartzman, C. M., Lehrbach, K., Castonguay, L. G., & Newman, M. G. (2020). Use of common and unique techniques in the early treatment phase for cognitive-behavioral, interpersonal/emotional, and supportive listening interventions for generalized anxiety disorder. *Psychotherapy*, *57*(3), 457–463. https://doi.org/10.1037/pst0000277

Ladany, N., Hill, C., Corbett, M. M., & Nutt, E. A. (1996). Nature, extent, and importance of what psychotherapy trainees do not disclose to their supervisors. *Journal of Counseling Psychology*, *43*(1), 10–24. https://doi.org/10.1037/0022-0167.43.1.10

Lapsley, D., & Woodbury, R. D. (2015). Social cognitive development in emerging adulthood. In J. J. Arnett (Ed.), *The Oxford handbook of emerging adulthood* (pp. 142–160). Oxford University Press. https://doi.org/10.1093/oxfordhb/9780199795574.013.16

Liu, E. T.-H. (2007). Dynamic sizing, multidimensional identities, & clinical supervision. *Pragmatic Case Studies in Psychotherapy*, *3*(3), 65–68. https://doi.org/10.14713/pcsp.v3i3.904

McLellan, L. F., Stapinski, L. A., & Peters, L. (2019). Pre-treatment CBT-mindedness predicts CBT outcome. *Cognitive Therapy and Research, 43*(2), 303–311. https://doi.org/10.1007/s10608-018-9977-7

McNealy, K. R., & Lombardero, A. (2019). Somatic presentation of mental health concerns, stigma, and mental health treatment engagement among college students. *Journal of American College Health, 68*(7), 774–781. https://doi.org/10.1080/07448481.2019.1590372

Mitchell, S. L., Oakley, D. R., & Dunkle, J. H. (2019). White paper: A multidimensional understanding of effective university and college counseling center organizational structures. *Journal of College Student Psychotherapy, 33*(2), 89–106. https://doi.org/10.1080/87568225.2019.1578941

Organista, K. C. (2019). Cognitive behavior therapy with Latinxs. In G. Y. Iwamasa & P. A. Hays (Eds.), *Culturally responsive cognitive behavior therapy: Practice and supervision* (2nd ed., pp. 79–104). American Psychological Association. https://doi.org/10.1037/0000119-004

Robinson, L., Delgadillo, J., & Kellett, S. (2020). The dose-response effect in routinely delivered psychological therapies: A systematic review. *Psychotherapy Research, 30*(1), 79–96. https://doi.org/10.1080/10503307.2019.1566676

Shefet, O. M. (2018). Ultra-brief, immediate, and resurgent: A college counseling paradigm realignment. *Journal of College Student Psychotherapy, 32*(4), 291–311. https://doi.org/10.1080/87568225.2017.1401790

Sue, D., & Sue, D. W. (Eds.). (2012). *Counseling the culturally diverse: Theory and practice* (6th ed.) John Wiley & Sons.

Williams, M. T., Chapman, L. K., Buckner, E. V., & Durrett, E. L. (2016). Cognitive behavioral therapies. In A. Breland-Noble, C. Al-Mateen, & N. Singh (Eds.), *Handbook of mental health in African American youth* (pp. 63–77). Springer. https://doi.org/10.1007/978-3-319-25501-9_4

Xiao, H., Carney, D. M., Youn, S. J., Janis, R. A., Castonguay, L. G., Hayes, J. A., & Locke, B. D. (2017). Are we in crisis? National mental health and treatment trends in college counseling centers. *Psychological Services, 14*(4), 407–415. https://doi.org/10.1037/ser0000130

Zigarelli, J. C., Jones, J. M., Palomino, C. I., & Kawamura, R. (2016). Culturally responsive cognitive behavioral therapy: Making the case for integrating cultural factors in evidence-based treatment. *Clinical Case Studies, 15*(6), 427–442. https://doi.org/10.1177/1534650116664984

12

Cognitive Behavior Therapy Consultation With Independent Practitioners

Dean McKay

The practice of psychological therapy is highly diverse. There are numerous theories, each with its own unique terminology and set of specialists. However, the vast majority of evidence-based practices are based on cognitive behavioral models of therapy (discussed in Tolin et al., 2015). Furthermore, while there are diverse theories and practitioners who endorse them, market forces have led to increasing numbers of providers to seek at least some consultation in cognitive behavior therapy (CBT; McKay, 2014). This means that, in order to deliver CBT, many independent practice providers seek professional consultation in this area.

In addition to the numerous theories that form the basis of therapeutic interventions, approximately 45% of all licensed or certificate-holding psychologists engage in independent practice, representing about 45,000 practitioners (Hamp et al., 2016). It has long been recommended that independent practitioners engage in consultation as a means to engage with colleagues and to avoid isolation (Greenburg et al., 1985; McGhee, 2017). Furthermore, it has been demonstrated that regular consultation improves treatment delivery (Edmunds et al., 2013).

At the present time, consumer demand for CBT is very high (Gaudiano & Miller, 2013). There are numerous reasons for this, including a public increasingly educated about mental health treatments, demand for outcomes in therapy, private sector insurance companies demanding outcomes from intervention, and a general increase in the proportion of practitioners who wish to

https://doi.org/10.1037/0000314-013
Training and Supervision in Specialized Cognitive Behavior Therapy: Methods, Settings, and Populations, E. A. Storch, J. S. Abramowitz, and D. McKay (Editors)

provide evidence-based approaches (even if they did not receive training in these methods). The demand for evidence-based approaches generally has been greatly aided by the efforts of professionals to promote and disseminate them, including through marketing appeals (e.g., Friedberg & Bayar, 2017). As a result, CBT consultation has also increased dramatically.

The aim of this chapter is to provide an overview of methods for providing CBT consultation to a wide array of independent practitioners. This includes identifying specific skills for the consultant, in consideration of the aforementioned fact that many practitioners seeking consultation may be minimally versed in the theoretical foundations for CBT. Two case examples demonstrate the consultation process, the first with a CBT practitioner and the second with a non-CBT practitioner.

OVERVIEW OF THE TECHNIQUE: THEORY AND PRACTICE

Consultation with established professionals from a wide range of theoretical perspectives requires extensive knowledge of the theories underlying CBT and being prepared to recommend approaches that will be appealing to the broadest swath of clinicians. Thus, the consultation process may be marked by diplomatically threading the needle on explicit education, while also being humble in the face of the other theoretical tradition of the consultee.

KEY CONCEPTS FOR TRAINEES TO LEARN

As this chapter examines consultation with established professionals, the engagement is about aiding professionals in integrating CBT methods into their existing daily practices. As a result, the consultation should proceed with particular sensitivity to the approach the consultee employs. This means both assessing for level of knowledge of CBT methods, while also considering the points of overlap and divergence between the approaches.

Most CBT consultants also provide this treatment to clients. Providers become known in their communities for the provision of specialized services, and, thus, are more likely to be attractive potential consultants. As a result, other practitioners may pursue consultation by contacting experts in their communities, even if consultation services are not advertised. When in this situation, the prospective consultant might consider the following checklist of questions that need to be addressed with the clinician seeking consultation.

- **What prompted this contact?** Akin to a referral question, gaining clarity of the reason(s) that led the clinician to contact a CBT consultant is essential. This will provide a frame of reference for how to begin developing goals for the consultation engagement. In addition to determining the scope of the consultation, at this point, it will be necessary for the consultant to provide clarity about their own scope of service. Issues around what the clinician can expect from the consultant need to be determined up front to manage expectations. For example, if a consultant is not prepared to educate and coach the clinician in how to adapt theoretical material into direct treatment models, but it is clear that is what the clinician needs to provide the service they seek to deliver, then the consultation relationship will not be satisfactory. However, the clinician may be seeking a limited scope of consultation, such as for a subset of problems in a case they are treatment, and the consultant feels comfortable providing the necessary oversight such that the clinician would be a technician.[1]

- **What kind of practice is this?** Just as CBT practitioners assess the environment in which their clients live, the CBT consultant should also assess the private practice environment to which they may consult. This leads to a number of important assessment questions regarding the practice itself, such as:

- **Is the practitioner engaged in solo practice, or a group practice?** If the practice is a true solo practice, then the consultant might be one of the few professional contacts for this person. This may lead to some additional recommendations for ongoing support, since the request for consultation could be motivated by an effort to overcome loneliness in addition to addressing questions about specific cases or the implementation of CBT. If it is a group practice, it is fair to inquire about how much contact the clinicians in the group have with one another, and if there are regular consultations among members of the group. Again, this serves as a useful frame of reference for the consultant in providing suggestions on implementing treatment.

- **Is the practice one that permits leaving the office with the client?** Many different evidence-based approaches benefit from in vivo practice. Exposure therapy for anxiety and obsessive–compulsive disorder, behavioral activation for depression, and social skills training for a wide array of problems, to name a few, can all be greatly enhanced by practicing live in the community while accompanied by the clinician. However, in some practices, as well as in some jurisdictions, engaging in treatment-related exercise can be challenging to orchestrate in the community. Furthermore, if the clinician is not accustomed to this kind of work, additional coaching

---

[1]The scope of the work sought by a clinician is typically for genuine treatment delivery reasons. However, CBT consultants should also beware clinicians seeking consultation for the sole purpose of completing paperwork that would create the impression of delivering CBT, when, in actuality, the intent is to continue providing non-evidence-based methods. Over the past 20 years, I have been approached by clinicians on over a dozen occasions in which the clinician stated, either initially or over the course of brief consultation, that they had no intention of delivering CBT. Instead, they wished to know "the language of CBT" to complete insurance precertification and ongoing treatment authorization forms. Upon learning this, in each case, I terminated consultation immediately.

to ensure that client privacy and Health Insurance Portability and Accountability Act (HIPAA) compliance is maintained may be necessary. In the event
that the clinician is simply uncomfortable with providing in vivo practice,
additional work-arounds may be recommended, such as between-session
client coaching via phone or other HIPAA-compliant platforms and detailed
consultation on imagery and role-play alternatives.

- **What is the theoretical orientation of the practitioner?** It is useful to
get to know the clinician before diving fully into CBT-based consultation.
This specifically includes their primary theoretical orientation, since some
recommendations may be counter to the theory espoused. For example,
in the New York area where I practice, there are still a large proportion
of traditional psychodynamically oriented practitioners. In recommending
exposure-based treatment, it has been also necessary to regularly discuss
the extremely low likelihood of adverse consequences that psychodynamic
theory otherwise predicts (i.e., symptom substitution; Tryon, 2008).

  Even if the clinician is a CBT-oriented practitioner, some important details
  are helpful to know before proceeding. For example, are they more comfortable with cognitive therapy or behavior therapy (colloquially, are they
  capital C, as in Cbt, or are they capital B, as in cBt?). If they are the former,
  the consultant may spend additional time providing guidance on behavioral
  interventions and their implementation (particularly in vivo in the community); if they are the latter, then additional focus on different cognitive
  distortions and cognitive processing biases will be essential for consideration
  in addressing the goals of the consultation. When consulting with CBT-
  oriented clinicians, opportunities to address specific, more detailed problem
  areas present themselves to the consultant, and they also may be more time
  limited than with clinicians of other theoretical orientations.

So You Think You Are Ready to Begin

With the background details established, and the goals of consultation determined, it's not quite yet time to consult. There's now a longer listening and
information-gathering phase around the specific problem for which consultation is sought. If it is a specific case, which, in my experience, it most often is,
then there is a clinical assessment by proxy that takes place, in which the
consultant evaluates the entire case up to that point through the eyes of the
clinician. This is a daunting task, and it is one that may lead the clinician to
need to gather additional information before any real interventions may be
recommended. This is most often the case for clinicians who practice in other
theoretical approaches. For example, psychodynamic clinicians often have very
detailed histories on their clients, but they might have far less on the granular
environment in which the client lives. When this is the case, the consultant
may need to coach the clinician on how to gather that additional highly specific environmental information, including basics such as antecedents, target

behaviors and consequences (as in behavior analysis), or environmental events, beliefs, and emotional outcomes (as in cognitive therapy).

WHAT MAKES FOR A GOOD CONSULTATION CASE?

Once an assessment of the clinician, clinician's goals, practice setting, and specifics of the case or broader consultation rationale has been set forth, actual consultation can begin. The task of consultation requires consideration of multiple levels of information throughout the process. Figure 12.1 provides a guide for conceptualizing the consultation process with CBT. The process moves from systems levels down to specific consultation "units," or recommendations that incorporate cognitive–behavioral principles.

A useful method for tailoring the consultation engagement to the needs of the clinician is to develop a "consultation plan" akin to a treatment plan that might be developed when engaged in direct clinical care. As can be seen from the process suggested thus far, the approach is comparable—the reason for consultation is identified, a structured assessment is undertaken, followed by an evaluation of the constraints around the administration of the interventions, and, then, interventions are implemented. As part of the implementation process, role play and behavioral rehearsal may be employed to ensure that the clinician can readily provide the intervention with their clients.

Ongoing Consultation

As with engagement in direct treatment delivery, each consultation session with the clinician should start with a review of the implementation of the tasks covered in the prior consultation, establishment of the goals for the session, and verification that the recommended interventions can be implemented with fidelity. This may result in new areas for additional assessment, as well

FIGURE 12.1. Independent Practitioner Consultation Process

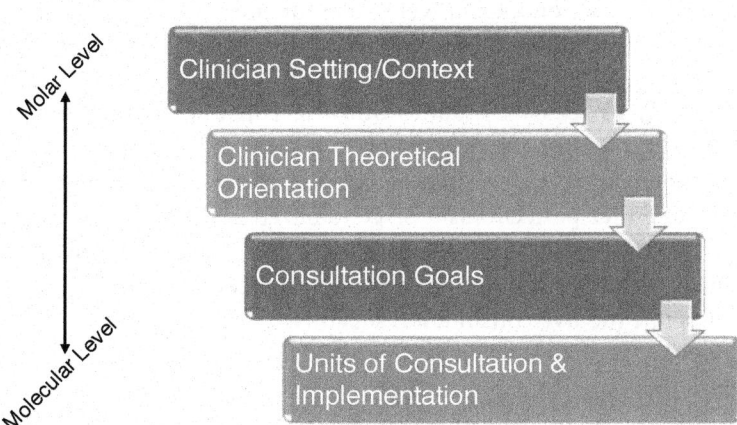

as potential revisions to the consultation conceptualization, given the introduction of new data points.

Illustrative Examples

To illustrate the consultation process, I provide two examples. One is with a CBT practitioner who had consultation needs for interventions outside her expertise. The second is with a clinician who practiced psychodynamic treatment, but who found a specific need for introducing cognitive behavioral procedures with a client he felt would best benefit from this approach. The demographic information related to the clinician, and their respective clinical consultation needs, have been altered to conceal their identities. For both consultations, meetings with the clinicians took place every two weeks for the course of the consultation.

Consultation With a CBT Clinician

Dr. Jones practiced CBT in a suburban area of a large metropolitan area. She was well-established as an expert in her community in the treatment of trauma, and for providing sex therapy for couples. She has been practicing for 15 years and has two colleagues in a small group practice. Dr. Jones sought consultation for implementing CBT for perfectionism and generalized anxiety, as, recently, several cases in her trauma caseload had co-occurring symptoms in these areas.

Practice Setting. As a group practice, Dr. Jones indicated that in vivo practice of behavioral skills was possible in her community. She further noted that her colleagues who shared the group practice were comfortable with going into the community with clients and that this was done periodically in the course of providing exposure-based intervention for trauma.

Consultation Goals. Dr. Jones stated that her goals were to (a) develop a repertoire in targeting perfectionism as a complicating factor in treatment for other problems and (b) develop skills in addressing generalized anxiety. She stated that she attended workshops on treatment for each of these problems at professional conferences and webinars, but she now needed assistance in specifically implementing these approaches with real clients.

Consultation Process. Dr. Jones and the consultant met on two prior occasions at professional conferences, but they did not know each other well. Dr. Jones also attended one webinar offered by the consultant on a topic unrelated to either perfectionism or generalized anxiety. As they resided in different geographic regions, the consultation meetings took place over secure video chat over the course of five consultation meetings. The following paragraphs describe the five consultation sessions.

Session 1. The first session covered an assessment of the practice and practitioner aims, as well as a further assessment of consultation needs and past experience of clinician in addressing problems similar to the ones for consideration in the consultation. This resulted in a preliminary consultation plan related to implementing interventions for perfectionism and generalized anxiety. Based on the discussion with Dr. Jones, she endorsed that she was a "Capital B cBt therapist." As a result, the consultant targeted perfectionism approaches first, since that would demand more work on cognitive interventions, an area Dr. Jones felt less confident in. Dr. Jones requested the area with lower confidence first, and she remarked that her clients needed this more urgently, and, thus, the imperative was greater.

Session 2. At the outset, this session covered a broad description of the clinical presentations of clients who would need perfectionism and generalized anxiety targeted. This included a verification that the targets were suitable to the client, and to further rule out potential alternative explanations for presenting conditions. This, in turn, led to the development of perfectionism interventions and verification of the ability to implement. The session concluded with a brief behavioral rehearsal of interventions.

Session 3. This session began with a follow-up assessment of the benefit of perfectionism interventions for the clients. As clients generally responded well, these approaches were expanded and connected to generalized anxiety. Following this, the consultant developed specific generalized anxiety intervention, with additional behavioral rehearsal for Dr. Jones to implement. The consultant also planned in vivo interventions, with an additional focus on behavioral interventions, including imagery for the clinician to develop and implement procedure practice.

Session 4. The consultant conducted a follow-up assessment of ongoing clinical procedures developed in prior sessions. At this point, given the advanced process in the consultation, the session covered additional troubleshooting of interventions, with anticipation of challenges in implementation with clients, and overcoming barriers to completing between session assignments by clients. The session concluded with additional behavioral rehearsal of client engagement with recommended interventions.

In this session, Dr. Jones reported high levels of confidence in administering the procedures. In behavioral rehearsal, they practiced role reversal, whereby Dr. Jones enacted the role of instructing the consultant in the interventions recommended, as a verification that she mastered the approach.

Session 5. This session covered an assessment of ongoing clinical procedures. The consultant and Dr. Jones discussed advanced coverage of the procedures developed and implemented to this point and reviewed planning for additional intervention development. Dr. Jones reported a high degree of confidence in implementing perfectionism and generalized anxiety interventions, and the consultant recommended additional clinical resources for her to continue to develop these clinical skills.

Summary of Consultation With a CBT Clinician. When working with self-identified CBT independent-practice clinicians, it remains useful to assess for specific CBT skills, granular orientation within CBT (i.e., more behavioral, more cognitive), and then proceed to address the goals for the consultation arrangement. These engagements are potentially more targeted in scope, as the consultation does not necessarily require as much education around the anticipated clinical response to interventions, as well as, potentially, the need for dispelling some misunderstandings around the fundamentals of CBT, as will be demonstrated in the next illustration with a non-CBT oriented clinician.

Consultation With a Non-CBT Clinician

Dr. Smith operated a solo practice in an urban area, describing himself as eclectic, but leaning more psychodynamic. The specific reason for consultation was that a long-time client who initiated treatment for depression also recently reported to Dr. Smith debilitating panic symptoms. Dr. Smith first attempted to address these symptoms in the context of the ongoing treatment he was delivering, but after several sessions concluded that cognitive behavioral methods were more likely necessary.

Practice Setting. The solo practice Dr. Smith operated was in his apartment, which he reported was fairly common among independent solo clinicians in his community. He had never considered going to any public places with clients as part of treatment and did not feel comfortable with doing so as part of integrating CBT into treatment for his client's panic symptoms.

Consultation Goals. In discussing the aims of consultation with Dr. Smith, he reported interest in addressing his client's panic symptoms, and he felt it could be integrated with other facets of treatment. He was familiar with other psychodynamic thinkers who endorsed what could be construed as exposure-based treatment (i.e., Davenloo, 1995). As the client also reported that they were not interested in seeking treatment with a different therapist, Dr. Smith narrowed the aims of consultation to focus solely on establishing the means for him to address his client's panic symptoms. It was also recommended that, in the event the client's symptoms did not resolve with the consultation, Dr. Smith would again broach the idea of the client seeking treatment with a specialist and returning after the panic symptoms remit.

Consultation Process. Efficacious treatment for panic involves a combination of interoceptive exposure with cognitive therapy (Pompoli et al., 2018). While Dr. Smith reported openness to exposure, when confronted with the prospect of engaging in specifically interoceptive exposure, he began to report hesitation. One of the concerns he raised was that, from his theoretical perspective, it was axiomatic that such intense anxiety was dangerous (for a general discussion, see Barber et al., 2013). This led to an in-depth discussion of comparative efficacy of treatments for panic and how the hypotheses of the theory did not result in the anticipated adverse consequences (e.g., symptom substitution; Tryon, 2008).

In the session-by-session consultation process with Dr. Smith, the overall structure was consistent from meeting to meeting. Specifically, each session began with a review of the prior meeting, followed by an update on the client who initiated consultation, a series of recommendations for interventions, and rehearsal with Dr. Smith for practicing exposure and cognitive interventions. Dr. Smith also wove detailed consideration of the mechanisms of action, and how the client might be expected to respond to each intervention, into each of the sessions. This was done to address anxiety Dr. Smith had regarding implementing exposure (i.e., Deacon et al., 2013). Dr. Smith reported that his client benefited rapidly from interoceptive exposure that involved quickly running up and down stairs, enacting lightheadedness by quickly moving the head up from between the legs, and, ultimately, hyperventilation using a paper bag.

The consultation engagement with Dr. Smith required eight sessions. As part of this consultation, some additional goals emerged in which Dr. Smith began to consider incorporating cognitive behavioral approaches with other clients who reported significant anxiety. In the course of these discussions, Dr. Smith realized he would be better served by enrolling in workshops and other formal advanced trainings, and then contact the consultant again in order to more efficiently use consultation work to integrate with treatment for his clients. In fact, Dr. Smith recontacted the consultant two years after the initial consultation for his client with panic after he completed several workshops and intensive training programs.

Summary of Consultation With a Non-CBT Clinician. The illustration with Dr. Smith shows that the nature of CBT consultation with a non-CBT oriented clinician may require a narrower focus in order to ensure that a specific set of skills are conveyed that can be competently administered with fidelity. It also suggests that it could require more time to accomplish the same goal that might be articulated with a CBT-oriented clinician. This is a reasonable expectation, one that might be given at the outset with non-CBT clinicians so that they are prepared for the additional cost and time commitment. In the case of Dr. Smith, who had a positive experience with the consultant and whose interest in CBT was further stimulated by the work, it led him to pursue additional training. As consultants, while this is a desirable indirect outcome, it is also one that should not be expected. Clinicians of all theoretical orientations are typically very busy, and the effort necessary to learn a significantly new clinical skill is a considerable undertaking, one most clinicians neither have the time nor resources to do.

COMMON MISTAKES, OBSTACLES, AND ETHICAL ISSUES

Practitioners of CBT who turn to consultation may be tempted to assume that a consultee who expresses interest in the approach are ready to "convert" to using it for all cases. This is a result of the zeal with which many CBT practitioners embrace the theories. And this is a mistake, as most professionals seeking consultation are looking to apply the approach for one or a few of the clients on their overall caseload. Thus, it is better to fully engage with the practitioner for the cases on which they are seeking consultation rather than view this as an opportunity to proselytize about the virtues of CBT.

In my experience, engagement with non-CBT oriented clinicians often benefits from acknowledging points of convergence between approaches as a means to facilitate integrating CBT methods into practice. Naturally, the consultant is in an advantageous position, since they are usually sought by the clinician; but, nonetheless, the temptation to "convert" the non-CBT clinician can be great and might be best avoided to ensure that the consultation goals and treatment needs of clients can be accomplished.

CONCLUSION

Consultation with independent practice clinicians is extremely rewarding, whether it is with practitioners who are well-versed in CBT and need specific refinements in skills, or non-CBT clinicians who express an openness to integrating these approaches in their practice. The approach to consultation illustrated in this chapter mirrors specific aspects of CBT delivery with clients—determine goals of treatment, provide education regarding the rationale for the intervention, rehearse the approach, and implement it outside of the consultation session.

Given that there is a highly diverse array of psychotherapy approaches, CBT consultation with independent practice clinicians means encountering many methods that may fall well outside the knowledge base of the consultant. As a result, in the consultation assessment, it is often useful to determine whether a specific approach being practiced would be counter to the goals of the consultation itself. As most CBT practitioners, who would, thus, be the potential consultants, adhere to evidence-based practice standards, there is a temptation to address broader issues in treatment by the clinician, such as the perception that some interventions not only lack an evidence base, but they might not be scientifically grounded. Consultants are urged to tamp down this temptation, as the likelihood of positive engagement with the clinician will diminish.

The research base on consultation with independent practice clinicians is limited. Accordingly, the general model for consultation engagement described in this chapter is based on a translation of cognitive behavioral methods, but this warrants investigations into the efficacy of the process, as well as the acceptability of different CBT interventions.

REFERENCES

Barber, J. P., Muran, J. C., McCarthy, K. S., & Keefe, J. R. (2013). Research on dynamic therapies. In M. J. Lambert (Ed.), *Bergin and Garfield's handbook of psychotherapy and behavior change* (pp. 443–494). Wiley.

Davenloo, H. (1995). *Unlocking the unconscious*. Wiley.

Deacon, B. J., Farrell, N. R., Kemp, J. J., Dixon, L. J., Sy, J. T., Zhang, A. R., & McGrath, P. B. (2013). Assessing therapist reservations about exposure therapy for anxiety disorders: The Therapist Beliefs about Exposure scale. *Journal of Anxiety Disorders, 27*(8), 772–780. https://doi.org/10.1016/j.janxdis.2013.04.006

Edmunds, J. M., Beidas, R. S., & Kendall, P. C. (2013). Dissemination and implementation of evidence-based practices: Training and consultation as implementation strategies. *Clinical Psychology: Science and Practice, 20*(2), 152–165. https://doi.org/10.1111/cpsp.12031

Friedberg, R. D., & Bayar, H. (2017). If it works for pills, can it work for skills? Direct-to-consumer social marketing of evidence-based psychological treatments. *Psychiatric Services, 68*(6), 621–623. https://doi.org/10.1176/appi.ps.201600153

Gaudiano, B. A., & Miller, I. A. (2013). The evidence-based practice of psychotherapy: Facing the challenges that lie ahead. *Clinical Psychology Review, 33*(7), 813–824. https://doi.org/10.1136/ebmh.11.1.5

Greenburg, S. L., Lewis, G. J., & Johnson, M. (1985). Peer consultation groups for private practitioners. *Professional Psychology: Research and Practice, 16*(3), 437–447. https://doi.org/10.1037/0735-7028.16.3.437

Hamp, A., Stamm, K., Lin, L., & Christidis, P. (2016). *2015 APA survey of psychology health service providers.* American Psychological Association. https://www.apa.org/workforce/publications/15-health-service-providers

McGhee, J. (2017). *Isolation, disconnection, and burnout: The importance of staying connected in private practice.* Routledge. https://doi.org/10.4324/9781315673035-7

McKay, D. (2014). "So you say you are an expert": False CBT identity harms our hard earned gains (President's Column). *The Behavior Therapist, 37*, 213–216.

Pompoli, A., Furukawa, T. A., Efthimiou, O., Imai, H., Tajika, A., & Salanti, G. (2018). Dismantling cognitive-behaviour therapy for panic disorder: A systematic review and component network meta-analysis. *Psychological Medicine, 48*(12), 1945–1953. https://doi.org/10.1017/S0033291717003919

Tolin, D. F., McKay, D., Forman, E. M., Klonsky, E. D., & Thombs, B. D. (2015). Empirically supported treatment: Recommendations for a new model. *Clinical Psychology: Science and Practice, 22*, 317–338.

Tryon, W. W. (2008). Whatever happened to symptom substitution? *Clinical Psychology Review, 28*(6), 963–968. https://doi.org/10.1016/j.cpr.2008.02.003

13

Supervising the Delivery of Cognitive Behavior Therapy in Medical Settings

Livia Guadagnoli, Jason J. Washburn, and Zeeshan Butt

Delivering cognitive behavior therapy (CBT) in a medical setting provides trainees with a rich training experience in adapting behavioral interventions to a unique environment. While rooted in the foundational principles of CBT, the application of CBT is often adjusted to incorporate the medical disease and meet the demands of the medical setting. Treatment goals can include addressing both physical and psychological symptoms, health behavior change, and disease management (Kazak et al., 2017; Magidson & Weisberg, 2014). Treatment structure may differ from traditional outpatient therapy and require flexibility on the part of the trainee. Finally, the amount of integration and interdisciplinary communication between psychological services and the medical setting varies. For example, in some models, psychologists are housed in a department of psychiatry, whereas in other systems, they are embedded in primary care or another specialty medical clinic (Hong & Robiner, 2016; Kazak et al., 2017; Kinsinger et al., 2015).

All of these factors—adapting CBT to complement the medical condition, navigating the medical environment, and working on an interdisciplinary team—underscore the unique and dynamic nature of CBT in medical settings and the need to provide high-quality training for the next generation of mental health practitioners. This chapter provides an overview of training and supervision of CBT in medical settings. We review key concepts and techniques important for delivering therapy in this setting, discuss the characteristics for appropriate and inappropriate training cases, and explore ethical issues related

https://doi.org/10.1037/0000314-014
Training and Supervision in Specialized Cognitive Behavior Therapy: Methods, Settings, and Populations, E. A. Storch, J. S. Abramowitz, and D. McKay (Editors)

to delivering CBT in a medical setting. We also highlight common mistakes trainees make and how to address them, as well as obstacles that affect supervision with trainees.

KEY CONCEPTS FOR TRAINEES TO LEARN

Providing training and supervision in CBT in the context of a medical settings may be different than in traditional mental health settings. It is critical that supervisors help trainees to understand that mental health is unlikely to be the primary concern in a medical setting. Treatment targets are diverse and can include managing psychological symptoms in the context of a medical condition (e.g., depression in the context of a cancer diagnosis), addressing the medical symptoms themselves (e.g., decreasing abdominal pain in patients with irritable bowel syndrome), or fostering health behavior change and disease management (Magidson & Weisberg, 2014). Behavioral health assessments may also stray from the traditional psychodiagnostic evaluations, as psychologists in medical settings are tasked with assessing psychosocial factors and readiness for medical procedures such as bariatric surgery, organ transplants, and gender-affirming hormone therapy (Kazak et al., 2017). Regardless, trainees will need to adjust to the understanding that mental health concerns in a medical context are likely to be perceived by medical professionals as a complication that interferes with their ability to provide medical care effectively and efficiently. Given the centrality of the physical condition in medical contexts, supervisors need to emphasize to trainees the importance of delivering brief psychological services that address current and identifiable symptoms, especially those symptoms that have a direct impact on either the patient's medical condition or the ability of the medical provider to deliver treatment (Cully et al., 2012).

Although CBT may be used in a medical context to treat common mental health disorders, trainees also need to be prepared to address a wider range of problems beyond those that are directly linked to mental health concerns. In medical settings, particularly integrated care settings, CBT is used to address behavioral, cognitive, and emotional concerns that may worsen, complicate, or interfere with medical conditions and treatment but, in isolation, may not necessarily rise to the level of a mental disorder (Magidson & Weisberg, 2014). For example, trainees may use CBT to address the side effects of medical treatment (Poort et al., 2019), to manage the fear of recurrence of a medical condition (Luberto et al., 2019), to supplement treatment of chronic pain (Darnall, 2019), or to target dysfunctional beliefs about insulin in the treatment of diabetes (Gherman et al., 2017).

Trainees may be appropriately trained in traditional mental health contexts to maintain fidelity to a specific CBT intervention; however, in medical contexts, flexibility is critical (Gatchel & Oordt, 2003). Flexibility is especially required as trainees experience barriers to implementing CBT in medical contexts. For example, a trainee may arrive to conduct a brief intervention with a patient in the intensive care unit, only to find that the patient is sleeping, under sedation, or undergoing a procedure. Flexibility is also required with regard to how the CBT intervention is implemented. For example, a patient experiencing severe anxiety while undergoing inpatient treatment for COVID-19 requires CBT interventions that minimize talking and do not involve breathing techniques. Trainees also need to be prepared to work with patients who can't speak at all and pivot to interventions that don't require verbal interaction, such as behavioral activation (Santo Pietro et al., 2019). Flexibility is also required for patients who would benefit from cultural adaptations of CBT. For example, trainees need to be nimble in assessing and incorporating a patient's cultural values, environmental context, and cultural preferences into CBT strategies and techniques (Landa-Ramírez et al., 2020). In managing flexibility in the delivery of CBT, it is important for supervisors to help their trainees differentiate between essential and nonessential components of a CBT intervention so they can maintain fidelity to the model, but also flexibly adapt the intervention to the unique medical setting or the needs of the patient (Mignogna et al., 2018).

Trainees need to be prepared for the possibility that CBT may be less efficacious with some medical populations. For example, some evidence suggests that using brief CBT with medical patients with greater physical functioning limitations and lower self-efficacy results in more modest outcomes for depression and anxiety (Hundt et al., 2018). Supervisors may need to work with their trainees to enhance CBT interventions, such as directly addressing low participation and adherence (Kerns et al., 2014), as well as manage expectations of the trainees, the patients, and the medical providers.

Given that medical conditions may be primary in mind for the patient and the other providers, trainees must be taught to understand and emphasize the interplay between physical health, well-being, and behavioral, cognitive, and emotional functioning. Delivering CBT interventions that quickly and directly address medical concerns, such as how to improve exercise and nutrition, negotiate with a medical doctor, manage their medications, or cope with distress associated with their medical conditions, may open the door for strategies that then address more significant mental health concerns (Brandt et al., 2020).

KEY TECHNIQUES FOR TRAINEES TO LEARN

There are several techniques for trainees to learn, in the context of both the content and the delivery of the CBT intervention, as well as in terms of communication and functioning within a medical setting. As discussed, treatment in a medical setting can differ greatly from treatment in a traditional mental health setting, which can be overwhelming for trainees. However, the key techniques for trainees to learn are rooted in foundational principles of CBT. Thus, training should focus on promoting competency in CBT, while developing flexibility in their ability to adapt the individual intervention points to the presenting problem, within the context of a medical condition and setting.

Psychoeducation

Providing psychoeducation equips the patient with information necessary to understand their medical condition, while also providing evidence and justification for engaging in a mental health treatment. A course of CBT-focused treatment typically includes providing education on the biopsychosocial model of health (Engel, 1980), a fundamental model in behavioral medicine that underscores the connection between biological (e.g., genetic predisposition, physical health), psychological (e.g., attitudes/beliefs, coping), and social (e.g., socioeconomic status, social support) factors affecting health. Trainees should become comfortable in delivering specific education about the medical condition itself, such as reviewing disease processes and treatment options, as well as highlighting the impact of stress and psychosocial factors on disease experience and management (e.g., diet, medication adherence). Additionally, trainees should explain how the CBT model is adapted to medical conditions through expanding the multidirectional impact of our cognitions, emotions, and behaviors to include physiology and symptom experience.

Relaxation Training

Chronic stress can negatively impact health and exacerbate chronic disease, from physically affecting the body itself to interfering with an individual's ability to effectively manage their condition (Cohen et al., 2007; Tabibian et al., 2015). Relaxation training consists of a variety of techniques, including diaphragmatic breathing, progressive muscle relaxation, guided imagery, body scan, and autogenic training, that can reduce stress (Esch et al., 2003; Hopper et al., 2019). These techniques are optimal for trainees delivering therapy within a medical setting, as they can be taught relatively quickly, are tailored to the individual patient, and are practiced to build self-efficacy (Bandura, 1997). While relaxation is an excellent tool, trainees may need to work with the patient and/or medical providers to modify relaxation strategies to be appropriate for their specific medical condition (e.g., avoiding a certain body part that may be painful for a patient during a body scan, confirming with the medical team that diaphragmatic breathing is safe in a patient with respiratory illness).

Self-Monitoring

A common goal in CBT is to increase a patient's awareness of their cognitions, emotions, and behaviors. Self-monitoring can bring into awareness patterns of behavior that occur before, during, or after the onset of symptoms. This can provide insight into how the patient responds when they experience a symptom, as well as help to better understand how these responses affect their overall disease experience. A patient can log the situation in which a symptom occurs (e.g., time of day, place, event) as well as the resulting cognitions, emotions, and behaviors over the course of a designated period of time (e.g., 1 week). The trainee can then review this information together with the patient in session to identify cognitive, emotional, and behavioral patterns. Increased self-awareness can lead to better management of these reactions, which in turn can lead to decreased symptoms and health care utilization (Barker et al., 2018; Hevey et al., 2020).

Cognitive Strategies

As a tenet of CBT, cognitive skills are crucial techniques for trainees to learn when working with patients in medical settings. The first key technique is identifying automatic thoughts and/or cognitive distortions, both helpful and unhelpful. The act of simply noticing thoughts as "just thoughts" or identifying patterns of thinking can be an intervention within itself. Using cognitive restructuring to replace unhelpful thoughts with more balanced or rational thoughts is another excellent technique that can be applied to the medical condition. Not only can it help patients cope more effectively, but also it reinforces the underlying message that, while physical symptoms may not always be avoided, patients can learn to manage how to respond to those symptoms (Reigada et al., 2014).

However, it is important to note that when working with patients in a medical setting, a thought that might be considered "negative" could very much be justified. For example, the thought "I can no longer eat my favorite meals" may be accurate for a patient who made a major lifestyle change due to diabetes. In these instances, intervention should be less focused on changing the thought itself and more on cultivating acceptance of the situation, fostering gratitude and resilience, and living a high-quality life despite the disease (Kangas et al., 2014; Levin & Applebaum, 2014; Reigada et al., 2014). In circumstances in which there is excessive worry related to a realistic thought, trainees should aim to address the disproportionate distress, without invalidating the thoughts (Levin & Applebaum, 2014).

Behavioral Strategies

Finally, there are several important behavioral techniques for trainees to learn when working with patients in a medical setting. Exposure can be used with patients who have anxiety and phobias that are interfering with a medical condition. For example, exposure can help with a patient with diabetes experiencing difficulty taking insulin due to a needle phobia, or a patient with a history of a stroke who is now afraid to drive in the car alone. Exposure can increase the tolerance of uncertainty and teach patients to effectively regulate themselves in the context of an anxiety-provoking situation (Weisman & Rodebaugh, 2018).

Behavioral activation is another technique trainees should use when working with patients in a medical setting (Hopko et al., 2011). Behavioral activation enables patients to engage in pleasurable and values-consistent activities to improve their mood and overall quality of life. Engaging in rewarding activities can not only reinforce positive engagement and behavior but also modify unhelpful illness or avoidance behaviors, resulting in improved mood and quality of life (Fernández-Rodríguez et al., 2019). However, behavioral exercises may need to be modified depending on the patient, disease, or situation. For example, in patients with inflammatory bowel disease, an exposure may need to be adapted depending on whether the patient is in remission or experiencing a disease flare (Reigada et al., 2014). Thus, trainees should work with the patient to develop safe and effective alternatives to exposures and behavioral activation exercises.

PATIENT CHARACTERISTICS FOR IDEAL TRAINING CASES

It is important for the CBT-focused supervisor to be thoughtful in selecting cases for their trainees. This thoughtfulness can take many forms and will likely change over the course of the supervision relationship and as the student demonstrates increases in both competence and confidence in their therapeutic skills (Henderson, 1999; Morgan et al., 2008). Ideally, as a rough guide, the supervisor outlines expectations of the trainee and their trajectory over the course of the supervision relationship, along with milestones the trainee should expect to reach by the end of the rotation or experience. In an overarching sense, all cases are good training cases for the CBT trainee working in a medical setting, as long as there is a clear line of discussion and collaboration between the supervisor and trainee (Magidson & Weisberg, 2014). That said, there are characteristics of a good training case that may be useful to consider.

Every trainee comes to their first medical setting placement with some form of clinical experience, even if quite limited. When possible, it can be affirming for the trainee to get a diagnostically straightforward case, from an assessment perspective, with empirically supported treatments available, from an intervention perspective. These are not necessarily "easy" cases, but they may be easier for the trainee than a case with more complexity. Of course, some settings do not lend themselves to this type of cherry-picking of cases, but when possible, it can be helpful for the trainee to have early successes to build confidence and to help establish the supervision relationship.

On a related note, sometimes patients get access to the psychologist by virtue of their medical condition or their treatment, but the presenting psychological issues have very little to do with their medical diagnoses (Robiner et al., 2014). In fact, many patients have their first-ever interaction with a psychologist because there is an integrated provider on their medical team (Nash et al., 2012). These cases can be useful for the trainee because the medical condition exists in the background and not in the fore. Further, the trainee has the opportunity to dispel myths about mental health treatment and can focus on a case where their psychological knowledge may be more important than their biomedical knowledge.

Of course, though, the goal of the supervision experience is not to provide trainees with easy cases. Trainees can and should fully absorb the service line in which they find themselves by attending didactic sessions, completing self-driven readings of source material provided by the supervisor, and developing collegial relationships with the other health providers they will interact with on a regular basis. That exposure puts trainees in a good position to work with the more diagnostically complex patient, who may experience psychological sequelae of their medical condition or even psychological disorders related to medical treatment. These tend to be rich cases from the perspective of both the supervisor and the trainee. So, while it may be easier to treat a patient without personality pathology, it is more realistic to accept that for these patients, cognitive and behavioral interventions may be most successful (Magidson & Weisberg, 2014; Matusiewicz et al., 2010). Careful CBT assessment and intervention of these cases can be incredible learning opportunities for the trainee, can allow the patient to more successfully receive their necessary medical treatment, and can relieve the medical team from trying to deliver behavioral management strategies (Chandler et al., 2019; van den Akker et al., 2018).

COMMON MISTAKES THAT TRAINEES MAKE AND HOW TO FIX THEM

As discussed throughout the chapter, medical settings provide trainees with complex and dynamic training experiences. It is common and often expected that trainees make mistakes as they navigate working in a medical setting. Thoughtful and effective supervision is important for strengthening the supervisor–supervisee relationship, increasing the trainee's clinical competency, and improving overall quality of patient care. In this section, we discuss common mistakes made by trainees, ways to effectively address them in supervision, and how to best fix them.

Assumptions About the Patient and Treatment

Trainees may be inclined to make assumptions about the patient and/or treatment, such as presuming to know how the patient is feeling, what their goals are for treatment, or their willingness to participate in a certain aspect of treatment. Another example is assuming that a patient with medically unexplained symptoms is relieved when given a negative test result. While likely well intentioned, assumptions about a patient's beliefs or feelings can be invalidating. Identifying and setting goals is another area where assumptions can interfere. This is particularly evident in a medical setting, when the trainee is tasked with navigating the patient's goals versus the goals of family members or the medical team and the initial reason for referral. It is important to remember that the goals of the medical team or family members may not always be aligned with the patient's personal goals. Finally, trainees may also hold assumptions about a patient's willingness to participate in a certain aspect of therapy. For example, a trainee may assume a patient with a needle phobia is not willing to participate in a "high anxiety" exposure, resulting in potential missed opportunities for learning and progress. On the other hand, assuming a patient is willing to participate in some aspect of treatment before consulting with them can negatively affect trust in the therapeutic relationship and undermine treatment.

While we are all at fault for making assumptions, trainees may be more susceptible, as it is desirable to want structure, certainty, and control when first beginning therapy. Fostering an open and flexible attitude as a supervisor can be helpful in navigating these complexities. As supervisors, it is important to regularly check in about assumptions during supervision. The goal should be to create a supervision environment where the trainee feels safe and comfortable discussing any assumptions they hold, the origins of the assumptions, and how to move forward better equipped to identify and challenge their own assumptions and biases. In addition, reviewing the patient–provider alliance, respecting the patient's boundaries, and setting goals and expectations with the patient are all excellent discussion topics and areas to explore with a trainee in didactic and supervision experiences.

Ineffective Patient–Provider Communication

Patient–provider communication is particularly important in medical populations, as many of the discussions may focus on delicate topics regarding the medical condition, disease course, and treatment expectations. Oftentimes these conversations can be difficult for both the provider and the patient. For example, in many chronic diseases, the symptoms and disease may not ever be "cured," which can evoke challenging discussions on disease course and treatment expectations. Conversations about death and dying are also not uncommon in medical settings. Trainees may find it difficult to engage in these conversations, given their relative newness to the field and lack of experience in working with certain medical populations. In turn, they may avoid direct or difficult conversations with patients in an attempt to mitigate their own discomfort or to prevent potential disruption of the therapeutic relationship. Supervisors should address this through acknowledging and normalizing the trainee's discomfort as well as their subsequent attempts to avoid the discomfort. Asking open and direct questions, while fostering an environment that promotes transparent conversation, is essential. Further, the supervisor and supervisee should engage in discussion on identifying, sitting with, and approaching discomfort as a way to increase trainees' tolerance of discomfort and self-regulation skills. Trainees can benefit from acknowledging their own limitations, while also learning how to ask the patient direct, genuine questions. For example, if a trainee is unfamiliar with a certain aspect of the patient's condition, acknowledging this to the patient and asking for clarification can be a helpful skill in effective communication with a patient. The supervisor should also be willing to acknowledge their own limitations and effectively model how to appropriately proceed (e.g., seek consultation, review the literature).

Lack of Interprovider Communication

Effective communication is a vital skill when operating on a team within a medical setting, as it offers a multidisciplinary approach to the patient's care and ensures that the different providers are on the same page (Hong & Robiner, 2016; Kirch & Ast, 2017). Effective communication can include consulting with other providers, conceptualizing care from a biopsychosocial framework, and promoting psychological intervention where appropriate (Kazak et al., 2017; Levin & Applebaum, 2014). From a trainee's perspective, lack of communication with a medical team can arise for several reasons. The trainee may feel anxious or intimidated about speaking with another provider on the medical team, particularly one they do not communicate with often or who is in a position of power (e.g., a medical attending). Addressing this with a trainee involves discussing the complexity of interdisciplinary communication, particularly when power dynamics are involved, as well as skills training. Supervisors should emphasize that effective communication is a learned skill that takes practice. Examples of ways to foster this skill may include role plays in supervision, modeling effective communication with other providers in front of the trainee, and "scaffolding," where the supervisor is initially involved in interdisciplinary communications and slowly gives the trainee more autonomy as competency is developed (Alfonsson et al., 2018). Similar issues may arise when communicating with a supervisor. In a supervisor–supervisee relationship, there is an established power differential between the trainee and their supervisor, which is elevated by the evaluative role a supervisor has. Trainees may be hesitant to discuss in-session difficulties or areas they feel they need improvement for fear of a negative evaluation by their supervisor. Thus, it is imperative that supervisors create a space within supervision that welcomes mistakes and establishes trust. Supervisors should acknowledge the power differential while also assuring the trainee that they can and should come to supervision with any "mistakes" or difficulties.

Over- and Underadherence to the CBT Model

Trainees may experience more difficulty staying "on task" or adherent to CBT in medical settings. Depending on the referral question, presenting problem, and patient's goals, session content may include addressing both mental health and medical conditions. In addition, other environmental and social stressors will inevitably occur over the course of treatment that can affect session structure and content. The trainee may find themselves being "pulled" in different directions, trying to effectively treat and address several targets. Supervisors can help trainees by creating a clear and encompassing case conceptualization. Case conceptualization is a skill in CBT practice that is extremely helpful in medical populations, as it can help to identify and understand all of the factors— biological, psychological, and social—that are affecting the patient at one time. In addition, it can aid in developing a treatment plan for how to best address the underlying, transdiagnostic problems. Another helpful skill is reinforcing agenda setting. This can be done through discussion and/or modeling by setting an agenda at the beginning of supervision. Finally, advocating for the trainee to bring up what they are noticing in session to the patient and being willing to discuss and problem-solve the issue together can be helpful in establishing trust in the relationship and buy-in for the treatment itself.

On the other hand, trainees may be too adherent to the CBT structure. As noted previously, delivering psychological interventions on a medical team and/or within a medical setting requires a significant amount of flexibility and adaptability by the provider. Treatment in a traditional mental health setting typically looks like 45- to 50-minute sessions in an outpatient therapy room. This is not the case in medical settings. First, session structure and timing can vary depending on the medical setting. For example, in the case of dialysis, rehabilitation, and inpatient hospitalizations, treatment is often delivered bedside while the patient is receiving medical care and can last as little as 5 to 10 minutes. This shifts the dynamic from the patient engaging in treatment in the trainee's space to the trainee entering the patient's room or the patient's place of care. Similarly, referrals may come in the form of "warm handoffs," and trainees must be willing and ready to assess, plan, and potentially treat someone they meet that same day. This is often the case in primary care psychology or consultation liaison service. Such consultation requests are common between physician peers, and that culture of rapid collaboration extends to other health providers in the system. This type of referral and treatment requires a great deal of flexibility. Given these changes, trainees may feel the urge to adhere closely to the structure of CBT. However, traditional CBT is not always feasible or appropriate, and there are nuances when delivering CBT to different medical populations, as previously discussed. Supervisors can address this issue through promoting the core CBT skills and techniques, while fostering flexibility in their adaptation. A provider who feels confident in their understanding and delivery of these skills will be better able to apply them in an unfamiliar setting.

ETHICAL ISSUES IN TREATMENT APPLICATION

Supervisors must address ethics in the context of their supervision with trainees. Medical settings often present with ethical issues that differ from those found in traditional mental health settings. For example, the brief nature of many inpatient and outpatient visits in medical settings raises concerns with Principle A of the American Psychological Association's *Ethical Principles of Psychologists and Code of Conduct* (APA Ethics Code; American Psychological Association, 2017), Beneficence and Nonmaleficence. Supervisors should assist their trainees in weighing the benefits and potential for harm in providing CBT to outpatients or inpatients who may have limited time to devote to the treatment and prepare for patients being unexpectedly discharged or transferred. Trainees may also face situations in which providing CBT in a medical context results in other medical professionals stigmatizing the patient for having mental health problems (Hanson et al., 2005). In these situations, the supervisor and the trainee must weigh the potential for harm in providing CBT in the medical context versus focusing on medical care and waiting to treat the mental condition in a mental health setting.

Principle B: Fidelity and Responsibility is another critical ethical principle to consider when providing CBT in medical settings. Trainees need to have a clear understanding of their role in medical contexts, not only when working with patients, but also when consulting and interacting with other medical professionals. Although some medical professionals are well versed in the roles and competencies of mental health providers, others are less knowledgeable and may ask trainees to provide services or opinions that are outside of the trainees' role or competencies. As such, the supervisor needs to help the trainee to develop interprofessional skills that allow the trainee to initiate and maintain positive relationships with other medical professionals while making the trainee's role and boundaries of competence clear.

A well-defined presentation of roles and boundaries to other medical professionals may also stave off potential complications with Principle C: Integrity, when providing CBT in medical contexts. Given that medical professionals are understandably focused on treating the medical condition of a patient, they may desire a trainee to magically remove any complications to treatment that are presented by a mental health condition. Trainees must be taught to be accurate in presenting the efficacy of their interventions and avoid making commitments to other providers or patients that they cannot keep. Given that trainees are often not in the medical setting full-time, they also need to be clear about the limits of what they can provide with regard to CBT treatment. Indeed, in many medical settings, full CBT treatment is unlikely, and even brief CBT protocols may be difficult to implement when the trainee is on-site only a few days a week.

Trainees may find themselves in situations in which they are being asked by medical professionals, patients, or patients' friends or families to adjust the intensity or type of CBT services that they provide. Principle D: Justice makes it clear that trainees need to provide CBT services that are equitable to all patients, and that their approach to delivery of CBT does not unfairly privilege or disadvantage one patient over another patient. Trainees need to be made aware of any "VIP" services that are established within a medical setting, and to have the skills to resist pressures to privilege VIP patients in the services they provide. Additionally, supervisors should work with and support trainees in developing and using advocacy skills to argue for care for patients who may not have the funding to cover their services.

Principle E: Respect for People's Rights and Dignity is frequently employed when providing CBT in medical settings. Indeed, confidentiality and privacy are very different in a medical setting than in a traditional mental health setting, making it challenging for trainees to navigate the delivery of CBT in the former. Supervisors need to prepare trainees for potential pitfalls in maintaining confidentiality and privacy, such as what to disclose to whom, and what to document and where. Ideally, trainees will be working in medical contexts in which policies and practices for delivering CBT have already been developed and implemented by psychologists working in that context. Outside of standard policies and practices for protecting confidentiality and privacy in what information they document and release to others, trainees need to be prepared for complications associated with the physical structure of the medical context, and the flow of care in these contexts. For example, trainees need to be prepared for how to manage privacy and confidentiality with patients in shared rooms, when medical professionals interrupt the intervention, or when the patient has visitors. Specifically, supervisors should work with trainees on how to introduce themselves, particularly when consent to release information to the patient's family or friends has not been established. The trainee must also be aware of the need to inform the patient about their rights to privacy and confidentiality and help the patient to identify the benefits and harms of disclosing their treatment of a mental health condition to family or friends. Supervisors also need to discuss with their trainees the ethical considerations of including, or excluding, sensitive information from the medical record, particularly when the release of such information—intentional or unintentional— to the public may be harmful to the patient.

COMMON OBSTACLES IN SUPERVISION AND WAYS OF OVERCOMING THEM

Supervision of CBT trainees presents some unique challenges for both the supervisor and the supervisee in the medical setting (Henderson, 1999). The good news is that most of these challenges are predictable and can be addressed proactively throughout the supervision relationship. Among the challenges commonly encountered are a need for trainees to get up to speed on medical diagnoses and their presentation, the impact of medical/surgical treatment on the mental well-being of patients, medications commonly used in the medical setting, the need for optimal communication with other health care providers, and the need to layer these new skills onto existing competencies.

Many psychology trainees receive their training in an arts and sciences environment and, as such, are not embedded within a medical school or other academic health center setting. This puts many trainees at a disadvantage when they first come to a medical setting (Robiner et al., 2014). Not only is the culture and environment an adjustment but also, most importantly, so are the patients. Trainees working in either generalist or specialized medical settings will need to get up to speed on the most common medical diagnoses and their presentation. The most effective way for supervisees to meet this need is a combination of didactic and clinical experience (Ludwigsen & Albright, 1994). Supervisors should prepare trainees with appropriate readings prior to initiating clinical work and then reinforce those readings with focused discussion of unique medical aspects of individual cases, as students encounter them (Robiner & Schofield, 1990). It is unrealistic for students to learn all they need from medical primers, but such exposure is invaluable for providing a framework for how commonly encountered cases may present from a cognitive, behavioral, and affective perspective. Supervisors can then help students hone that new knowledge to gauge their biopsychosocial assessment of new cases.

It is not enough for trainees to understand the presentation and course of diagnoses they will encounter in the medical setting (Evans & Carpenter, 2019). They must also get up to speed on the medications and interventions used to treat those conditions. This can be a substantive stumbling block: Initially, many CBT trainees are not well versed in psychotropic medications, let alone the broad array of medications used to treat medical conditions. This is simply a nonstarter in the medical environment. While trainees will not prescribe medications, they may be asked to weigh in on the potential benefit of starting psychotropic medications or even weaning patients off these medications (VandenBos & Williams, 2000). While it is important for the trainee to appreciate (and be able to communicate) the limits of their scope of practice, that does not mean a trainee should expect to be mute on such matters (Shahidullah et al., 2018). This is true for both optimal interprofessional communication and patient education. With time and experience, trainees should increase their familiarity with not only generic and brand names of common drugs but also dosing ranges. This can be accomplished, in part, by using helpful smartphone applications like Epocrates, MedScape, and Micromedex (Lau & Kolli, 2017). Far too often, for example, patients are started on very small doses of a selective serotonin reuptake inhibitor and never increased into therapeutic range, remaining on such medications for months, if not years. Careful interview and discussion with a patient on such matters can be helpful motivation for a patient to discuss their medications more carefully with their primary care provider or other prescriber (Aston et al., 2021).

Communication skills are critical for CBT trainees regardless of setting or patient population. But in no setting is this need clearer than in the medical setting (Henderson, 1999; Robiner et al., 2014). Supervisors must stress this critical skill on day one of the trainee's rotation; the psychologist must not be a passive consultant but must gather information from other providers and communicate their findings back to the team in an efficient, timely, and comprehensible manner (Kaslow et al., 2015). Team cultures do vary, but it is not uncommon for a consultation to the psychologist to include either no or very vague referral information. Ideally, the supervisor will facilitate the trainee having clarity on the referral before beginning the initial meeting. This information gathering is best done transparently, so that the trainee learns from the supervisor who and how to connect to obtain this clarity.

An additional challenge that comes up in the supervision of CBT skills in a medical environment is how to layer new knowledge on top of existing skills (Morgan et al., 2008). When the trainee enters into the medical environment, they need to assimilate a new lexicon, new culture, and a biopsychosocial framework, but they also need to learn how to incorporate what they already know about psychological principles and interventions, while learning how to augment and adapt those skills in a new population (Henderson, 1999; Robiner et al., 2014; Robiner & Schofield, 1990). Conducting CBT in the medical environment necessitates the trainee being flexible and tenacious by stretching and growing their CBT muscles, as well as incorporating it into a medical model that may be different from other settings in which they've worked (Magidson & Weisberg, 2014). This requires a unique partnership between the supervisor and the trainee. Ideally, the supervisor makes these challenges clear at the outset of the training relationship, checks in frequently with the student about the supervision process, and solicits ways to improve their knowledge and skills. The trainee, in turn, comes prepared for supervision, asks questions as they come up, and seeks out supplemental knowledge in the form of readings, experiences, and other venues (Henderson, 1999; Morgan et al., 2008).

CONCLUSION

There is little doubt that the adaptation and application of CBT in medical settings has led to enhanced quality of care for patients. As the fields of psychology and medicine continue to integrate, the demand for psychologists and other mental health practitioners in these settings will increase. For trainees, this creates a host of important training goals, from adapting CBT interventions to meet the needs of the medical disease to learning how to operate on an interdisciplinary team in a new setting. Meanwhile, supervisors are tasked with providing a space and the skill set to help trainees learn and grow within this unique and challenging environment. Through understanding key concepts and techniques, characteristics for training cases, and challenges that can arise for the trainee both individually and within supervision, supervisors can ensure high-quality training for the next generation of mental health practitioners.

REFERENCES

Alfonsson, S., Parling, T., Spännargård, Å., Andersson, G., & Lundgren, T. (2018). The effects of clinical supervision on supervisees and patients in cognitive behavioral therapy: A systematic review. *The Cognitive Behaviour Therapist, 47*(3), 206–228. https://doi.org/10.1080/16506073.2017.1369559

American Psychological Association. (2017). *Ethical principles of psychologists and code of conduct* (2002, Amended June 1, 2010, and January 1, 2017). http://www.apa.org/ethics/code/index.aspx

Aston, A., Smith, S., De Boos, D., & Tickle, A. (2021). Do clinical psychologists have a role in clients' use of psychotropic medication? A mixed methods investigation exploring current forms of involvement. *Psychology and Psychotherapy: Theory, Research and Practice, 94*(Suppl. 2), 359–377.

Bandura, A. (1997). *Self-efficacy: The exercise of control.* W H Freeman/Times Books/Henry Holt & Co.

Barker, I., Steventon, A., Williamson, R., & Deeny, S. R. (2018). Self-management capability in patients with long-term conditions is associated with reduced healthcare utilisation across a whole health economy: Cross-sectional analysis of electronic health records. *BMJ Quality & Safety, 27*(12), 989–999. https://doi.org/10.1136/bmjqs-2017-007635

Brandt, C. P., Deavers, F., Hundt, N. E., Fletcher, T. L., & Cully, J. A. (2020). The impact of integrating physical health into a brief CBT approach for medically ill veterans. *Journal of Clinical Psychology in Medical Settings, 27*(2), 285–294. https://doi.org/10.1007/s10880-019-09634-2

Chandler, M. J., Locke, D. E., Crook, J. E., Fields, J. A., Ball, C. T., Phatak, V. S., Dean, P. M., Morris, M., & Smith, G. E. (2019). Comparative effectiveness of behavioral interventions on quality of life for older adults with mild cognitive impairment: A randomized clinical trial. *JAMA Network Open, 2*(5), e193016. https://doi.org/10.1001/jamanetworkopen.2019.3016

Cohen, S., Janicki-Deverts, D., & Miller, G. E. (2007). Psychological stress and disease. *Journal of the American Medical Association, 298*(14), 1685–1687. https://doi.org/10.1001/jama.298.14.1685

Cully, J. A., Armento, M. E., Mott, J., Nadorff, M. R., Naik, A. D., Stanley, M. A., Sorocco, K. H., Kunik, M. E., Petersen, N. J., & Kauth, M. R. (2012). Brief cognitive behavioral therapy in primary care: A hybrid type 2 patient-randomized effectiveness-implementation design. *Implementation Science, 7*(1), 64. https://doi.org/10.1186/1748-5908-7-64

Darnall, B. D. (2019). *Psychological treatment for patients with chronic pain*. American Psychological Association. https://doi.org/10.1037/0000104-000

Engel, G. L. (1980). The clinical application of the biopsychosocial model. *The American Journal of Psychiatry, 137*(5), 535–544. https://doi.org/10.1176/ajp.137.5.535

Esch, T., Fricchione, G. L., & Stefano, G. B. (2003). The therapeutic use of the relaxation response in stress-related diseases. *Medical Science Monitor, 9*(2), RA23–RA34.

Evans, S. M., & Carpenter, K. M. (Eds.). (2019). *APA handbook of psychopharmacology*. American Psychological Association. https://doi.org/10.1037/0000133-000

Fernández-Rodríguez, C., Villoria-Fernández, E., Fernández-García, P., González-Fernández, S., & Pérez-Álvarez, M. (2019). Effects of behavioral activation on the quality of life and emotional state of lung cancer and breast cancer patients during chemotherapy treatment. *Behavior Modification, 43*(2), 151–180. https://doi.org/10.1177/0145445517746915

Gatchel, R. J., & Oordt, M. S. (2003). *Clinical health psychology and primary care: Practical advice and clinical guidance for successful collaboration*. American Psychological Association. https://doi.org/10.1037/10592-000

Gherman, A., Alionescu, A., & Sucală, M. (2017). Cognitive restructuring for psychological insulin resistance: A randomized clinical intervention. *Journal of Evidence-Based Psychotherapies, 17*(1), 129–137. https://doi.org/10.24193/jebp.2017.1.8

Hanson, S. L., Kerkhoff, T. R., & Bush, S. S. (2005). *Health care ethics for psychologists: A casebook*. American Psychological Association. https://doi.org/10.1037/10845-000

Henderson, P. (1999). Supervision in medical settings. In M. Carroll & E. Holloway (Eds.), *Counselling supervision in context* (pp. 85–103). Sage Publications.

Hevey, D., Wilson O'Raghallaigh, J., O'Doherty, V., Lonergan, K., Heffernan, M., Lunt, V., Mulhern, S., Lowry, D., Larkin, N., McSharry, K., Evans, D., Morris Roe, J., Kelly, M., Pardoe, P., Ward, H., & Kinsella, S. (2020). Pre-post effectiveness evaluation of Chronic Disease Self-Management Program (CDSMP) participation on health, well-being and health service utilization. *Chronic Illness, 16*(2), 146–158. https://doi.org/10.1177/1742395318792063

Hong, B. A., & Robiner, W. N. (2016). Psychologists in academic health centers and medical centers: Being visible, relevant and integral. *Journal of Clinical Psychology in Medical Settings, 23*(1), 11–20. https://doi.org/10.1007/s10880-016-9450-2

Hopko, D. R., Armento, M. E., Robertson, S. M., Ryba, M. M., Carvalho, J. P., Colman, L. K., Mullane, C., Gawrysiak, M., Bell, J. L., McNulty, J. K., & Lejuez, C. W. (2011). Brief behavioral activation and problem-solving therapy for depressed breast cancer patients: Randomized trial. *Journal of Consulting and Clinical Psychology, 79*(6), 834–849. https://doi.org/10.1037/a0025450

Hopper, S. I., Murray, S. L., Ferrara, L. R., & Singleton, J. K. (2019). Effectiveness of diaphragmatic breathing for reducing physiological and psychological stress in adults: A quantitative systematic review. *JBI Database of Systematic Reviews and Implementation Reports, 17*(9), 1855–1876. https://doi.org/10.11124/JBISRIR-2017-003848

Hundt, N. E., Renn, B. N., Sansgiry, S., Petersen, N. J., Stanley, M. A., Kauth, M. R., Naik, A. D., Kunik, M. E., & Cully, J. A. (2018). Predictors of response to brief CBT in patients with cardiopulmonary conditions. *Health Psychology, 37*(9), 866–873. https://doi.org/10.1037/hea0000595

Kangas, M., Milross, C., & Bryant, R. A. (2014). A brief, early cognitive-behavioral program for cancer-related PTSD, anxiety, and comorbid depression. *Cognitive and Behavioral Practice, 21*(4), 416–431. https://doi.org/10.1016/j.cbpra.2014.05.002

Kaslow, N. J., Kapoor, S., Dunn, S. E., & Graves, C. C. (2015). Psychologists' contributions to patient-centered medical homes. *Journal of Clinical Psychology in Medical Settings, 22*(4), 199–212. https://doi.org/10.1007/s10880-015-9445-4

Kazak, A. E., Nash, J. M., Hiroto, K., & Kaslow, N. J. (2017). Psychologists in patient-centered medical homes (PCMHs): Roles, evidence, opportunities, and challenges. *American Psychologist, 72*(1), 1–12. https://doi.org/10.1037/a0040382

Kerns, R. D., Burns, J. W., Shulman, M., Jensen, M. P., Nielson, W. R., Czlapinski, R., Dallas, M. I., Chatkoff, D., Sellinger, J., Heapy, A., & Rosenberger, P. (2014). Can we improve cognitive-behavioral therapy for chronic back pain treatment engagement and adherence? A controlled trial of tailored versus standard therapy. *Health Psychology, 33*(9), 938–947. https://doi.org/10.1037/a0034406

Kinsinger, S. W., Ballou, S., & Keefer, L. (2015). Snapshot of an integrated psychosocial gastroenterology service. *World Journal of Gastroenterology, 21*(6), 1893–1899. https://doi.org/10.3748/wjg.v21.i6.1893

Kirch, D. G., & Ast, C. E. (2017). Health care transformation: The role of academic health centers and their psychologists. *Journal of Clinical Psychology in Medical Settings, 24*(2), 86–91. https://doi.org/10.1007/s10880-016-9477-4

Landa-Ramírez, E., Greer, J. A., Sánchez-Román, S., Manolov, R., Salado-Avila, M. M., Templos-Esteban, L. A., & Riveros-Rosas, A. (2020). Tailoring cognitive behavioral therapy for depression and anxiety symptoms in Mexican terminal cancer patients: A multiple baseline study. *Journal of Clinical Psychology in Medical Settings, 27*(1), 54–67. https://doi.org/10.1007/s10880-019-09620-8

Lau, C., & Kolli, V. (2017). App use in psychiatric education: A medical student survey. *Academic Psychiatry, 41*(1), 68–70. https://doi.org/10.1007/s40596-016-0630-z

Levin, T. T., & Applebaum, A. J. (2014). Acute cancer cognitive therapy. *Cognitive and Behavioral Practice, 21*(4), 404–415. https://doi.org/10.1016/j.cbpra.2014.03.003

Luberto, C. M., Hall, D. L., Chad-Friedman, E., & Park, E. R. (2019). Theoretical rationale and case illustration of mindfulness-based cognitive therapy for fear of cancer recurrence. *Journal of Clinical Psychology in Medical Settings, 26*(4), 449–460. https://doi.org/10.1007/s10880-019-09610-w

Ludwigsen, K. R., & Albright, D. (1994). Training psychologists for hospital practice: A proposal. *Professional Psychology: Research and Practice, 25*(3), 241–246. https://doi.org/10.1037/0735-7028.25.3.241

Magidson, J. F., & Weisberg, R. B. (2014). Implementing cognitive behavioral therapy in specialty medical settings. *Cognitive and Behavioral Practice, 24*(4), 367–371. https://doi.org/10.1016/j.cbpra.2014.08.003

Matusiewicz, A. K., Hopwood, C. J., Banducci, A. N., & Lejuez, C. W. (2010). The effectiveness of cognitive behavioral therapy for personality disorders. *The Psychiatric Clinics of North America, 33*(3), 657–685. https://doi.org/10.1016/j.psc.2010.04.007

Mignogna, J., Martin, L. A., Harik, J., Hundt, N. E., Kauth, M., Naik, A. D., Sorocco, K., Benzer, J., & Cully, J. (2018). "I had to somehow still be flexible": Exploring adaptations during implementation of brief cognitive behavioral therapy in primary care. *Implementation Science, 13*(1), 76. https://doi.org/10.1186/s13012-018-0768-z

Morgan, C. D., Soetaert, D. K., & Heinrichs, R. J. (2008). Supervision in medical settings. In A. K. Hess, K. D. Hess, & T. H. Hess (Eds.), *Psychotherapy supervision: Theory, research, and practice* (2nd ed., pp. 450–470). John Wiley & Sons.

Nash, J. M., McKay, K. M., Vogel, M. E., & Masters, K. S. (2012). Functional roles and foundational characteristics of psychologists in integrated primary care. *Journal of Clinical Psychology in Medical Settings, 19*(1), 93–104. https://doi.org/10.1007/s10880-011-9290-z

Poort, H., Onghena, P., Abrahams, H. J. G., Jim, H. S. L., Jacobsen, P. B., Blijlevens, N. M. A., & Knoop, H. (2019). Cognitive behavioral therapy for treatment-related fatigue in chronic myeloid leukemia patients on tyrosine kinase inhibitors: A mixed-method study. *Journal of Clinical Psychology in Medical Settings, 26*(4), 440–448. https://doi.org/10.1007/s10880-019-09607-5

Reigada, L. C., McGovern, A., Tudor, M. E., Walder, D. J., & Warner, C. M. (2014). Collaborating with pediatric gastroenterologists to treat co-occurring inflammatory bowel disease and anxiety in pediatric medical settings. *Cognitive and Behavioral Practice, 21*(4), 372–385. https://doi.org/10.1016/j.cbpra.2014.03.004

Robiner, W. N., Dixon, K. E., Miner, J. L., & Hong, B. A. (2014). Psychologists in medical schools and academic medical centers: Over 100 years of growth, influence, and partnership. *American Psychologist, 69*(3), 230–248. https://doi.org/10.1037/a0035472

Robiner, W. N., & Schofield, W. (1990). References on supervision in clinical and counseling psychology. *Professional Psychology: Research and Practice, 21*(4), 297–312. https://doi.org/10.1037/0735-7028.21.4.297

Santo Pietro, M. J., Marks, D. R., & Mullen, A. (2019). When words fail: Providing effective psychological treatment for depression in persons with aphasia. *Journal of Clinical Psychology in Medical Settings, 26*(4), 483–494. https://doi.org/10.1007/s10880-019-09608-4

Shahidullah, J. D., Hostutler, C. A., & Stancin, T. (2018). Collaborative medication-related roles for pediatric primary care psychologists. *Clinical Practice in Pediatric Psychology, 6*(1), 61–72. https://doi.org/10.1037/cpp0000207

Tabibian, A., Tabibian, J. H., Beckman, L. J., Raffals, L. L., Papadakis, K. A., & Kane, S. V. (2015). Predictors of health-related quality of life and adherence in Crohn's disease and ulcerative colitis: Implications for clinical management. *Digestive Diseases and Sciences, 60*(5), 1366–1374. https://doi.org/10.1007/s10620-014-3471-1

van den Akker, L. E., Beckerman, H., Collette, E. H., Knoop, H., Bleijenberg, G., Twisk, J. W., Dekker, J., de Groot, V., & the TREFAMS-ACE study group. (2018). Cognitive behavioural therapy for MS-related fatigue explained: A longitudinal mediation analysis. *Journal of Psychosomatic Research, 106*, 13–24. https://doi.org/10.1016/j.jpsychores.2017.12.014

VandenBos, G. R., & Williams, S. (2000). Is psychologists' involvement in the prescribing of psychotropic medication really a new activity? *Professional Psychology: Research and Practice, 31*(6), 615–618. https://doi.org/10.1037/0735-7028.31.6.615

Weisman, J. S., & Rodebaugh, T. L. (2018). Exposure therapy augmentation: A review and extension of techniques informed by an inhibitory learning approach. *Clinical Psychology Review, 59*, 41–51. https://doi.org/10.1016/j.cpr.2017.10.010

14

Supervising the Delivery of Cognitive Behavior Therapy in School Settings

Kristin A. Gansle and George H. Noell

Children and youth commonly spend most of the day in school, making it a critical setting in which mental and behavioral health (MBH) services are needed (Burns et al., 1995; Eklund et al., 2020; Farmer et al., 2003). Over 20% of children and youth experience mental health or behavioral concerns that warrant intervention (Centers for Disease Control and Prevention, 2013; Kazdin, 2017; Merikangas et al., 2010; Weist et al., 2003), and more than seven in 10 do not receive needed intervention (Greenberg et al., 2003; Weist et al., 2003). Considering the many hurdles to securing services in the community, such as cost, availability, transportation, and stigma (Eklund et al., 2020; Hanchon & Fernald, 2013), the bulk of youth who receive services will do so in schools (Farmer et al., 2003; Jacob & Coustasse, 2008; Juszczak et al., 2003). Given that the American Psychological Association's *Ethical Principles of Psychologists and Code of Conduct* mandate psychologists to practice only within areas in which they are skilled (American Psychological Association, 2017), it is essential that school-based clinicians receive supervision that allows them to gain and improve skills to provide quality services to children and youth.

Public schools are governmental institutions; a diverse array of civil rights follow students into schools. These include protections against unreasonable discipline, unnecessary segregation, and the right to supports that allow them to meaningfully access education (Yell, 2019). Due to schools' responsibility to act *in loco parentis*, typical clinical protections such as privilege typically cannot apply. Schools are inherently social service systems in which many layers of

https://doi.org/10.1037/0000314-015
Training and Supervision in Specialized Cognitive Behavior Therapy: Methods, Settings, and Populations, E. A. Storch, J. S. Abramowitz, and D. McKay (Editors)

services are available without regard for the ability to pay, which makes them unique clinical settings. Further, schools are required under law to act for the welfare of all students; therefore, intervention and service are inevitably layered. Clinicians may also find themselves working with children in private, religious, and other school or school-like settings. These private institutions may not be bound by the same civil rights provisions that apply to public schools. However, the fundamental principles of effective treatment remain the same. Typically, a clinician engaging in cognitive behavior therapy (CBT) will not be the first or even the second intervention. On the contrary, multiple types of intervention may be implemented by several different educators before the case is promoted in queue to the clinician. Not all referring concerns may be appropriate to a school-based clinician. Referral concerns must affect school functioning. If a student has a problem that is affecting their social relationships but is not affecting their ability to make good progress in school, they would not necessarily be entitled to services. Although this may change as mental health clinics become more available in schools, until that time, effects on school functioning should be apparent.

KEY CONCEPTS FOR TRAINEES TO LEARN

Within the school setting, trainees must master several important concepts prior to practicing independently.

Goal Setting

When supervising school clinicians implementing CBT, it is imperative to consider the goals of therapy first so that the quality and outcomes of the process may be measured, evaluated, and improved (Fixsen et al., 2005). Within schools, this may happen at three levels: the child, or outcome of treatment; the clinician, or growth in CBT skills; and the school/organization, or management of resources and prioritization of cases. The first two require measurement of child and clinician behavior; the third requires measurement of school outcomes. These levels of outcome are important dimensions in the success of clinical as well as administrative supervision of CBT programs in schools (Flanagan, 2015).

Treatment Outcomes

Due to the time demands on clinicians in schools and the impracticality of providing direct service to all who need it (Eklund et al., 2020; McNamara et al., 2019), consultation provides a framework through which interventions for MBH concerns may be developed, implemented, monitored, and improved (Noell & Gansle, 2014). Consultation is the provision of indirect service to the client, in this case the student, by providing support to an intermediate service provider. In schools, it is typically the classroom teacher who receives support, but it can be a classroom aide or other school professional who is providing direct service. A clinical psychologist, a school psychologist, a social worker, or another professional with expertise in MBH service provision will direct CBT. The clinician may act as the immediate therapist, may consult with educators in the environment, or may blend these roles. A supervisor may manage the case load and provide support to the therapist.

Therapist Growth

Supervision is a combination of teaching therapeutic technique and providing corrective feedback; it may be described as an opportunity for the supervisor to assess competence, help the clinician develop competence through objective feedback, and share knowledge between them (Flanagan, 2015). As in CBT itself, supervision sessions should be structured and focused, but both participants should feel free to bring their concerns to the sessions (Liese & Beck, 1997). Within the school setting, other variables that will have an impact on the success of CBT include the size of caseloads and other demands on the clinician's time in addition to their skills.

Managing Resources and Prioritizing Cases

Supervision in CBT addresses the relationship between clinician and client, as well as the successful application of the therapeutic process. In their jobs, however, school clinicians commonly require an additional level of assessment. School clinicians are often the individuals receiving referrals for students with MBH concerns as members of school-level teams that may provide assessment, intervention, and progress monitoring services. As a consultant in that hierarchy, they may be responsible to determine which cases have priority. In this role they must commonly make decisions surrounding the intensity of intervention provided across cases. Once that has been determined, the consultant may act as an intermediary, determining whether the resources are available to put an intervention plan in place. For example, would a student with a school avoidance issue have priority over another who engages in self-injury? Obviously, this would depend on the specifics of the cases, but some assessment and data gathering would be necessary before a decision could be made.

A heuristic for prioritizing cases should focus first on whether there is a threat of danger or harm to the student or others; clinicians in school settings are ethically required to provide those services (Barnett et al., 1996; Noell et al., in press). These might include asthma management or aggressive behavior that has led to student or teacher harm or could reasonably be predicted to lead to harm. Next, if CBT has been written into the individualized education program (IEP), the Individuals With Disabilities Education Improvement Act (IDEA; 2004) requires that those services be provided to them as a matter of law. Failing to provide IEP-mandated services is a violation of students' civil rights and can serve as the predicate for litigation (Yell, 2019). Priority in additional student concerns may be determined according to the judgment of the clinician, but typically, those concerns that will have the greatest impact on student functioning will take precedence (Noell et al., 2009). For example, a student whose hand-washing behavior is preventing them from accessing curriculum might be prioritized over one whose fidgeting is irritating the teacher in the classroom. A competent supervisor should take the time to review cases with the clinician to assist them in developing the skills to allow them to allocate resources appropriately. This is best accomplished as an active process in which the scope of cases and available resources are actively managed in a planful way, rather than in a reactive, adjunct fashion.

KEY TECHNIQUES FOR SUPERVISORS AND TRAINEES TO LEARN

There are additional skills that supervisors must master as they work with their trainees to provide quality services within the schools.

Supervisor Competencies

Clinical supervision can be an essential element of the provision of effective, evidence-based CBT that improves client outcomes and enhances learning (Milne et al., 2011; Moeller et al., 2020; Pugh & Margetts, 2020). It is obviously necessary in contexts in which clinicians are themselves receiving training. Many studies have evaluated the effectiveness of clinician training within CBT, including activities such as treatment planning, instruction and rehearsal, affective processing, and self-reflection (Pugh & Margetts, 2020; e.g., Liese & Beck, 1997). *Action-based supervision* includes those activities that simulate thera-peutic interaction; role play may be the most familiar of these, and chair work is a more creative action-based approach that is supported by data (Pugh & Margetts, 2020). In chair work, the clinician holds a conversation with either an imagined client or imagined parts of the self, symbolized by an empty chair or chairs (Milne & Reiser, 2017). Such activities allow experiential learning: The supervisor demonstrates the technique, and the clinician practices with expert feedback given by the supervisor. Although these methods have been shown to be valued by clinicians and preferred to discussion (Bennett-Levy et al., 2009; Johnston & Milne, 2012; Rakovshik & McManus, 2013), modeling, role play, and practice with feedback are used much less often than talk-based activities such as discussion during supervision (Milne, 2008; Townend et al., 2002). To the extent that it is pragmatic, clinical supervision should include action-based activities. For maximum effect, the rationale for using these activ-ities should be introduced into the supervisory relationship at the outset, the activities themselves practiced, and corrective and positive feedback given until skills are mastered (Pugh & Margetts, 2020). The clinician should also be asked to provide feedback as to the supervisor's performance of responsibilities. Although many quality instruments have not been available for measuring supervision, preliminary evidence for a new evaluation tool for clinical super-vision (Moeller, Moerch, Rosenberg Supervision Scale, or MMRSS) has been promising (Moeller et al., 2020); future supervision dyads should use technically sound instruments to evaluate the quality of the supervision provided, and to improve practice as needed.

Therapist Competencies

There is a vast literature that addresses CBT training (e.g., Boswell & Constantino, 2022; Wenzel, 2021). Many of these therapeutic choices, such as decreasing anxiety, differential reinforcement of other behaviors, and check in/check out procedures, may be successfully used in the school setting. It is important to acknowledge, however, that not all CBT is equally relevant within the school setting or appropriate to students of all ages and functioning levels. When determining which referral concerns are appropriate for CBT at school, consider whether amelioration of the concern will help the student function better in terms of academics or behavior in the school setting. School-based CBT might appropriately address school avoidance, aggression, negative thoughts that contribute to poor test performance, or tantrums that prevent academic skills from being gained. However, issues like phobias of flying (aviophobia) or of heights (acrophobia) that may cause stress in students when they are with their families but that are not directly education related might not be an appropriate fit for CBT in schools. In addition, therapy for issues like substance use, severe eating disorders, and sleep disorders might better employ an off-site clinical therapist to work with those concerns in the times and places that are relevant to the concerns. Finally, there are students whose current level of intellectual functioning would make them poor candidates for CBT and who have referral concerns, such as reading deficits, that are more appropriately addressed by different types of interventions.

SELECTING CASES FOR SUPERVISION

Making active choices about whether cases are appropriate for a clinician they are supervising is an important part of the supervisor's ethical responsibilities. There is no single meaningful rule for this process, as it is inevitably a match-to-need process. Early in a clinician's training, typically cases cannot be too simple; complexity in cases creates problems for inexperienced clinicians who are unable yet to distinguish relevant features and provide targeted therapy for difficult cases. Ideally, early cases should have limited complexity. Generally, these should be low-risk students who can be treated so that the supervised clinician can master the CBT process with little risk of doing harm and without the need to negotiate extra complexity and adjunctive procedures. As the clinician's proficiency increases, progressively more complex cases become appropriate learning opportunities, presuming the clinician possesses requisite competencies and can receive appropriately close supervision. It is important as this progression toward increasingly independent complex practice proceeds that the supervisor remains vigilant about the match between the student's specific need and the clinician's skills. Depending on their competencies and previous experience, an intermediate or advanced therapist may or may not be prepared for a client with suicide risk, obsessive–compulsive disorder, or violent aggression.

ETHICAL ISSUES IN ESTABLISHING SUPERVISORY RELATIONSHIPS

Although it may be possible in other therapeutic settings, it is not common in schools for a clinician to select their own supervisor. At the start of the CBT supervisory process, an understanding should be reached between the supervisor and clinician regarding the supervisory relationship. This understanding typically takes the form of a contract between the two parties, otherwise known as a Document of Informed Consent to Supervise. Pratt and Lamson (2012) provided a detailed structure for this contract that informs all parties of their responsibilities within the relationship. Typically, the contract includes the parties' names and contact information, including emergency contact information; when, where, and how the supervisory sessions will occur (e.g., in person, via Zoom, on the phone); how often the sessions will occur and for how long they will last; the beginning and ending dates of supervision; and who will provide supervision or assistance if the primary supervisor is unavailable in an emergency. Disclosures regarding the entities to whom the clinician is responsible, with whom information may be shared, and the boundaries of confidentiality in the school session are included, as well as the roles that all supervisors will take, if there is more than one supervisor. Finally, a contract should specify the conditions under which it may be terminated, such as if the supervisor or clinician moves out of the area, an ethical complaint is levied, or if the clinician chooses not to attend scheduled supervision sessions. Numerous examples of supervision contracts may be accessed online.

Any supervisory contract and relationship will need to attend to the ethical and legal dimensions of the complex multiple relationships between the supervisor, clinician, child/youth client, teacher, and parents. It will be critically important for the supervisor and clinician to be aware of the bounds of confidentiality and privilege in the context of their work. Depending on who is employing them, it is possible that their work would be covered by privilege, and it is possible that it would not (Yell, 2019). Failing to clarify whether the relationships are privileged in schools and acting accordingly is one of the common pitfalls of practice in schools. Similarly, ensuring that clinicians disclose the supervisory relationship to clients at the outset and providing contact information for the supervisor is necessary (Pratt & Lamson, 2012). Additionally, supervision creates unique challenges in the relationship between the supervisor and clinician in that the supervisor is expected to be concerned for the growth, development, and well-being of the clinician in a broad sense while balancing this against their supervisory relationship. This creates unique challenges surrounding maintaining boundaries and not falling into an inappropriate dual relationship (see Vasquez, 1992). This concern also parallels the challenge of concern for the clinician's development while maintaining the primacy of the clients' rights and needs in the supervisory relationship.

In addition to numerous and complex ethical considerations, work in schools will bring supervisors and clinicians into contact with legal considerations as well. Supervisors and, to a lesser degree, clinicians should be familiar with a wide range of laws to meet standards of competency. These include the Americans With Disabilities Act (1990, 2008), the Rehabilitation Act of 1973, the Family Educational Rights and Privacy Act of 1974, and IDEA, as well as relevant state provisions of the enactment of IDEA. Obviously, comprehensive review of these laws is beyond the scope of this chapter, but they are critical elements of practice in schools.

Building Supervisor–Trainee Rapport

When supervising, consider that clinicians may be anxious about being evaluated and can make the supervisor uncomfortable as a result, possibly leading to less productive supervision. Establishing rapport is an important part of the supervisory relationship. Although there is rarely a cookbook method for establishing rapport, taking time to have discussions with the therapist about non-work-related topics in a nonthreatening environment may work toward creating a pleasant and nurturing relationship. For example, taking the therapist out to lunch periodically and talking about family, hobbies, and/or interests has been known to have a positive impact on the supervisory relationship.

THE TREATMENT PLANNING PROCESS: DESIGN, EVALUATION, AND CLOSURE

A natural progression of treatment within schools typically involves clinicians working directly with teachers or parents to design an intervention based on data collected during assessment, to evaluate its outcomes, to revise the intervention if necessary, and to wrap up the treatment process.

Designing Treatment Plans

A teacher or parent generally provides the clinician with a referral concern regarding a student. A combination of direct and indirect assessment is typically used to determine more specific information about student needs. This assessment may include meeting with the client to determine their perspective on their needs for therapy, direct observation of the student in the relevant setting(s), interviews with involved educators, interviews with parents, and behavior rating scales or objective instruments that may be used to collect data on the target behaviors for therapy. Once this has been completed, a meeting with the individual who made the referral is typically held, and target behaviors are identified, treatment goals specified, and a treatment plan or intervention designed. Important outcomes of this meeting are to determine the specific form of CBT to be implemented and what data can be collected to indicate success of CBT or a need to modify the plan.

There are, however, several decision points to negotiate before outcomes may be measured. The behavior goal and the type, intensity, and frequency of CBT must be determined (Noell & Gansle, 2006), as well as who will provide direct service and what kind of supervision will be necessary. What evaluation would be appropriate to make decisions about the success of CBT? Depending on the consultative process and the choice of intervention (which are beyond the scope of this chapter), the teacher, the MBH service provider, an aide in the classroom, or some combination may provide pieces of CBT, collect data, and evaluate them to inform the intervention course.

Measuring Treatment Plan Implementation

The implementation of a therapeutic plan is rarely assured due to the number of other demands on clinicians' and teachers' time, as well as the fact that changing both adult and child behavior is a challenging undertaking (Schwarzer, 2008). Measurement of outcomes is a critical issue in evaluating therapist growth, and the evaluation of data coupled with feedback from supervisory interactions is the primary method for improving practice. The target variable for the focus of CBT should be objectively defined. The success of CBT should be determined using measurable products as evidence for the outcomes of the therapeutic relationship between the therapist and the student. A substantial part of supervising clinicians who provide direct or consultative service for MBH concerns may be conceptualized as the evaluation of treatment plan implementation (TPI; Noell et al., 2017). In other words, are those who provide treatment doing so as designed?

Two methods for enhancing TPI may be considered antecedent and consequent approaches. Implementation planning (Hagermoser Sanetti et al., 2015) includes meeting and reviewing the plan and modifying it to improve the probability that it will be implemented prior to its enactment (Sanetti et al., 2014). For example, if teachers do not have the necessary skills to complete the part of the plan to which they are assigned, instruction might be necessary before the plan can be implemented with any expectation of success. Despite some methodological issues (Noell et al., 2017), increased levels of treatment adherence have been found following implementation planning (Fallon et al., 2016; Sanetti et al., 2014).

There is an extensive research base supporting that after treatment has been implemented, performance feedback (PFb) leads to improvements in TPI (Noell & Gansle, 2014). In PFb, the data produced by implementation of the treatment plan are reviewed with the treatment agent(s) and evaluative feedback is given about the clinician's performance in treatment compliance. The clinician may also receive assistance in determining whether the treatment requires revision, whether this treatment should be abandoned in favor of another, or whether additional treatment elements should be added to the treatment package. PFb has been shown successful with a spacing of twice per week to 2 weeks, as well as contingent on incomplete intervention delivery (Noell et al., 2017). The general process of defining what treatment should look like, clarifying how it will be measured, and providing feedback on its performance can be used both with supervisors to clinicians and with clinicians to consultees (generally parents and educators). A critical challenge is deciding how to measure implementation, whether through live or recorded observations, permanent products, or self-report. Generally, the utility of the assessment process and feedback is enhanced by maximizing direct measurement to the extent it is practical.

Measurement of Treatment Outcomes

Measurement of the treatment plan's target variables is important in determining next steps in treatment planning. If the target variables have been defined objectively, determining progress of treatment should follow logically. For example, if anxiety is the referral concern, and an anxiety rating scale score is the measure, completing the rating scale before and after intervention and comparing them is a reasonable approach. The student, teacher, or clinician may be asked to complete rating scales that measure target behaviors. The Strengths and Difficulties Questionnaire (SDQ; Goodman, 1997) is a commonly used brief screening measure of behavior of individual students that may be completed by parents, caregivers, or teachers generally to evaluate the success of CBT (McSherry et al., 2019). It has a relatively extensive history of use in assessing treatment outcomes. Although the Children's Global Assessment Scale (C-GAS; Shaffer et al., 1983) was normed in the 1980s, current research indicates that it is still a useful measure of disturbance and severity of clinical concerns (Lundh et al., 2016; White et al., 2014). The Child Behavior Checklist (Achenbach & Edelbrock, 1991) is another quality instrument that is commonly used in schools and research to evaluate a variety of symptoms that may be targets for CBT.

Depending on the size of the caseload, practitioners in schools at times may need to rely on less direct measures. Permanent product data are often helpful and have lower time costs than direct observation. If self-monitoring is part of homework from CBT, the student can be involved in the measurement of their own outcomes by monitoring and then recording that which they monitor. A natural progression would be to involve the student in their own intervention plan and follow up with self-evaluation of the target concern. Alternatively, if the CBT plan requires that the student record negative thoughts on a worksheet (Yoshino et al., 2019), the worksheets that are completed as a part of the plan can be collected, the negative thoughts counted, and the results used to evaluate success of the intervention. Additionally, use of permanent products may decrease reactivity to measurement that can result from direct observation (Foster & Cone, 1986).

Treatment Plan Evaluation and Revision

Once data are collected, they can be used to monitor the progress of CBT. If the data demonstrate progress toward treatment goals, obviously the supervisor and clinician would choose to stay the course. If the trend is negative or has plateaued, review the implementation data from all the treatment agents, and assess whether the plan is being implemented as designed. If it is not, institute another check on implementation, or change the contingencies for treatment implementation. Revising a plan that is ineffective because it is not being implemented can lead to a series of futile program revisions. A critical consideration under these conditions is improving implementation. If the program is being implemented but no positive effects are seen, it is time to reassess and determine whether the intervention is appropriate to the target concern.

Aside from measuring whether treatment was implemented, decisions should be made regarding how to measure the variables that indicate the professional growth of the clinician. Direct observation is an established method for evaluating CBT skills (Lambert & Ogles, 1997; Liese & Beck, 1997); however, to be useful for planning for future behavior, a valid and reliable observation instrument should be employed (Milne & Reiser, 2011). Although several instruments exist, there is some concern that effective operationalization of the relevant treatment components to address in clinical supervision has yet to be achieved (Milne & Reiser, 2011; Olds & Hawkins, 2014). Most evaluate the efficacy of supervision using anecdotal evidence. This is an area for future research.

Closing Therapeutic Cases and Supervisory Relationships

The closure of therapeutic cases and that of supervisory relationships have similar general structure, goals, and processes. In both instances, they should be active, planful processes that reflect purposeful work by the supervisor or clinician to add a final contribution to the supervisory or therapeutic process. Generally, the focus is to review and share goals, progress, achievements, and remaining challenges. Effective closure sessions leave participants with a strong sense of their interpersonal bond, shared work, and achievements. Additionally, an effective closure session should provide a chance to discuss remaining growth opportunities and whether and under what conditions follow-up contact with the supervisor would be appropriate. Finally, a well-structured closure session should provide space to ensure that supervisors, clinicians, and clients (if appropriate) have the opportunity to share their thoughts and feelings about therapy in what may be a final interaction.

APPROACHES TO COMMON CHALLENGES FOR SUPERVISORS AND TRAINEES

Implementing either CBT or clinical supervision in schools is complex, and their intersection can yield challenges that are both common and idiosyncratic. In this section, we identify six common challenges and describe approaches that may prove helpful in navigating them. One of the most common and natural challenges for all supervisory relationships is reluctance on the part of the trainee or supervised clinician to admit mistakes (Williams & Sommer, 2002).

Reluctance to Admit Mistakes

It is virtually universal that trainees want their supervisor to have a positive view of them, and they perceive mistakes as a barrier to achieving this end. As a result, they can be expected quite naturally to try to hide or minimize mistakes. It is critical for supervisors to address this at the outset of the relationship. Clarify that mistakes are part of learning, are expected, and within reasonable bounds, are welcome as part of the learning process. It can be quite helpful to relate stories of mistakes from previous trainees' experiences and how they were an opportunity to improve practice. This can be especially powerful in group supervision if more advanced trainees are willing to share how they grew professionally from sharing mistakes and that the process was not aversive for them.

Struggling With Boundaries

It is natural for clinicians to struggle with establishing appropriate closeness and rapport with clients, consultees, and supervisors without drifting into overly intimate relationships that are unproductive and may become dual or multiple relationships to some degree (Gottlieb et al., 2009). The critical challenge for supervisors is to be direct and honest about this struggle, acknowledging that it is always a work in progress and that errors in degree are part of the process. Supervisors should be certain to reflect on boundaries and carefully monitor the process against a desired goal.

Time Management

A third common challenge for both parties is to reasonably consider the management of time in the supervised therapeutic relationship. For CBT to be effective, it needs to move forward at a reasonable pace. Excessive delays between intake interviews, assessments, design of treatment plans, and treatment initiation can all be demoralizing for the client. However, a clinician is almost always slower at all these processes as they train: Acclimating to a new environment, locating resources, and developing skills take time. It is critical that supervisors actively manage caseloads to make good use of clinician time without overloading them so the quality of treatment is undermined by a caseload that is too heavy for the clinician's current skills.

Complexity

Complexity in presenting problems is difficult for anyone learning a new skill. For clinicians in schools, it is relatively easy to become highly focused on the skills and resources they are trying to bring to students without sufficiently appreciating the extent to which they need to adapt their approach to the student they serve. The following adage applies here: "When the only tool you have in your toolbox is a hammer, everything looks like a nail." This can be particularly true for clinicians using primarily verbal procedures within CBT across students who vary widely in developmental level due to either age or developmental challenges. It is important for supervisors to remain cognizant of the challenges and capacities of the students referred for services and ensure they are appropriate for the CBT model the clinician is learning and that appropriate developmental adaptations are made. In the absence of this meta-cognitive aspect of therapy, clinicians may lack the perspective to avoid dead-end approaches with students who will end up ill served and highly frustrated.

Appropriate Data

One of the core challenges of behavior therapy in schools is obtaining appropriate data about outcomes and treatment implementation (Noell et al., 2017). This is likely to be an ongoing frustration for both the supervisor and the clinician. The key challenge is that resources are almost always stretched, and more elaborate data collection may draw resources away from treatment. The critical challenge of the supervisor in this regard is modeling and teaching appropriate creativity in getting the best data possible, appropriate humility and skepticism about what is and can be known based on data quality, and how to negotiate a path forward. Having a supportive guide and role model for these issues can be invaluable for clinicians. Talking through these issues with clinicians in a tell–show–do manner will allow them to learn how to think about these in a productive manner.

Don't Assume Everyone Will Do What They're Asked to Do

An additional challenge that is virtually ubiquitous in behavior therapy in schools and its supervision is for clinicians and supervisors to assume that other people will follow directions. This is particularly surprising given CBT therapists' rich understanding of the effortful nature of change; the deep, reciprocal, ecological patterns sustaining current behavior; and the common disconnect between saying and doing (Karlan & Rusch, 1982). It is as if we know this but assume it does not apply to people who are working with us. The critical task for supervisors is to acknowledge the issue, promote professional skepticism about what people say about their behavior, and teach clinicians how to get better estimates of actual treatment compliance and behavior change. It would be wise for supervisors to adopt a similar worldview about their work with clinicians.

CONCLUSION

In a world in which the cost of private provider mental health services makes them functionally unavailable to many families, the school setting is an excellent one in which to provide CBT for students' mental and behavioral health concerns. Students already spend many hours per day in the setting in which services can be provided by clinicians who are available for their needs. Providing quality supervision to clinicians is an important method of ensuring students in need receive excellent service. Through the arrangement of a supervision contract, setting goals, implementing CBT, monitoring implementation and outcomes, and revising therapy as necessary, students will receive the valuable service they deserve.

REFERENCES

Achenbach, T. M., & Edelbrock, C. S. (1991). *Manual for the Child Behavior Checklist and Revised Parent Report Form for child behavior profile.* University of Vermont.

American Psychological Association. (2017). *Ethical principles of psychologists and code of conduct* (2002, Amended June 1, 2010, and January 1, 2017). http://www.apa.org/ethics/code/index.aspx

Americans With Disabilities Act Amendments Act of 2008. Pub. L. No. 110-325 (2008).

Americans With Disabilities Act of 1990. Pub. L. No. 101-336, § 2, 104 Stat. 328 (1990).

Barnett, D. W., Bauer, A. M., Ehrhardt, K. E., Lentz, F. E., & Stollar, S. A. (1996). Keystone targets for change: Planning for widespread positive consequences. *School Psychology Quarterly, 11*(2), 95–117. https://doi.org/10.1037/h0088923

Bennett-Levy, J., McManus, F., Westling, B. E., & Fennell, M. (2009). Acquiring and refining CBT skills and competencies: Which training methods are perceived to be most effective? *Behavioural and Cognitive Psychotherapy, 37*(5), 571–583. https://doi.org/10.1017/S1352465809990270

Boswell, J. F., & Constantino, M. J. (2022). *Deliberate practice in cognitive behavioral therapy.* American Psychological Association. https://doi.org/10.1037/0000256-000

Burns, B. J., Costello, E. J., Angold, A., Tweed, D., Stangl, D., Farmer, E. M. Z., & Erkanli, A. (1995). Children's mental health service use across service sectors. *Health Affairs, 14*(3), 147–159. https://doi.org/10.1377/hlthaff.14.3.147

Centers for Disease Control and Prevention. (2013). Mental health surveillance among children: United States, 2005–2011. *Morbidity and Mortality Weekly Report, 62*(Suppl. 2), 1–35. https://www.cdc.gov/mmwr/pdf/other/su6202.pdf

Eklund, K., DeMarchena, S. L., Rossen, E., Izumi, J. T., Vaillancourt, K., & Kelly, S. R. (2020). Examining the role of school psychologists as providers of mental and behavioral health services. *Psychology in the Schools, 57*(4), 489–501. https://doi.org/10.1002/pits.22323

Fallon, L. M., Collier-Meek, M. A., Sanetti, L. H., Feinberg, A. B., & Kratochwill, T. R. (2016). Implementation planning to promote parents' treatment integrity of behavioral interventions for children with autism. *Journal of Educational & Psychological Consultation, 26*(1), 87–109. https://doi.org/10.1080/10474412.2015.1039124

Family Educational Rights and Privacy Act of 1974, P.L. 93-380, 88 Scat. 57 (1974).

Farmer, E. M. Z., Burns, B. J., Phillips, S. D., Angold, A., & Costello, E. J. (2003). Pathways into and through mental health services for children and adolescents. *Psychiatric Services, 54*(1), 60–66. https://doi.org/10.1176/appi.ps.54.1.60

Fixsen, D. L., Naoom, S. F., Blase, K. A., Friedman, R. M., & Wallace, F. (2005). *Implementation research: A synthesis of the literature* (FMHI Publication No. 231). University of South Florida, Louis de la Parte Florida Mental Health Institute, The National Implementation Research Network. https://nirn.fpg.unc.edu/resources/implementation-research-synthesis-literature

Flanagan, R. (2015). Professional issues in cognitive and behavioral practice for school psychologists. In R. Flanagan, K. Allen, & E. Levine (Eds.), *Cognitive and behavioral interventions in the schools* (pp. 307–321). Springer. https://doi.org/10.1007/978-1-4939-1972-7_15

Foster, S. L., & Cone, J. D. (1986). Design and use of direct observation. In A. R. Ciminero, K. S. Calhoun, & H. E. Adams (Eds.), *Handbook of behavioral assessment* (pp. 253–324). Wiley.

Goodman, R. (1997). The Strengths and Difficulties Questionnaire: A research note. *Journal of Child Psychology and Psychiatry, 38*(5), 581–586. https://doi.org/10.1111/j.1469-7610.1997.tb01545.x

Gottlieb, M. C., Younggren, J. N., & Murch, K. B. (2009). Boundary management for cognitive behavioral therapies. *Cognitive and Behavioral Practice, 16*(2), 164–171. https://doi.org/10.1016/j.cbpra.2008.09.007

Greenberg, M. T., Weissberg, R. P., O'Brien, M. U., Zins, J. E., Fredericks, L., Resnik, H., & Elias, M. J. (2003). Enhancing school-based prevention and youth development through coordinated social, emotional, and academic learning. *American Psychologist, 58*(6-7), 466–474. https://doi.org/10.1037/0003-066X.58.6-7.466

Hagermoser Sanetti, L. M., Collier-Meek, M. A., Long, A. C., Byron, J., & Kratochwill, T. R. (2015). Increasing teacher treatment integrity of behavior support plans through consultation and implementation planning. *Journal of School Psychology, 53*, 209–229. https://doi.org/10.1016/j.jsp.2015.03.002

Hanchon, T. A., & Fernald, L. N. (2013). The provision of counseling services among school psychologists: An exploration of training, current practices, and perceptions. *Psychology in the Schools, 50*(7), 651–671. https://doi.org/10.1002/pits.21700

Individuals With Disabilities Education Improvement Act of 2004, 20 U.S.C. § 1400 (2004).

Jacob, S., & Coustasse, A. (2008). School-based mental health: A de facto mental health system for children. *Journal of Hospital Marketing & Public Relations, 18*(2), 197–211. https://doi.org/10.1080/15390940802232499

Johnston, L. H., & Milne, D. L. (2012). How do supervisees learn during supervision? A grounded theory study of the perceived developmental process. *The Cognitive Behaviour Therapist, 5*(1), 1–23. https://doi.org/10.1017/S1754470X12000013

Juszczak, L., Melinkovich, P., & Kaplan, D. (2003). Use of health and mental health services by adolescents across multiple delivery sites. *The Journal of Adolescent Health, 32*(6, Suppl.), 108–118. https://doi.org/10.1016/S1054-139X(03)00073-9

Karlan, G. R., & Rusch, F. R. (1982). Correspondence between saying and doing: Some thoughts on defining correspondence and future directions for application. *Journal of Applied Behavior Analysis, 15*(1), 151–162. https://doi.org/10.1901/jaba.1982.15-151

Kazdin, A. E. (2017). Addressing the treatment gap: A key challenge for extending evidence-based psychosocial interventions. *Behaviour Research and Therapy, 88*, 7–18. https://doi.org/10.1016/j.brat.2016.06.004

Lambert, N. J., & Ogles, B. M. (1997). The effectiveness of psychotherapy supervision. In C. E. Watkins (Ed.), *Handbook of psychotherapy supervision* (pp. 421–446). Wiley.

Liese, B. S., & Beck, J. S. (1997). Cognitive therapy supervision. In C. E. Watkins (Ed.), *Handbook of psychotherapy supervision* (pp. 114–133). Wiley.

Lundh, A., Forsman, M., Serlachius, E., Långström, N., Lichtenstein, P., & Landén, M. (2016). Psychosocial functioning in adolescent patients assessed with Children's Global

Assessment Scale (CGAS) predicts negative outcomes from age 18: A cohort study. *Psychiatry Research, 242*, 295–301. https://doi.org/10.1016/j.psychres.2016.04.050

McNamara, K. M., Walcott, C. M., Hyson, D., Goforth, A., & Rossen, E. (2019). *Results from the NASP 2015 Membership Survey, Part two: Professional practices in school psychology* [Research report]. National Association of School Psychologists. https://www.nasponline.org/Documents/Research%20and%20Policy/Research%20Center/NRR_Mem_Survey_2015_McNamara_Walcott_Hyson_2019.pdf

McSherry, D., Malet, M. F., & Weatherall, K. (2019). The Strengths and Difficulties Questionnaire (SDQ): A proxy measure of parenting stress. *British Journal of Social Work, 49*(1), 96–115. https://doi.org/10.1093/bjsw/bcy021

Merikangas, K. R., He, J. P., Burstein, M., Swanson, S. A., Avenevoli, S., Cui, L., Benjet, C., Georgiades, K., & Swendsen, J. (2010). Lifetime prevalence of mental disorders in U.S. adolescents: Results from the National Comorbidity Survey Replication—Adolescent Supplement (NCS-A). *Journal of the American Academy of Child & Adolescent Psychiatry, 49*(10), 980–989. https://doi.org/10.1016/j.jaac.2010.05.017

Milne, D. (2008). CBT supervision: From reflexivity to specialization. *Behavioural and Cognitive Psychotherapy, 36*(6), 779–786. https://doi.org/10.1017/S1352465808004773

Milne, D. L., & Reiser, R. P. (2011). Observing competence in CBT supervision: A systematic review of the available instruments. *The Cognitive Behaviour Therapist, 4*(3), 89–100. https://doi.org/10.1017/S1754470X11000067

Milne, D. L., & Reiser, R. P. (2017). *A manual for evidence-based CBT supervision*. John Wiley and Sons. https://doi.org/10.1002/9781119030799

Milne, D. L., Reiser, R. P., Cliffe, T., Breese, L., Boon, A., Raine, R., & Scarratt, P. (2011). A qualitative comparison of cognitive-behavioural and evidence-based clinical supervision. *The Cognitive Behaviour Therapist, 4*(4), 152–166. https://doi.org/10.1017/S1754470X11000092

Moeller, S. B., Rosenberg, N. K., Hvenegaard, M., Straarup, K., & Austin, S. F. (2020). A new tool for rating cognitive behavioural supervision: Preliminary findings in a clinical setting. *The Cognitive Behaviour Therapist, 13*. https://doi-org.proxy.lib.odu.edu/10.1017/S1754470X2000001X

Noell, G. H., Ardoin, S. P., & Gansle, K. A. (2009). Academic assessment. In J. L. Matson, F. Adrasik, & M. L. Matson (Eds.), *Assessing childhood psychopathology and developmental disabilities* (pp. 311–340). Springer. https://doi.org/10.1007/978-0-387-09528-8_11

Noell, G. H., & Gansle, K. A. (2006). Assuring the form has substance: Treatment plan implementation as the foundation of assessing response to intervention. *Assessment for Effective Intervention, 32*(1), 32–39. https://doi.org/10.1177/15345084060320010501

Noell, G. H., & Gansle, K. A. (2014). Research examining the relationships among consultation procedures, treatment integrity, and outcomes. In W. P. Erchul & S. M. Sheridan (Eds.), *Handbook of research in school consultation: Empirical foundations for the field* (2nd ed., pp. 386–408). Lawrence Erlbaum Associates.

Noell, G. H., Gansle, K. A., & Long, A. C. J. (in press). Behavioral consultation: Linking referral concerns, intervention, and outcomes. In L. Theodore, M. Bray, & B. Bracken (Eds.), *Desk Reference in School Psychology*. Oxford University Press.

Noell, G. H., Volz, J. R., Henderson, M. Y., & Williams, K. L. (2017). Evaluating an integrated support model for increasing treatment plan implementation following consultation in schools. *School Psychology Quarterly, 32*(4), 525–538. https://doi.org/10.1037/spq0000195

Olds, K., & Hawkins, R. (2014). Precursors to measuring outcomes in clinical supervision: A thematic analysis. *Training and Education in Professional Psychology, 8*(3), 158–164. https://doi.org/10.1037/tep0000034

Pratt, K. J., & Lamson, A. L. (2012). Supervision in behavioral health: Implications for students, interns, and new professionals. *The Journal of Behavioral Health Services & Research, 39*(3), 285–294. https://doi.org/10.1007/s11414-011-9267-6

Pugh, M., & Margetts, A. (2020). Are you sitting (un)comfortably? Action-based supervision and supervisory drift. *The Cognitive Behaviour Therapist, 13*. https://doi.org/10.1017/S1754470X20000185

Rakovshik, S. G., & McManus, F. (2013). An anatomy of CBT training: Trainees' endorsements of elements, sources and modalities of learning during a postgraduate CBT training course. *The Cognitive Behaviour Therapist, 6*, 1–12.

Rehabilitation Act of 1973. P.L.105-220, 20 U.S. Code § 9201 (1973).

Sanetti, L. H., Collier-Meek, M. A., Long, A. J., Kim, J., & Kratochwill, T. R. (2014). Using implementation planning to increase teachers' adherence and quality to behavior support plans. *Psychology in the Schools, 51*(8), 879–895. https://doi.org/10.1002/pits.21787

Schwarzer, R. (2008). Modeling health behavior change: How to predict and modify the adoption and maintenance of health behaviors. *Applied Psychology, 57*(1), 1–29. https://doi.org/10.1111/j.1464-0597.2007.00325.x

Shaffer, D., Gould, M. S., Brasic, J., Ambrosini, P., Fisher, P., Bird, H., & Aluwahlia, S. (1983). A children's global assessment scale (CGAS). *Archives of General Psychiatry, 40*(11), 1228–1231. https://doi.org/10.1001/archpsyc.1983.01790100074010

Townend, M., Iannetta, L., & Freeston, M. (2002). Clinical supervision in practice: A survey of cognitive behavioural psychotherapists accredited by the BABCP. *Behavioural and Cognitive Psychotherapy, 30*(4), 485–500. https://doi.org/10.1017/S1352465802004095

Vasquez, M. J. (1992). Psychologist as clinical supervisor: Promoting ethical practice. *Professional Psychology: Research and Practice, 22*(3), 196–202. https://doi.org/10.1037/0735-7028.23.3.196

Weist, M. D., Goldstein, A., Morris, L., & Bryant, T. (2003). Integrating expanded school mental health programs and school-based health centers. *Psychology in the Schools, 40*(3), 297–308. https://doi.org/10.1002/pits.10089

Wenzel, A. (Ed.). (2021). *Handbook of cognitive behavioral therapy: Two-volume set.* American Psychological Association.

White, S. W., Smith, L. A., & Schry, A. R. (2014). Assessment of global functioning in adolescents with autism spectrum disorders: Utility of the Developmental Disability-Child Global Assessment Scale. *Autism, 18*(4), 362–369. https://doi.org/10.1177/1362361313481287

Williams, M. B., & Sommer, J. F. (2002). Some final thoughts on competence. In M. B. Williams & J. F. Sommer Jr. (Eds.), *Simple and complex post-traumatic stress disorder: Strategies for comprehensive treatment in clinical practice* (pp. 387–398). Haworth Maltreatment and Trauma Press/The Haworth Press.

Yell, M. L. (2019). *The law and special education* (5th ed.). Pearson Education.

Yoshino, A., Okamoto, Y., Jinnin, R., Takagaki, K., Mori, A., & Yamawaki, S. (2019). Role of coping with negative emotions in cognitive behavioral therapy for persistent somatoform pain disorder: Is it more important than pain catastrophizing? *Psychiatry and Clinical Neurosciences, 73*(9), 560–565. https://doi.org/10.1111/pcn.12866

15

Cognitive Behavior Therapy Supervision of Multidisciplinary Teams in Intensive Levels of Care

Bradley C. Riemann, Nicholas R. Farrell, and Rachel C. Leonard

Cognitive behavior therapy (CBT) is a structured, skills-oriented approach to psychotherapy that has empirical support for addressing a variety of common mental health disorders (e.g., Hofmann et al., 2012). It has well-established efficacy for disorders, including anxiety disorders (Olatunji et al., 2010), obsessive–compulsive disorder (OCD) and related disorders (McKay et al., 2015), eating disorders (EDs; Linardon et al., 2017), and depression (DeRubeis et al., 2008), among others.

Two factors that drive patient response to CBT are the quality and quantity of the care delivered. Quality is commonly considered when discussing treatment response. The more a clinician adheres to the CBT model, the higher the quality of treatment they will deliver, which will result in better treatment response (Miller & Binder, 2002). While commonly discussed regarding medication, quantity or "dose" is rarely considered when discussing psychosocial treatment response. Nevertheless, there appears to be a dosage effect between the severity and complexity of a patient's presentation and how much high-quality CBT is needed to obtain a response (e.g., Stewart et al., 2005). Due in large part to this dosage effect, "intensive" CBT levels of care (LOC) have been developed. These include intensive outpatient (6–15 hours per week), partial hospital (16–30 hours per week), residential (24 hours per day, treatment model), and inpatient LOC (24 hours per day, stabilization model).

The objective of this chapter is to provide readers with a comprehensive description of the unique training and supervision needed within intensive LOC. We describe the training and supervision model used with the CBT

https://doi.org/10.1037/0000314-016
Training and Supervision in Specialized Cognitive Behavior Therapy: Methods, Settings, and Populations, E. A. Storch, J. S. Abramowitz, and D. McKay (Editors)
Copyright © 2022 by the American Psychological Association. All rights reserved.

Academy at Rogers Behavioral Health System (RBH) for the past 20 years (Farrell et al., 2019). RBH is a large, not-for-profit behavioral health care system with 18 locations in seven different states. At these locations, RBH offers 251 intensive programs, including intensive outpatient, partial hospital, residential and inpatient programs. Within these LOC, RBH offers specialty programs, including (a) OCD and anxiety disorders, (b) EDs, (c) depressive disorders, (d) trauma and related disorders, and (e) co-occurring mental health and substance use disorders. Over this time frame, thousands of staff members have been trained and supervised utilizing CBT Academy.

IDENTIFYING APPROPRIATE TRAINEES

All prospective trainees are interviewed to determine their goodness of fit for the training program and ultimate role. It is important to establish consistency between a prospective trainee's theoretical treatment approach and the program model they will be required to follow. Even though this is not unique to intensive levels of care, we believe this is such a critical piece that we will review several basic steps used at RBH. First, we ask about the extent to which the individual believes in the CBT model by asking questions such as, "Do you believe that maladaptive thoughts and behaviors cause emotional disturbances?" and "Do you believe the targets of treatment should be those maladaptive thoughts and behaviors?" If a trainee can answer "yes" to these questions, they may be a good candidate for training. If not, it has been our experience that they will not be.

We also ask specific questions to identify goodness of fit for the specific role or program for which we are interviewing. This is especially important when interviewing individuals to work in our OCD programs. For these programs, we also ask prospective trainees to assess whether they would be able, without hesitation, to conduct exposures, including those targeting contamination (e.g., touch a toilet seat and not wash their hands) or religious obsessions (e.g., write the number 666 in red ink). The premise here is that not everyone is cut out for this type of work. It is critical that prospective employees in OCD programs can effectively work with all types of OCD symptoms and engage in any necessary exposures. Similarly, we ask about experience and comfort level with tasks specific to other programs, such as assessing one's comfort level with guiding patients in trauma-focused exposure therapy and assessing for endorsement of a "diet culture mentality" for individuals seeking to work in ED programs.

Next, we evaluate the potential trainee's ability to work in an intensive treatment environment. There are several key questions to note here. First, are they a team player or do they prefer to have autonomy in providing treatment services? It is important to discuss the high levels of severity and the corresponding levels of disability and impairment they will routinely see in higher LOC and evaluate their fit for these settings. Working in higher LOC can be challenging for some individuals, especially at the residential level of care. Examples of impairment are given (e.g., incontinence, suicidal threats), and each trainee is asked to assess their comfort level with these scenarios.

KEY TRAINING CONCEPTS

All trainees in intensive LOC need to learn several key concepts. These include the treatment components and goals in different LOC, the importance of working within a multidisciplinary team (MDT), and the need to adhere to the standardized treatment delivered.

Treatment Components and Goals of Different LOC

Trainees in intensive LOC need to learn the differences between each LOC and how this impacts their responsibilities. Intensive LOC differ in terms of the number of hours of treatment delivered each day, the components of treatment, the level of support provided after the treatment day concludes, and the goals for treatment. Each trainee needs to understand and stay within the respective program parameters. Trainees need to understand the importance of starting and stopping programming on time. They need to know what components of treatment to include and when, how, and why to include them (i.e., scope of treatment). For example, is family therapy part of the treatment day? If so, at what time during the program hours can and should it occur? Can it be done after program hours when it is more convenient for the family? The importance of homework assignments (i.e., self-directed therapeutic work), including what to assign and how much to assign, also needs to be covered.

Intensive outpatient and partial hospital programs do not provide support after regular program hours offered in residential or inpatient treatment. Patients are generally instructed to list questions that may arise on evenings and weekends and bring these the next treatment day. It is also critical that all patients in intensive outpatient and partial hospital programs are told that, in the case of an emergency, they should go to the nearest emergency department, call 911, or call a local designated emergency line. Trainees need to be aware of these important issues and what to instruct their patients to do in each case. In contrast, in residential and inpatient LOC, the program is staffed 24 hours per day, seven days per week. Trainees need to know what they should be doing and what their responsibilities are during nonprogramming times (e.g., visitation hours, therapeutic outings) and how to handle a psychiatric crisis or emergency, including who to contact.

Different LOC also have very different goals for the treatment experience. Inpatient care is built to stabilize a psychiatric crisis in a short period of time (i.e., average duration of treatment may be 5–7 days). Compared with inpatient care, residential treatment is a longer term treatment model. Patients will have high levels of symptom severity and complexity, and, thus, high levels of disability as well. As a result, average duration of treatment may vary widely, but it is not unusual for a patient to be treated for 45 to 60 days. The goal for residential treatment is reduction of symptoms to the point at which the corresponding disability has been reduced so that 24-hour support is no longer needed. The treatment goal for partial hospitalization depends on if the patient is going to discharge to intensive outpatient or straight to traditional outpatient treatment (i.e., 1–2 hours per week), as the treatment goals would vary depending on the discharge plan. It is crucial for trainees to understand these important differences in intensive LOC. Additionally, intensive LOC trainees need to learn and accept that they will never get to "finish what they start." Although significant reductions in symptoms and disability are routinely achieved, patients are still often symptomatic, even when discharging from an intensive outpatient program to a traditional one. This is a unique aspect of intensive LOC, and preparing clinicians for this through training is critical.

Working Within a Multidisciplinary Team

Due to the nature of intensive LOC, MDTs are necessary, and, as a result, issues and concepts related to MDTs and the need to work within a team structure need to be included in any training and supervision experience. Team members may include psychologists, psychiatrists, nurses, master's-degree-holding therapists and/or social workers, paraprofessionals, and dieticians. Training should include role clarification, as well as key theoretical concepts and techniques to provide a standard treatment experience and ensure that all are on the same philosophical page and using the same nomenclature while interacting with patients and their families.

An important aspect of an MDT is the professional hierarchy within it. Understanding each person's role and responsibility, as well as who makes the final decisions, is an important training component. This includes using professional titles when communicating to or referring to a member of the team to a patient or their family (e.g., "Dr. Smith"), fully supporting the treatment decisions made by the team leader(s), and generally following the chain of command (i.e., resolving differences in opinion as a team and agreeing to defer to recognized clinical and medical program leaders if these differences cannot be resolved).

Depending on the intensity of the LOC, ancillary staff such as clinic receptionists, teachers, and, perhaps, even housekeeping staff need to provide support consistent with the treatment messages provided by the team. Thus, they also need to have a basic understanding of the verbiage and treatment principles used.

Adherence to the Standardized Treatment Delivered

Finally, the importance of providing and adhering to standardized treatment protocols within an intensive LOC is reviewed. Although each patient follows an individualized treatment plan, intensive programs at RBH implement strict empirically supported, manualized treatment protocols. We discuss "treatment rails" that providers need to stay on enabling us to provide the best care possible (i.e., variability in treatment delivery leads to poorer outcomes). Any deviation from these protocols needs to be discussed with and approved by members of the MDT before initiating. All treatment components need to be offered to each patient without fail. To ensure all staff have sufficient knowledge of the standardized treatment protocols used at RBH, a robust training program, CBT Academy, was developed (see the next section for more information).

In addition to the tactical aspects of training, we also emphasize the importance of understanding and communicating the "why" behind those tactics. Spending time explaining the rationale behind these key concepts is a wise investment of time and resources, as it greatly increases staff buy-in and adherence to the model. Furthermore, staff understanding of the theoretical underpinnings of the treatment interventions likely enhances the quality of their delivery, thereby improving treatment response (Abramowitz, 2013).

Any negative beliefs related to CBT must also be addressed. These can commonly include the belief that treatments adhering to a protocol or manual compromise the therapeutic relationship and stifle therapist creativity (Addis et al., 1999) or the belief that exposure therapy poses unreasonable risk for harm to patients (Deacon et al., 2013). Often, discussing the rationale for the techniques being used assists in uncovering and countering these beliefs. If a trainee is unable to align themselves with the CBT model, they are directed to seek employment elsewhere, possibly within a different department within the system.

KEY TRAINING TECHNIQUES: CBT ACADEMY COMPONENTS

Many of the key CBT techniques that trainees in intensive LOC need to learn overlap with standard evidence-based outpatient therapy, so we do not review these techniques here (e.g., exposure and response prevention for OCD, behavioral activation [BA] for depression; see Chapters 1 and 8, this volume, for more information on these topics). Instead, we focus on providing more detail on the components of CBT Academy and techniques that are more unique to intensive LOC. CBT Academy is a required, comprehensive training program consisting of three components: didactic instruction, required readings, and job shadowing.

Core Components of CBT Academy

The first component involves intensive didactic instruction, which includes approximately 10 days of workshop-based instruction on specific CBT strategies most often utilized in the CBT-based treatment programs within RBH (e.g., exposure therapy). Many of the workshops require participants to engage in role-playing activities and other experiential tasks (e.g., creating an exposure hierarchy) to further facilitate skills acquisition. In addition to learning specific CBT strategies, trainees are also taught about the self-report assessment instruments given to patients, including information about scoring interpretation, basic psychometric properties of the instruments, and how patients' scores inform treatment decisions. The presenters are licensed clinical psychologists with considerable training and experience within their topic areas, often including published academic articles related to the topics on which they present. Trainees complete a quiz on each of the content areas and are given two opportunities to pass each quiz with a score of 80% or higher.

The second component of training includes required readings from a collection of manuals, books, and journal articles on CBT-based treatment interventions utilized across our programs. With guidance from their clinical supervisor, trainees are expected to integrate key aspects of these readings into their clinical practice of CBT (e.g., discouraging avoidance of scheduled BA activities).

Finally, the third component of the training program involves shadowing trained staff members working within different CBT-based treatment programs. General trainees, or those who would like to provide this care but for whom there is not yet a specific role identified, shadow within diverse programs to gain experience with different levels of care and patient populations. This includes shadowing within inpatient, residential, partial hospital program, and intensive outpatient LOC; shadowing within programs that provide treatment to children, adolescents, and adults; and shadowing within programs that provide the specialized treatment RBH delivers for OCD and other anxiety disorders, EDs, mood disorders, posttraumatic stress disorder, and substance use disorders. At times, trainees have already been identified to fill specific roles, pending their performance throughout the training process. For these individuals, their shadowing schedule may be more targeted toward their eventual role. As the course of shadowing progresses, trainees are encouraged to increase their involvement in facilitating various CBT techniques as their skill proficiency allows.

Trainees are required to complete a skills checklist indicating which skills they have performed, whether they were observed performing the skill, and any additional notes or questions they had about the skill. Some examples of skills included on this checklist are providing psychoeducation (e.g., rationale for exposure therapy), developing an exposure or BA hierarchy, and "coaching" a patient during an exposure task. Trainees provide a confidence rating for how well they feel they can perform each of the skills included in the checklist. Further, trainers complete a corresponding survey to evaluate trainees' skills. The supervising psychologist may then review these evaluations to determine additional training needs.

Therapeutic Homework

An additional part of CBT Academy's training is developing and assigning therapeutic homework. Homework is a critical part of any CBT LOC (Kazantzis et al., 2010). Treatment-related homework is an essential component in acquiring new CBT learning and skills, generalizing new learning to existing and novel situations, and, ultimately, maintaining learning after formal treatment has ceased. Trainees are taught the role homework plays in the treatment process (e.g., definition of homework, outcomes, benefits), including the importance of homework adherence on outcomes (e.g., Simpson et al., 2011), how to communicate this role to patients and their families, and the different types of homework assignments. Homework types include behavioral interventions (e.g., in vivo exposure, imaginal exposure, BA, prolonged exposure), cognitive techniques (e.g., reappraising maladaptive thoughts), and self-monitoring of symptoms. We emphasize the individualized nature of homework, as well as the collaborative process of creating homework assignments, including the developmental appropriateness of those assignments (e.g., using concrete, understandable language when working with youth). We also emphasize homework adherence, which is the extent to which patients complete the recommended homework (Kazantzis et al., 2016), including the quantity completed (i.e., time spent, number of trials), and the quality of homework (e.g., completing exposure trials as prescribed). Clear expectations of the time spent each day completing homework are necessary. Other areas covered include the benefits of using a homework coach and the role family can play, identifying barriers to homework completion (e.g., safety behaviors, motivation), strategies to enhance compliance, goal setting, and use of rewards systems.

LOC-Specific Techniques

There are also important techniques that trainees need to learn that are unique to intensive LOC. Due to the severity and complexity of patient presentations in intensive LOC, these primarily center on staff and patient safety, and team members receive annual training on these skills. Trainings include distress management, nonviolent crisis intervention, and self-defense. Other trainings focused on ensuring safety in a psychiatric setting include safety searches, hospital code systems, infection control, fire safety, milieu management, and basic lifesaving, including first aid, choking, and cardiopulmonary resuscitation. Other trainings related to regulatory guidelines and compliance include the Emergency Medical Treatment and Labor Act and medication administration.

Post-CBT Academy Supervision

In addition to the training described previously, once a trainee has completed CBT Academy, they receive weekly group and individual supervision from a licensed psychologist or experienced master's-level clinician working within their program. Individual supervision covers a range of topics but typically includes discussion of patients' progress, including relevant assessment scores and progress in the exposure or BA hierarchy; any additions or subtractions to those hierarchies; additional skills training (e.g., providing additional information about a technique, role playing, modeling); discussion of any legal, ethical, cultural, or safety concerns; and overall clinical direction (i.e., which strategies to use with specific patients). Patients in higher LOC often have multiple diagnoses, so case conceptualization and assistance in prioritizing different treatment needs are other important aspect of the supervision process. Also, if relevant, discussions on problem solving related to noncompliance with the treatment plan (i.e., motivation, secondary gains) occur.

Group supervision occurs during multidisciplinary, weekly team meetings in which specific cases are discussed, and clinical direction and guidance regarding use of specific interventions is provided. Each member of the MDT reports on their work with each patient. Consistent with measurement-based care, patients' progress measures and the hierarchy completion percentage are also reviewed to help guide discussion, direct any changes in the treatment plan, and assist with discharge planning.

Intensive LOC also provide ample opportunity for supervising psychologists to directly observe staff interactions with patients. Supervisors can prioritize new trainees to assist or gauge fidelity, or cases that are not responding to treatment as usual.

PATIENT CHARACTERISTICS THAT MAKE GOOD AND POOR TRAINING CASES

By the very nature of intensive LOC, patients presenting for treatment tend to be severe and complex. As a result, trainees should be exposed to all cases within a clinical program, including severe and complex cases, during their training shadow shifts. We do not implement a hierarchy of training cases starting with more straightforward cases and then working our way up over time. In intensive LOC, there are not many of these cases as acute ones; complex patients with multiple diagnoses are the rule rather than exception. We want our trainees to be exposed to a variety of cases, including patients who are not responding to treatment as usual, so they learn to pivot treatment plans and utilize the MDT to course correct. Rather, we emphasize getting new trainees to shadow our most experienced providers. RBH has developed a preceptor program in which seasoned staff are vetted and trained on how to train others during shadow shifts. Once the preceptor course is completed, staff are then eligible to train others and are compensated at a higher rate when engaged in precepting tasks. Preceptor training includes how to switch "hats" from coworker to coach, specific skills needed to coach someone else and provide feedback, guidance on how to determine priorities for shadow shifts, and information about the importance of serving as a role model.

COMMON MISTAKES MADE BY TRAINEES AND HOW TO FIX THEM

In this section, we review common mistakes that we observe in our intensive LOC trainees. Areas of concern include issues related to implementing treatment protocols and balancing staff or patient effort.

Protocol Drift

One common mistake we observe is lack of fidelity when implementing treatment protocols. RBH provides highly manualized treatment within our intensive LOC. As discussed earlier, trainees are instructed on implementing these protocols within CBT Academy. Fidelity to these treatment protocols is measured in a variety of ways, including formal assessments conducted by the trainee's supervisor. A common phenomenon is protocol drift (e.g., Waller, 2009). Over time, some providers begin to adhere less and less to the treatment protocol they should be utilizing. This fact illustrates the importance of ongoing maintenance monitoring, in addition to initial monitoring to establish competence. Adherence to treatment protocols is of particular importance within intensive LOC to limit patient and staff confusion and maximize patient outcomes.

At times, this drift seems to be deliberate. Despite vetting trainee candidates in terms of goodness of fit, some staff members with different therapeutic perspectives slip through the training gate. Once in a patient care position, they may revert to what their previous training may have taught them and veer away from the established protocol. In these cases, some trainees are required to repeat CBT Academy or certain elements of it. They may also receive more supervision and more frequent fidelity monitoring. In other cases, formal human resources–related interventions are necessary, including performance improvement plans and, at times, reassignment or dismissal.

Protocol drift, however, generally takes place with less awareness or intent on the part of the provider. Over time, erosion from the model happens slowly, and the provider may not even be aware of the drift. Subtle comments made in supervision or observations made during fidelity monitoring may not seem to be violations of the treatment protocol, but they could be an indicator that drift is occurring and should be addressed (i.e., the old saying of "give an inch and they will take a mile" is very relevant when it comes to protocol drift). At times, trainees may need to repeat certain elements of CBT Academy, but, most commonly, this is managed within supervision and is quickly corrected, especially if caught early. Specific areas of erosion-related protocol drift we commonly observe include pairing arousal reduction techniques (e.g., diaphragmatic breathing) with exposures, permitting safety behaviors, and not responding quickly or skillfully to lack of cooperation with treatment assignments.

Focusing Too Much on Protocol

Although protocol drift is common, another mistake we see is focusing exclusively on protocol implementation and not on other key therapeutic constructs such as rapport building. At times, well-intended clinicians can get so wrapped up in following the protocol that they can deliver it in a sterile, robotic fashion with limited patient engagement. Each trainee is asked to work on developing their own style of delivery. They shadow with multiple preceptors and are asked to take elements of strength from each and combine into their own delivery "package." Shadowing their clinical preceptors should also allow them to see how to interact with their patients on a more personal, yet professional, manner. Given the nature of intensive CBT and the compressed, frequent interactions between staff and patients, this is even more critical than in traditional outpatient LOC.

Another common mistake is the lack of balance between provider and patient effort within intensive LOC. We often observe trainees and new staff not "pushing" patients far enough. As discussed previously, for a patient to be appropriate for intensive CBT LOC, a high degree of severity and complexity needs to be present. Well-meaning staff may be reluctant to ask someone who is suffering to engage in certain treatment elements (e.g., exposing the patient to feared situations and circumstances). This may occur in isolated incidents (e.g., not assigning as much work because a patient was having a bad day) or for an entire treatment episode (e.g., not establishing complete response prevention for OCD before discharging). We discuss trainees "pushing patients too far" in terms of specific assignments later in the ethics section.

Imbalance Between Staff Effort and Patient Effort

This issue of balance can also be related to overall treatment effort exerted by the staff and patient. Staff often expend considerable energy at the beginning of treatment with their patients on rapport building and identifying motivation for treatment. The didactic phase of CBT Academy includes training in motivational interviewing strategies. If, though, after these efforts have continued for some time and the patient has not increased engagement in treatment to the point where they will likely benefit, then it may be necessary to examine alternatives.

There may be instances in which "you can't work harder than your patient and expect a good outcome." We must work as hard as our patients and their families, but if we are consistently putting in more effort than they are, it is unlikely they will respond to treatment. It is important to determine if the timing is not right or if an alternative approach or focus of treatment may needed before the patient will benefit from the treatment being provided. This balance is a difficult but important element to training and needs to be connected to rapport building, as discussed previously. This area is a focus for ongoing supervision with most of our trainees and is a common source of burnout for intensive clinicians, given the types of patients they treat.

The lack of balancing provider and patient effort can also occur when a trainee asks their patients to do too much. A common error we observe is a provider attempting to treat all diagnoses and symptoms simultaneously. In intensive LOC, it is not uncommon for a patient to have multiple diagnoses that cause significant impairment. An advantage to intensive LOC is being able to address most, if not all, symptom areas prior to discharge but not necessarily at the same time. Trainees need to learn to assess each patient's treatment capacity and how much they can handle (i.e., therapeutic "bandwidth"). Based on this assessment, a provider can form an individualized case conceptualization and prioritize what to work on and when. The issue of "timing is everything" related to what and when to therapeutically address is a focus of training and ongoing supervision.

ETHICAL ISSUES IN TREATMENT APPLICATION

A common ethical issue related to CBT and, particularly with exposure therapy, is "how far to go" with a patient. This is a significant problem but, obviously, not unique to intensive LOC and, therefore, is discussed only briefly. Our training instructs trainees to not ask patients to do anything they would not do themselves, anything illegal, or anything that is dangerous. Discussion also includes being sensitive to a patient's cultural background in determining therapeutic endpoints. As a general rule of thumb, our trainees are encouraged to follow the guidelines of Olatunji et al. (2009), who advocated that clinicians must carefully consider patient safety and well-being in designing exposures but can proceed confidently if the exposure task in consideration involves stimuli that at least some people routinely encounter without an unreasonably high risk for harm or serious misfortune.

Intensive LOC are unique treatment settings and, therefore, pose unique ethical concerns. Patients spend between three and 24 hours per day with MDTs for weeks, if not months, at a time. This allows staff to gain a thorough understanding of the patient's treatment needs and to provide much-needed care to help alleviate their suffering. Intensive LOC allow time to discuss not only their diagnostic-related issues but help support other life areas such as relationships, school, and work, or unemployment. In residential and inpatient LOC, staff may need to assist with activities of daily living, such as getting out of bed, completing bathing or grooming routines, or plating a meal. All this time and energy spent together creates a unique bond between staff and patient. In the majority of cases, this bond helps propel the patient to achieve life-changing progress. It is quite common to have patients and their families tell team members that you "saved my life" and "I will be forever grateful." Patients and their families will routinely send holiday cards, school pictures, and graduation and wedding announcements. These reminders of the positive impact MDTs can have on a patient's life are rewarding and reinforcing of all the effort that is put into patient care. However, this bond can also pose some unique ethical issues related to intensive treatment application.

Therapeutic boundary setting is an example of an ethical issue that can arise in intensive LOC. Strong empathetic and supportive relationships are necessary to maximize therapeutic gains, but these relationships must not progress any further. Staff and patients need to be reminded that we are not family or friends. We cannot accept gifts or take pictures with one another. All team members receive extensive, annual trainings on boundaries and ethics, and this is a focal point for administrative, medical, and clinical leadership oversight on all units. Additional annual trainings are conducted on regulatory compliance, Health Insurance Portability and Accountability Act (HIPAA), cultural diversity, and patient rights, concerns, and grievances.

COMMON OBSTACLES IN SUPERVISION AND STRATEGIES TO ADDRESS THEM

As discussed previously, supervision with a licensed psychologist is a key component of RBH's intensive LOC. A common mistake we see is staff, at times, not taking advantage of supervision by not bringing up areas of growth related to their treatment skills. In some cases, it seems to be related to a lack of insight (i.e., they do not know what they do not know). An effective countermeasure to this is ongoing maintenance fidelity monitoring. This allows supervisors to see for themselves what "blind spots" are present. Another reason for not taking advantage of supervision is a reluctance to admit gaps or areas where they may need more skill building. At times, this can be related to not wanting to disappoint their supervisors or even concerns over their continuing employment. It is imperative for supervisors to encourage open discussion and reinforce trainees for their disclosures. The spirit of these meetings should be continuous improvement related to patient care. Reluctance to admit gaps can, at times, be exacerbated if supervision is conducted in group format, as trainees may not only not want to avoid disappointing their supervisor but also may be embarrassed to admit these gaps in front of peers. A solution we have found helpful is to require a trainee to come to individual or group supervision with at least two questions each week. This establishes a teaching environment and normalizes asking questions.

CONCLUSION

Intensive CBT LOC are necessary for some individuals due to the severity and complexity of diagnoses and the subsequent impairment they cause. Intensive LOC have many of the same training needs that traditional outpatient programs have. However, several areas appear to be more unique to intensive LOC. The CBT Academy training program at RBH was used as the model for this discussion. It focuses on providing a standard training experience that includes didactic education, readings, clinical shadow shifts, annual supportive trainings, and ongoing supervision to effectively implement the standard treatment protocols used in over 250 intensive CBT programs across the country.

Several unique conceptual trainings include readiness to work in an intensive LOC, differences between levels related to logistics and treatment goals, working as a member of an MDT, and the need for adherence to standardized therapeutic practices. Specific techniques requiring training in intensive LOC center primarily on patient safety and the need for ongoing supervision and mentorship regardless of how long one has practiced. CBT Academy is a training model that provides a wealth of diverse training opportunities such that trainees develop an impressively well-rounded skill set.

Common mistakes seen in intensive LOC are clinical drift, both strategic and otherwise, as well as an imbalance in therapeutic effort between the MDT and the patient. Fidelity monitoring can greatly reduce the occurrence of these issues. Although supervision is a key component to providing care in intensive LOC, not all trainees take full advantage of it due to a lack of insight and, at times, embarrassment to admit skill deficits. An area of particular concern for intensive LOC is boundary issues. At times, the time and energy spent between team members and patients seem to blur the line for some between a strong therapeutic relationship and something beyond. There needs to be constant boundary vigilance, and regular discussions within supervision related to boundaries and ethics is imperative.

REFERENCES

Abramowitz, J. S. (2013). The practice of exposure therapy: Relevance of cognitive-behavioral theory and extinction theory. *Behavior Therapy, 44*(4), 548–558. https://doi.org/10.1016/j.beth.2013.03.003

Addis, M. E., Wade, W. A., & Hatgis, C. (1999). Barriers to dissemination of evidence-based practices: Addressing practitioners concerns about manual-based psycho-therapies. *Clinical Psychology: Science and Practice, 6*(4), 430–441. https://doi.org/10.1093/clipsy.6.4.430

Deacon, B. J., Farrell, N. R., Kemp, J. J., Dixon, L. D., Sy, J. T., Zhang, A. R., & McGrath, P. B. (2013). Assessing therapist reservations about exposure therapy for anxiety disorders: The Therapist Beliefs about Exposure scale. *Journal of Anxiety Disorders, 27*(8), 772–780. https://doi.org/10.1016/j.janxdis.2013.04.006

DeRubeis, R. J., Siegle, G. J., & Hollon, S. D. (2008). Cognitive therapy versus medication for depression: Treatment outcomes and neural mechanisms. *Nature Reviews Neuroscience, 9*(10), 788–796. https://doi.org/10.1038/nrn2345

Farrell, N. R., Leonard, R. C., & Riemann, B. C. (2019). The 'behavioral specialist' model of training novice paraprofessional clinicians: An innovative, cost-effective approach for increasing the scalability of CBT. *Behavior Therapist, 42*(4), 111–117.

Hofmann, S. G., Asnaani, A., Vonk, I. J., Sawyer, A. T., & Fang, A. (2012). The efficacy of cognitive behavioral therapy: A review of meta-analyses. *Cognitive Therapy and Research, 36*(5), 427–440. https://doi.org/10.1007/s10608-012-9476-1

Kazantzis, N., Whittington, C., & Dattilio, F. (2010). Meta-analysis of homework effects in cognitive and behavioral therapy: A replication and extension. *Clinical Psychology: Science and Practice, 17*(2), 144–156. https://doi.org/10.1111/j.1468-2850.2010.01204.x

Kazantzis, N., Whittington, C., Zelencich, L., Kyrios, M., Norton, P. J., & Hofmann, S. G. (2016). Quantity and quality of homework compliance: A meta-analysis of relations with outcome in cognitive behavior therapy. *Behavior Therapy, 47*(5), 755–772. https://doi.org/10.1016/j.beth.2016.05.002

Linardon, J., Wade, T. D., de la Piedad Garcia, X., & Brennan, L. (2017). The efficacy of cognitive-behavioral therapy for eating disorders: A systematic review and meta-analysis. *Journal of Consulting and Clinical Psychology, 85*(11), 1080–1094. https://doi.org/10.1037/ccp0000245

McKay, D., Sookman, D., Neziroglu, F., Wilhelm, S., Stein, D. J., Kyrios, M., Matthews, K., & Veale, D. (2015). Efficacy of cognitive-behavioral therapy for obsessive–compulsive disorder. *Psychiatry Research, 225*(3), 236–246. https://doi.org/10.1016/j.psychres.2014.11.058

Miller, S. J., & Binder, J. L. (2002). The effects of manual-based training on treatment fidelity and outcome: A review of the literature on adult individual psychotherapy. *Psychotherapy: Theory, Research, & Practice, 39*(2), 184–198. https://doi.org/10.1037/0033-3204.39.2.184

Olatunji, B. O., Cisler, J. M., & Deacon, B. J. (2010). Efficacy of cognitive behavioral therapy for anxiety disorders: A review of meta-analytic findings. *The Psychiatric Clinics of North America, 33*(3), 557–577. https://doi.org/10.1016/j.psc.2010.04.002

Olatunji, B. O., Deacon, B. J., & Abramowitz, J. S. (2009). The cruelest cure? Ethical issues in the implementation of exposure-based treatments. *Cognitive and Behavioral Practice, 16*(2), 172–180. https://doi.org/10.1016/j.cbpra.2008.07.003

Simpson, H. B., Maher, M. J., Wang, Y., Bao, Y., Foa, E. B., & Franklin, M. (2011). Patient adherence predicts outcome from cognitive behavioral therapy in obsessive-compulsive disorder. *Journal of Consulting and Clinical Psychology, 79*(2), 247–252. https://doi.org/10.1037/a0022659

Stewart, S. E., Stack, D. E., Farrell, C., Pauls, D. L., & Jenike, M. A. (2005). Effectiveness of intensive residential treatment (IRT) for severe, refractory obsessive-compulsive disorder. *Journal of Psychiatric Research, 39*(6), 603–609. https://doi.org/10.1016/j.jpsychires.2005.01.004

Waller, G. (2009). Evidence-based treatment and therapist drift. *Behaviour Research and Therapy, 47*(2), 119–127. https://doi.org/10.1016/j.brat.2008.10.018

16

Supervising the Delivery of Cognitive Behavior Therapy for Children and Adolescents

Amanda Palo

Cognitive behavior therapy (CBT) has been heavily studied in the last half-century and is a mainstay in the psychotherapy world. It has been adapted for several mental health concerns, populations, and modalities. Given the evidence base in favor of CBT when it comes to effectively treating various mental health disorders in child or adolescent populations (Weisz & Kazdin, 2017), it follows that most psychology training programs strive for trainees to develop a solid foundation in delivering this intervention. Thus, there is a call for qualified supervisors who can provide effective training in CBT interventions.

In brief, CBT is based on the cognitive behavioral model (Beck, 1964), which proposes that an individual's perception or interpretation of a situation has a significant impact on the way the individual is affected by the situation (e.g., emotional reactions, behavior). Beck (1976) proposed three levels of cognition central to the cognitive model: core beliefs or cognitive schemas, dysfunctional assumptions, and negative automatic thoughts. The latter two components operate together to filter information in such a way that it remains consistent with an individual's core beliefs. This cognitive model underscores the importance of cognitive processes in the ways in which individuals interpret, react, and make meaning from experiences. CBT incorporates the cognitive model while also acknowledging the important role behavior has in impacting emotional experiences. The cognitive behavioral model proposes that thoughts, behaviors, and emotions all influence one another; therefore, we can influence emotions by intervening at the level of our thoughts and/or behaviors. Of note, thoughts, feelings, and behaviors do not occur in isolation; the environmental

https://doi.org/10.1037/0000314-017
Training and Supervision in Specialized Cognitive Behavior Therapy: Methods, Settings, and Populations, E. A. Storch, J. S. Abramowitz, and D. McKay (Editors)

context must be considered when developing a formulation and implementing CBT interventions. For children in particular, this includes the family, school, and social contexts.

CBT is an evidence-based intervention for a variety of presenting problems in childhood (Weisz & Kazdin, 2017). While specific strategies implemented may depend on the presenting problem (e.g., anxiety, depression, behavioral difficulties), each intervention is grounded in CBT theory and focuses on addressing problematic thoughts and behaviors. In general, CBT focuses on teaching clients how to change the ways they think and behave in an effort to more positively impact their emotions. Given the importance of the family context, as well as the child's developmental level, the practice of CBT with children often heavily involves the child's parents. At the cognitive level, treatment may involve helping a child identify "thinking traps" that can contribute to feelings of anxiety, anger, or sadness and learn ways of becoming "detectives with their thoughts" in order to restructure unhelpful cognitions. At the behavioral level, treatment can involve teaching the child emotion regulation or social skills, encouraging them to reduce avoidance and, instead, face their fears (i.e., exposure therapy), as well as teaching the child's parents effective behavioral strategies to manage behavioral difficulties.

KEY CONCEPTS FOR TRAINEES TO LEARN

Supervisors who are working with trainees should ensure that the trainees develop an understanding of several key concepts integral to effectively implementing CBT with children and families. Beck (2011) provided a good summary of these concepts, which are outlined next.

CBT is a present-focused, time-limited treatment that is structured, goal oriented, and problem focused. To this end, trainees benefit from introduction to the notion that CBT sessions typically have a specific structure, usually involving setting the agenda, briefly checking in with the patient regarding their homework from the previous session, introduction to or practice of skills, and assigning new homework.

The therapeutic alliance is of critical importance in delivering CBT, like any form of psychotherapy. Therapists must develop a strong working alliance with their child patients, as well as the patient's family, in order to effectively implement the treatment, which requires the therapist to be both collaborative and directive. This is particularly critical in exposure-based treatment involving confronting feared triggers. The stance of the therapist channels collaborative empiricism, in which the therapist and the child are a team working together to investigate the beliefs that the child has in an open, curious manner (Friedberg & McClure, 2002).

Another vital skill trainees must learn is case conceptualization, which facilitates the selection of appropriate CBT interventions, given the patient's unique characteristics and presentation. In addition, trainees should become well-versed in the CBT model, with a clear understanding that treatment involves applying techniques focused on changing a child's behavior and thinking. These characteristics and concepts of CBT provide the framework in which trainees can begin implementing treatment techniques with children and their families.

KEY TECHNIQUES FOR TRAINEES TO LEARN

CBT for youth involves various techniques that therapists must learn and master. These may be categorized in terms of cognitive techniques (e.g., cognitive restructuring, guided discovery) and behavioral techniques (e.g., exposure therapy, breathing and relaxation techniques). Specific techniques are designed for specific presenting problems, for instance, use of exposure therapy with anxiety and obsessive–compulsive disorders, behavioral activation with depressive disorders, and behavioral parent training with disruptive behavior disorders. Additional techniques that are appropriate for a wide variety of presenting problems in youth include mindfulness, problem solving or social-skills training, and behavioral experiments. A more detailed discussion of these techniques is beyond the scope of this chapter, but readers can consult earlier chapters within this volume for additional information (Murphy & Christner, 2006).

PATIENT CHARACTERISTICS THAT MAKE FOR A GOOD CBT TRAINING CASE

Research suggests that various CBT interventions are effective treatments for essentially the full spectrum of mental health concerns among children and adolescents, including anxiety disorders, depression, disruptive behavior disorders, attention-deficit/hyperactivity disorder, autism spectrum disorder, eating disorders, and elimination disorders (Weisz & Kazdin, 2017). However, various patient factors can complicate CBT implementation. A good training case for a clinician new to implementing CBT might involve the following: a youth patient with no comorbid diagnoses, who regularly attends sessions, completes homework assignments, is engaged in the therapy process, and has parents or caregivers who are motivated and engaged in treatment. In contrast, a poor training case may have the following characteristics: a youth with a complex presentation, including multiple comorbid diagnoses; parents who are disengaged or do not see the value in therapy; and a youth who attends sessions irregularly and struggles to complete homework assignments.

COMMON MISTAKES THAT TRAINEES MAKE AND HOW TO ADDRESS THEM

When beginning to learn and implement CBT with children and families, it is common for trainees to experience a variety of different pitfalls. Surprisingly, there are few empirical data addressing this issue. An exception is a study by

Waltman and colleagues (2017), who identified several common pitfalls supervisors observed when supervising the implementation of CBT with adults among practitioners in community mental health settings. These included difficulties related to guided discovery, focusing on key content, strategy, agenda setting, application of CBT techniques, homework, feedback, and pacing. Clinical experience also allows for identifying additional common pitfalls for trainees implementing CBT with children and adolescents, including failure to attend to their developmental level, difficulty establishing a strong, collaborative therapeutic alliance, difficulty navigating family involvement in the therapy process, failing to attend to cultural considerations, and lack of a conceptualization to guide treatment. It is helpful for supervisors to anticipate and prepare for how to address these various pitfalls if they come up in supervision, as discussed next.

Pitfall 1: Failure to Attend to the Developmental Level of the Child or Adolescent Patient

It is misguided to assume that children and adolescents are "mini-adults" who will be responsive to interventions designed to be implemented with adults. Thus, taking into consideration a child or adolescent patient's developmental level is critical to a successful therapy outcome. This affects each aspect of the therapy process, from assessing the presenting problem, to rapport building, to language use in session, to selecting and implementing interventions in a way that the young person can understand, relate to, and learn from. Typically, consideration of a youth's developmental level may focus on cognitive, social, and emotional development, as well as developmental tasks the youth is presented with. When a trainee lacks attention to a youth's developmental level, they may struggle to develop a relationship with the patient, the patient may have difficulty understanding or relating to the therapist (e.g., a trainee using vocabulary, references, or metaphors that are beyond the understanding of the child), and the therapist may attempt interventions that are inappropriate and, therefore, ineffective.

Suggestions for Addressing Pitfall 1

Supervisors can provide feedback, support, and scaffolding to help trainees grow in their knowledge and application of child development and developmental psychopathology. At the assessment stage, supervisors can discuss developmental abilities a child the patient's age would typically have mastered and assess whether the patient appears to have any difficulties in these areas. The trainee can be taught to incorporate this information into the conceptualization and can learn to view a child and their presenting concerns through a developmental lens. When possible, supervisors should utilize direct observation or recordings to review the trainee's sessions with their youth patients to identify issues with a trainee's language or implementation of an intervention. Relying solely on a trainee's report of an intervention not working is useful but may not lead to knowledge of *why* an intervention does not work.

Supervisors can also engage with trainees to identify a variety of creative and flexible approaches to implementing a CBT intervention based on a child's developmental level. Furthermore, supervisors can provide guidance about not only what intervention to use, but also how to implement it effectively, given the child or adolescent's developmental level. Considerations for how to effectively implement various techniques include thinking about how to make the technique accessible to the youth, how to make the learning and practice process fun and engaging, and how to communicate the intervention to the youth in developmentally appropriate terms. For example, when identifying the strength or intensity of an emotion with young children, it is helpful to have a visual, concrete representation of intensity (e.g., feelings thermometer, clear cups filled with varying levels of gumballs). In contrast, when working with an adolescent with well-developed abstract thinking skills, such a presentation would be inappropriate.

Pitfall 2: Difficulty Establishing a Strong, Collaborative Therapeutic Alliance

Developing a collaborative therapeutic alliance with patients, regardless of their age, is seen as a necessary ingredient for facilitating change in therapy (Friedberg et al., 2009). Working with children and adolescents may require special attention to this element, given that youth are rarely self-referred for treatment and may not necessarily be motivated to engage in the therapy process. Trainees will likely be faced with youth patients with a variety of characteristics that may make rapport building somewhat difficult, including a hyperactive, difficult-to-corral preschooler, an extremely shy, timid school-aged child, or a defensive, disengaged adolescent. Each of these presentations requires a unique, individualized approach to rapport building.

Suggestions for Addressing Pitfall 2

The rapport-building process starts the moment the therapist meets their youth patient, and, indeed, building rapport with the parent may start even before then, when the therapist initially makes contact with the family by phone. When working with young children, trainees should be encouraged to take a calm, friendly approach in the initial meeting, introducing themselves to the youngster and orienting them to the session in a developmentally appropriate way. It is helpful to stage the therapy room with access to a variety of toys and games to help the child feel comfortable. When building rapport with small children, trainees should be encouraged to engage in play with the child in a nonthreatening manner, using humor and following the child's lead. Using board or card games can be helpful with young and school-aged children, as this provides a fun activity for the child, allows for interaction with the therapist, and may offer the therapist both useful clinical information about the child's behavior during game play (e.g., turn-taking, frustration tolerance), as well as an opportunity to ask the child questions about themselves while simultaneously providing a nonthreatening atmosphere. With adolescents, rapport building looks different. Trainees should be encouraged to meet the adolescent where they are at in terms of motivation and engagement in treatment and should work to help the adolescent feel comfortable talking about themselves, their social environment, and their concerns. Appropriate use of humor, as well as irreverence, can be helpful when working with adolescents, as well as basic clinical skills like validation and reflecting feelings.

Supervisors can also aid in the development of trainees' collaborative approach to therapy. This is particularly important with youth, as they are used to having an adult in charge, often with unilateral control. Trainees should work to develop a relationship that is clearly collaborative, inviting the youth to share their perspective and offering options for how to proceed, when possible, to help the youth demonstrate autonomy. When trainees push past the rapport-building phase, treatment can be impeded; thus, supervisors should assess rapport and ensure that a good, collaborative relationship exists before moving forward with treatment.

Pitfall 3: Difficulty Navigating Family Involvement in the Therapy Process

Working with youth involves working directly with the social context in which they are embedded. This may involve the youth's school, peer group, and community, and this most certainly involves the youth's family. Kendall (2012) noted that parents can play multiple roles in the treatment context, including consultants who share information about the child's history and presenting problems, coclients when targeting parent behavior that contributes to the child's presenting problem, and collaborators when they support their child's use of new skills in treatment. Proper involvement of the family is important both during the assessment and treatment stages. Often, several family factors directly affect the child's presenting problems, for instance, parenting behaviors that unintentionally reinforce misbehavior among children with behavioral difficulties, parental accommodation that unintentionally reinforces anxiety symptoms among anxious children, or parental invalidation that negatively impacts an adolescent with developing personality-related concerns. Therefore, embarking on treatment that does not include the youth's caregivers likely misses an important part of the picture.

Suggestions for Addressing Pitfall 3
Two aspects are noteworthy in addressing the issue of family involvement in the therapy process: The first is assessing and identifying the specific role the family may play in maintaining the child's presenting problems, and the second is engaging directly with the family in session. To address the first, supervisors should encourage initial assessment of family factors and discuss them with trainees when developing the initial conceptualization. To address the second, supervisors can help trainees attend to the therapeutic relationship with the parents or caregivers from the outset of treatment. Therapists can engage

with a youth patient's parents or caregivers collaboratively, noting that family members are "experts" when it comes to their children, while the role of the therapist is to help family members view their child and the child's presenting problems in a more adaptive, helpful way and provide them with tools to help their child address their presenting problems.

Trainees may feel uncomfortable in family sessions for a variety of reasons (e.g., lacking confidence in their role as therapist, difficulty managing potential conflict that can occur during family sessions, difficulty redirecting or setting boundaries with parents who may have strong personalities). Supervisors can help trainees anticipate potential difficulties during family sessions by planning for these in supervision, taking into consideration various factors, including those related to the parent, the child, the family dynamic, and the therapist's own interpersonal style and confidence in session. Strategies such as setting ground rules during family sessions regarding the use of active listening and acknowledging the therapist's role as moderator (or, at times, perhaps referee) can be helpful in setting the stage and empowering the therapist-in-training to manage the session effectively. Supervisors and trainees can also engage in role play to model effective responses to potentially challenging events which could occur during a family session. In addition, postsession debriefing may be helpful, as this presents an opportunity for the supervisor and trainee to explore aspects of the session that went well versus what could have gone better, allowing for additional learning and reflection to take place.

Pitfall 4: Lack of Attention to Cultural Considerations

Multicultural competence is an area of significant importance in training psychotherapists. An individual's cultural background influences their symptom presentation; perspectives about the etiology of their presenting problems; views about potential stigma of mental health conditions; verbal and non-verbal communication styles; and experiences such as systemic racism, oppression, and marginalization; among other important treatment-relevant factors (Friedberg & McClure, 2002; Schwab-Stone et al., 2001). Thus, consideration of cultural factors is integral to developing a strong working alliance and properly assessing, conceptualizing, and treating youth patients. Lack of attention to cultural factors can result in missing important information crucial to conceptualizing a patient's presenting problems, misapplication of interventions, and premature termination of services, which may lead to families failing to seek services in the future due to feelings that psychotherapy is not helpful or that they will not be understood and heard by their therapist.

Suggestions for Addressing Pitfall 4

The process of developing multicultural competence is one that continues throughout a psychotherapist's training and career (Brems, 2008). In addition to coursework encouraging self-exploration and building knowledge related to multicultural psychology, supervision is an important training ground in which trainees can develop cultural sensitivity. Supervisors should encourage trainees to assess cultural factors relevant for each patient during the intake process. Friedberg and McClure (2002) suggested actively assessing a child's or family's acculturation status, cultural identity, experiences with prejudice and marginalization, as well as the impacts these may have had on the youth's symptoms.

Brems (2008) identified three areas necessary for developing cultural sensitivity: awareness, knowledge, and skills. Awareness involves introspection and identification of one's own cultural background, beliefs, values, prejudices, stereotypes, and biases. Knowledge involves components, including, but not limited to, building knowledge about the beliefs and practices of different cultural groups, historical events and the impact these had and may continue to have on individuals from different cultural backgrounds, limitations and biases of mental health theories and interventions, and how to use and adapt therapeutic interventions in a culturally sensitive way. Finally, the third component involves helping the trainee build skills necessary to provide culturally sensitive services to youth and families, which may include skills related to proper attention to and assessment of cultural variables, flexibly tailoring therapeutic approaches and communication styles for each patient, and being careful to avoid applying cultural stereotypes to all individuals who share a given cultural background. Supervisors play an important role in helping trainees in all three of these areas.

Pitfall 5: Lack of a Conceptualization to Guide Treatment

Case conceptualization involves identifying the youth's presenting problems and developing hypotheses about how they developed and are maintained (Murphy & Christner, 2006). Rather than haphazardly implementing various CBT interventions with youth based only on knowledge of their presenting problem, case conceptualization helps therapists individually tailor treatment to youth based on their specific presentation. Various models of case conceptualization exist, though they generally involve consideration of predisposing, precipitating, perpetuating, and protective factors (Barker, 1988; Winters et al., 2007). Friedberg and McClure (2002) developed a case conceptualization model specifically for use with youth patients and suggest consideration of the following components when conceptualizing cases: presenting problem (in terms of physiological symptoms, mood, behavior, cognition, and interpersonal factors), cultural context variables, history and developmental milestones, cognitive variables, and behavioral antecedents and consequences.

Suggestions for Addressing Pitfall 5

Supervisors can take a structured, proactive approach to helping trainees develop case conceptualization skills. Following the intake assessment, supervisors can engage with trainees and encourage them to write out a formal case conceptualization, which they can review together. Trainees often struggle with appropriately identifying the relevant predisposing, precipitating, perpetuating, and protective factors for a given patient, and supervisors can provide support and guidance as needed. Supervisors should also encourage trainees to continuously reference and adjust their case conceptualization as appropriate throughout treatment, given that the case conceptualization involves hypotheses which may or may not turn out to be accurate (Friedberg & McClure, 2002). When trainees report to supervisors that their patient's presenting problems do not seem to be improving despite application of what seemed to be appropriate interventions, supervisors can direct the trainee to revisit the case conceptualization and engage with the trainee to reassess previous hypotheses.

Pitfall 6: Difficulty Implementing CBT Techniques

Elements of CBT that are commonly difficult for trainees to implement effectively include guided discovery, agenda setting, application of CBT techniques (e.g., exposure), homework, and feedback (Friedberg & Taylor, 1994; Waltman et al., 2017). These may be more challenging in the presence of clinically complex patients. Trainees may struggle with these elements for several reasons, including lack of confidence, the difficulty level of the skill itself, or if a trainee has traditionally used more nondirective approaches, to name a few. Supervisors can anticipate these difficulties and identify ways to help trainees build these skills.

Suggestions for Addressing Pitfall 6

Supervisors can use a variety of strategies to aid in trainees' learning of CBT techniques within the supervision context. More active strategies, including modeling and role playing during supervision meetings, may be beneficial tools for supervisors to help trainees strengthen their skills. For example, Bearman et al. (2017) found that after attending a workshop on cognitive restructuring for youth with depression, trainees who received supervision infused with more active approaches (e.g., role play, corrective feedback, and modeling) demonstrated greater improvement in CBT expertise, CBT competence, and greater fidelity in implementing cognitive restructuring than trainees who simply received standard "supervision as usual" without the active components. In addition, it has also been found that trainees perceive more active methods, such as role play and modeling, to be helpful learning methods to increase procedural knowledge of interventions (Bennett-Levy et al., 2009). Given this, supervisors should consider utilizing these more active methods, particularly when trainees demonstrate difficulty implementing specific CBT techniques.

There can be many reasons why a trainee may be struggling to master a CBT technique (Friedberg & Taylor, 1994); thus, it may be beneficial for a supervisor to engage with a trainee regarding the specific barriers they are experiencing and work together to address these appropriately. In doing so, a supervisor not only helps the trainee build skills but also models appropriate collaboration and problem solving. When it comes to guided discovery, one of the most difficult skills for trainees to learn, some have suggested encouraging trainees to observe or practice guided discovery within the supervision context, read articles, and watch videos of master clinicians demonstrating this skill (Friedberg & Clark, 2006; Friedberg & Taylor, 1994).

ETHICAL ISSUES IN TREATMENT APPLICATION

Attention to ethical issues is of paramount importance for trainees conducting clinical work with children and adolescents. All trainees should be familiar with the American Psychological Association's (APA's; 2017) *Ethical Principles of Psychologists and Code of Conduct* (APA Ethics Code) and, therefore, be attentive to potential ethical dilemmas that may become relevant during the course of their clinical work. Research suggests that both psychologists, as well as graduate student therapists, encounter a variety of ethical dilemmas, with some studies suggesting that issues related to confidentiality are among the most common issues for both of these groups (Fly et al., 1997; Pope & Vetter, 1992). When conducting clinical work with youth, issues related to both confidentiality, as well as informed consent, are of particular importance.

Children rarely initiate treatment on their own, and they are legally unable to consent for their own treatment. Despite, and, perhaps, because of these factors, involving the child in the informed consent process is critical. The APA Ethics Code stipulates that psychologists seek to obtain informed assent from individuals who cannot provide informed consent on their own, including children. As such, trainees discussing treatment consent with youth patients and their parents should strive to use developmentally appropriate language to explain information related to treatment. Involving the youth in the consent process is not only the ethical best practice, but it also sets the stage for treatment for the youth, emphasizing their active role and demonstrating a respect for the youth's autonomy. Furthermore, involving the child in the informed consent process may also have positive impacts on the development of the therapeutic alliance with the child (Ascherman & Rubin, 2008).

Part of the informed consent process involves discussion of confidentiality and its limits with youth and their families. Discussions of confidentiality can be challenging for a variety of reasons, including the potential developmental considerations necessary in order to ensure the child has a proper understanding of limits to confidentiality, as well as the fact that a youth's parents are involved in treatment. Student therapists should have a direct conversation about confidentiality and its limits with the youth and their parents during the first session. In my experience, it is helpful to provide the child and parent with concrete examples of information that will and will not be shared, and with whom such information could be shared (e.g., if a child says their parent hit them and left a bruise on their skin, this is information that would be reported to child protective services, while, in contrast, if a child indicates that they are angry with their mother for taking away their video game and they uttered a curse word at her after she left the room, this would not be shared with the parent).

In addition to the general limits of confidentiality (i.e., those related to harm of self and/or others), trainees should also discuss and clarify what information will be shared with parents during the course of treatment (Koocher, 2008). Brems (2008) noted that this can represent somewhat of a gray area in the treatment of youth, noting that, although providers may take various approaches to this issue, it is recommended to use good clinical judgment and balance the need to inform parents about the status of treatment with the need to protect the child's privacy. Similarly, Ascherman and Rubin (2008) suggested that therapists share general updates about treatment progress with parents rather than divulging specific details that could potentially affect the youth's trust in the therapist.

Issues related to confidentiality are also important when considering what information about the child's treatment is to be shared with others (e.g., the school, other providers). Although parents can legally authorize disclosure of their child's treatment-relevant information, the therapist should consider what information is necessary to disclose in order to address the request for information, as well as consider any potential negative impact that could come from releasing information about the youth (Ascherman & Rubin, 2008; Brems, 2008). In preparation for meeting with youth patients, trainees would benefit from supervisor discussion of these ethical issues, among others, to help trainees plan for appropriate ways to anticipate and address these concerns as they arise.

COMMON OBSTACLES IN SUPERVISION AND WAYS OF OVERCOMING THEM

Many potential difficulties can arise within the supervision context, which supervisors should be aware of and prepared to address. Although a comprehensive review of these possible difficulties is beyond the scope of this chapter, this section discusses a few common difficulties, along with suggestions for how supervisors can address them.

Ruptures in the Supervisory Relationship

A critical aspect of supervision is the supervisory relationship between the supervisor and the trainee, which is the foundation upon which activities of supervision take place. If the supervisory relationship becomes strained, this could negatively impact the supervision experience and, perhaps also, patient care. Issues related to the supervisory relationship have been cited as one of, if not the most common supervision issue reported by trainees (Ellis, 1991) and supervisors (Grant et al., 2012). There is an inherent power differential within the supervisory relationship, given that this relationship involves evaluation, and, as such, it is the supervisor's duty to establish a comfortable environment in supervision in which the trainee feels that they can trust the supervisor (Rosenbaum & Ronen, 1998). Falender and Shafranske (2004) noted that supervisors must balance and integrate both interpersonal skills and clinical skills and knowledge in order to develop a strong supervisory relationship with trainees.

Supervisors should regularly reflect on and attend to potential issues developing within the supervisory relationship; when problems emerge, supervisors should immediately attempt to address them with the trainee (Safran & Muran, 2001). In addition, supervisors should also express a willingness and interest in openly discussing issues related to supervision and the supervisory relationship with trainees (Mehr et al., 2010). Sellers and colleagues (2016) suggested that when a trainee is having difficulty, the supervisor should identify whether their own behavior or attitudes are contributing to the issue and also assess the degree to which the trainee's difficulty is skill-related versus related specifically to factors within the supervisory relationship. Skill-related difficulties can be addressed separately but, if the supervisor believes that their behavior is affecting the student's performance, Sellers et al. suggested that the supervisor apologize to the trainee, acknowledge how the supervisor's behavior has affected the supervisory relationship as well as the trainee, explicitly state how the supervisor plans to address their own behavior (e.g., what they will do differently), and regularly check in with the trainee about whether the change in the supervisor's behavior is having the desired effect. Other suggestions for supervisors include encouraging trainees to share feedback about supervision, working to establish a trusting relationship with the trainee, and consulting with a colleague or mentor about how to address an issue within the supervisory relationship (Ramos-Sánchez et al., 2002; Sellers et al., 2016).

Lack of Trainee Engagement in Supervision

Another obstacle that can arise in supervision occurs when a trainee struggles to meaningfully engage in supervision (e.g., reluctance to discuss cases in detail, defensiveness). Without trainee engagement in supervision, the supervisor struggles to provide adequate training, as well as clinical oversight, and this can result in trainees failing to benefit from supervision and patients potentially being provided with subpar care. Several potential reasons exist for trainee reluctance to disclose information related to patient care, including shame, embarrassment, feelings of incompetence, and fear of criticism or negative evaluation (Falender & Shafranske, 2004; Friedberg & Clark, 2006).

Fortunately, there are several ways supervisors can respond to this concern in order to encourage trainees to more actively participate in supervision and express vulnerability. First, they can normalize these feelings and empathically explore the trainee's reactions to receiving supervisor feedback (Falender & Shafranske, 2004). In addition, Friedberg and Taylor (1994) suggested that supervisors consider, as appropriate, sharing some of their own doubts, challenges, or shortcomings and how they addressed them in order to dispel the myth that advanced clinicians demonstrate perfect clinical skills without exception. When giving feedback, supervisors can be tactful and normalize feelings of incompetence or inadequacy, provide validation to the trainee, include a discussion of trainee strengths, and work to inoculate trainees to feedback by giving minor constructive feedback frequently (Grant et al., 2012; Mehr et al., 2010; Sellers et al., 2016). Supervisors can also encourage various exercises with trainees, such as asking the trainee to predict their supervisor's reaction or feedback following review of a session recording and comparing this with actual feedback provided, or helping trainees assess the accuracy of negative beliefs about their competence (Friedberg & Taylor, 1994).

Trainees' Difficult Personal Characteristics

Trainee personal characteristics, including arrogance, defensiveness, excessive seeking of validation or reassurance, general interpersonal skills, and difficulty responding to feedback, represent an additional factor that can serve as an obstacle to effective supervision (Grant et al., 2012; Sellers et al., 2016). Certainly, these trainee characteristics can elicit reactions from supervisors that can affect the supervisory relationship, as well as the supervisor's view of the trainee. Attention to this supervisor countertransference is important, and supervisors can engage in self-reflection or consultation with trusted colleagues to manage this.

When it comes to working effectively with trainees who demonstrate these more difficult personal characteristics, supervisors have several potential options. In one study assessing how supervisors managed difficulties in supervision, expert supervisors used four major strategies: relational (e.g., providing support, validation, acknowledging mistakes), reflective (e.g., monitoring, using patience and transparency, exploring countertransference, seeking consultation), confrontative (e.g., addressing an issue directly with the trainee, setting boundaries, or encouraging the trainee to seek personal therapy), and avoidant (e.g., not addressing the issue, withdrawing; Grant et al., 2012). It is recommended that supervisors engage in self-reflection to help individualize their approach to working with more challenging trainees, while attending to the supervisory relationship (e.g., acknowledging and managing countertransference, demonstrating empathy) and balancing support or praise with opportunities to provide constructive feedback to facilitate trainee growth (Kemer et al., 2017). When trainee interpersonal skills are of concern specifically, supervisors can gently provide feedback, help the trainee identify potential reasons for the behavior, and engage in role play or modeling to help the trainee develop more appropriate behaviors (Sellers et al., 2016). In addition, when it comes to trainee difficulty accepting feedback, Sellers and colleagues made several recommendations. First, they suggested that supervisors reflect on their own role in the process of giving feedback, discuss the educational importance of feedback, as well as the importance of accepting and responding to it appropriately, and encourage the trainee to reflect on the feedback they have received. They then suggested that supervisors can choose to engage the trainee in role play to demonstrate appropriate versus inappropriate responses to feedback.

Although several potential obstacles can arise in the context of supervision, a skilled supervisor can anticipate them, engage in self-reflection about their potential role when an obstacle arises, and work with the trainee in an open, nonjudgmental manner to immediately address the issue in order to prevent it from having a more significant impact on the supervision process.

CONCLUSION

A variety of evidence-based CBT interventions exist to treat the broad spectrum of mental health concerns among youth. In addition to proper didactic training in CBT, supervised practice of CBT with patients is a critical element of training for students, which allows therapists-in-training to bring interventions to life and individualize them based on each client's unique presentation. Although the research on what makes for effective CBT supervision lags far behind the evidence base supporting CBT interventions, it is clear that supervisors play a valuable role in training future psychotherapists. Supervising CBT for youth requires multiple competencies, including expertise in CBT interventions, the ability to establish strong, trusting working relationships with trainee therapists, navigation of various barriers to successful supervision experiences, and the ability to provide the trainee with opportunities to practice and hone their skills in a safe environment.

REFERENCES

American Psychological Association. (2017). *Ethical principles of psychologists and code of conduct* (2002, amended effective June 1, 2010, and January 1, 2017). https://www. apa.org/ethics/code/

Ascherman, L. I., & Rubin, S. (2008). Current ethical issues in child and adolescent psychotherapy. *Child and Adolescent Psychiatric Clinics of North America, 17*(1), 21–35, vii–viii. https://doi.org/10.1016/j.chc.2007.07.008

Barker, P. (1988). *Basic child psychiatry* (5th ed.). Blackwell Science Ltd.

Bearman, S. K., Schneiderman, R. L., & Zoloth, E. (2017). Building an evidence base for effective supervision practices: An analogue experiment of supervision to increase EBT fidelity. *Administration and Policy in Mental Health, 44*(2), 293–307. https://doi.org/ 10.1007/s10488-016-0723-8

Beck, A. T. (1964). Thinking and depression: II. Theory and therapy. *Archives of General Psychiatry, 10*(6), 561–571. https://doi.org/10.1001/archpsyc.1964.01720240015003

Beck, A. T. (1976). *Cognitive therapy and the emotional disorders*. International Universities Press.

Beck, J. S. (2011). *Cognitive behavior therapy: Basics and beyond* (2nd ed.). Guilford Press.

Bennett-Levy, J., McManus, F., Westling, B. E., & Fennell, M. (2009). Acquiring and refining CBT skills and competencies: Which training methods are perceived to be most effective? *Behavioural and Cognitive Psychotherapy, 37*(5), 571–583. https://doi.org/ 10.1017/S1352465809990270

Brems, C. (2008). *A comprehensive guide to child psychotherapy and counseling* (3rd ed.). Waveland Press.

Ellis, M. V. (1991). Critical incidents in clinical supervision and in supervisor supervision: Assessing supervisory issues. *Journal of Counseling Psychology, 38*(3), 342–349. https://doi.org/10.1037/0022-0167.38.3.342

Falender, C. A., & Shafranske, E. P. (2004). *Clinical supervision: A competency-based approach*. American Psychological Association. https://doi.org/10.1037/10806-000

Fly, B. J., van Bark, W. P., Weinman, L., Kitchener, K. S., & Lang, P. R. (1997). Ethical transgressions of psychology graduate students: Critical incidents with implications for training. *Professional Psychology: Research and Practice, 28*(5), 492–495. https://doi.org/10.1037/0735-7028.28.5.492

Friedberg, R. D., & Clark, C. C. (2006). Supervision of cognitive therapy with youth. In T. K. Neill (Ed.), *Helping others help children: Clinical supervision of child psychotherapy* (pp. 109–122). American Psychological Association. https://doi.org/10.1037/11467-006

Friedberg, R. D., & McClure, J. M. (2002). *Clinical practice of cognitive therapy with children and adolescents: The nuts and bolts*. Guilford Press.

Friedberg, R. D., McClure, J. M., & Garcia, J. H. (2009). *Cognitive therapy techniques for children and adolescents: Tools for enhancing practice*. Guilford Press.

Friedberg, R. D., & Taylor, L. A. (1994). Perspectives on supervision in cognitive therapy. *Journal of Rational-Emotive & Cognitive-Behavior Therapy, 12*(3), 147–161. https://doi.org/10.1007/BF02354593

Grant, J., Schofield, M. J., & Crawford, S. (2012). Managing difficulties in supervision: Supervisors' perspectives. *Journal of Counseling Psychology, 59*(4), 528–541. https://doi.org/10.1037/a0030000

Kemer, G., Borders, L. D., & Yel, N. (2017). Expert supervisors' priorities when working with easy and challenging supervisees. *Counselor Education and Supervision, 56*(1), 50–64. https://doi.org/10.1002/ceas.12059

Kendall, P. C. (2012). Guiding theory for therapy with children and adolescents. In P. C. Kendall (Ed.), *Child and adolescent therapy: Cognitive-behavioral procedures* (pp. 3–24). Guilford Press.

Koocher, G. P. (2008). Ethical challenges in mental health services to children and families. *Journal of Clinical Psychology, 64*(5), 601–612. https://doi.org/10.1002/jclp.20476

Mehr, K. E., Ladany, N., & Caskie, G. I. L. (2010). Trainee nondisclosure in supervision: What are they not telling you? *Counselling & Psychotherapy Research, 10*(2), 103–113. https://doi.org/10.1080/14733141003712301

Murphy, V. B., & Christner, R. W. (2006). A cognitive-behavioral case conceptualization approach for working with children and adolescents. In R. B. Mennuti, A. Freeman, & R. W. Christner (Eds.), *Cognitive-behavioral interventions in educational settings: A handbook for practice* (pp. 37–62). Routledge.

Pope, K. S., & Vetter, V. A. (1992). Ethical dilemmas encountered by members of the American Psychological Association: A national survey. *American Psychologist, 47*(3), 397–411. https://doi.org/10.1037/0003-066X.47.3.397

Ramos-Sánchez, L., Esnil, E., Goodwin, A., Riggs, S., Touster, L. O., Wright, L. K., Ratanasiripong, P., & Rodolfa, E. (2002). Negative supervisory events: Effects on supervision and supervisory alliance. *Professional Psychology: Research and Practice, 33*(2), 197–202. https://doi.org/10.1037/0735-7028.33.2.197

Rosenbaum, M., & Ronen, T. (1998). Clinical supervision from the standpoint of cognitive-behavior therapy. *Psychotherapy: Theory, Research, & Practice, 35*(2), 220–230. https://doi.org/10.1037/h0087705

Safran, J. D., & Muran, J. C. (2001). A relational approach to training and supervision in cognitive psychotherapy. *Journal of Cognitive Psychotherapy, 15*(1), 3–15. https://doi.org/10.1891/0889-8391.15.1.3

Schwab-Stone, M., Ruchkin, V., Vermeiren, R., & Leckman, P. (2001). Cultural considerations in the treatment of children and adolescents. Operationalizing the importance of culture in treatment. *Child and Adolescent Psychiatric Clinics of North America*, *10*(4), 729–743. https://doi.org/10.1016/S1056-4993(18)30027-0

Sellers, T. P., LeBlanc, L. A., & Valentino, A. L. (2016). Recommendations for detecting and addressing barriers to successful supervision. *Behavior Analysis in Practice*, *9*(4), 309–319. https://doi.org/10.1007/s40617-016-0142-z

Waltman, S., Hall, B. C., McFarr, L. M., Beck, A. T., & Creed, T. A. (2017). In-session stuck points and pitfalls of community clinicians learning CBT: Qualitative investigation. *Cognitive and Behavioral Practice*, *24*(2), 256–267. https://doi.org/10.1016/j.cbpra.2016.04.002

Weisz, J. R., & Kazdin, A. E. (Eds.). (2017). *Evidence-based psychotherapies for children and adolescents* (3rd ed.). Guilford Press.

Winters, N. C., Hanson, G., & Stoyanova, V. (2007). The case formulation in child and adolescent psychiatry. *Child and Adolescent Psychiatric Clinics of North America*, *16*(1), 111–132. https://doi.org/10.1016/j.chc.2006.07.010

17

Supervising the Delivery of Cognitive Behavior Therapy With Spiritual and Religious Patients

Moses Appel and David H. Rosmarin

The terms "spirituality" and "religion" are often used interchangeably because of their considerable overlap, but they have different meanings. While spirituality refers to any relation to what is regarded as sacred, religion, specifically, refers to institutionalized or culturally bound ways of relating to something sacred (Hill et al., 2000). For the purpose of this chapter, we will combine the terms as *spirituality/religion* (S/R) because in the United States, where we are located, the vast majority of the population is either spiritual and religious, or neither (Marler & Hadaway, 2002). Furthermore, the issues discussed in this chapter are equally relevant to both constructs.

S/R is one of many aspects of human diversity, similar to culture, race, ethnicity, and sexual orientation, in that there are many different religious and spiritual beliefs among the general population. Even within religious and spiritual groups, there is considerable diversity regarding specific traditions, beliefs, rituals, and customs. However, while such diversity exists, there is an abundance of commonality as well. Given the commonality among spiritual and religious groups, clinicians can gain skills in assessing and incorporating S/R into treatment, regardless of the breadth of their S/R knowledge, personal S/R affiliation, or lack thereof (Rosmarin & Pirutinsky, 2020).

A majority of Americans maintain S/R beliefs and practices. In fact, almost three quarters of the American population professes "certain" belief in God, and more than half report that religion is "very important" in their lives (Gallup, 2011). Furthermore, more than half of Americans engage in daily prayer

https://doi.org/10.1037/0000314-018
Training and Supervision in Specialized Cognitive Behavior Therapy: Methods, Settings, and Populations, E. A. Storch, J. S. Abramowitz, and D. McKay (Editors)

(Pew Research Center, 2014b), and 36% attend religious services weekly (Pew Research Center, 2014a). With these numbers, it is not surprising that more than half of patients are interested in addressing S/R in their treatment. This is true for both inpatient and outpatient settings (Rose et al., 2001; Rosmarin et al., 2015). In contrast, in a survey of 262 cognitive behavior therapy (CBT) practitioners, participants reported substantially lower levels of S/R belief and practice than the general population. Along with this, 36% of respondents reported some discomfort in addressing religious issues with clients, with 19% even reporting that they never, or rarely, inquire about religion in a session (Rosmarin et al., 2013). One of the contributing factors to this disparity between patients' and clinicians' desire to address S/R in therapy is that most clinicians have had little to no experience approaching S/R topics with patients. In fact, Rosmarin et al. (2013) found that 71% of participants reported little to no training in how to assess and address religious issues in treatment. Given this lack of training, most CBT therapists are ill-equipped to handle almost any S/R issues that arise in therapy. This chapter provides a guide for supervisors in how to help trainees assess for patients' S/R in the practice of CBT and (to a lesser degree) incorporate S/R in CBT treatment.

KEY CONCEPTS FOR TRAINEES TO LEARN

The first, and most important, concept for trainees in CBT to learn is the importance of assessing S/R with *all* of their patients. As mentioned earlier, S/R is a major part of life for so many people, and it often plays a role in mental health. It can be directly related to a patient's psychological symptoms or used a resource for patients to cope with their psychopathology. While most trainees have not had specific training in this area, they need not be disheartened, as this requires little more than the skills most clinicians already possess, such as asking questions and engaging in experimentation and critical thinking. Second, given that many facets of S/R are present across multiple traditions, clinicians assessing for S/R do not need to have an in-depth knowledge about every religious and spiritual group in order to be helpful. Rather, they can approach this domain similarly to how they would approach other domains of a patient's life, such as personal relationships. Clinicians should begin by opening the topic for discussion using broad questions about the patient's S/R, such as "Do you consider yourself to be part of any S/R group?" or "Do you engage in any S/R practices?" and then narrow their questioning based on the patient's responses.

The role of the CBT clinician in assessing S/R in therapy is not to promote or discourage S/R but, rather, determine whether any facets of the patient's S/R beliefs or practices (a) are contributing to the presenting problem or (b) have the potential to be used to improve psychological functioning. In order to be effective at assessing S/R with patients, the clinician does not need to share the patient's faith. It is more important for the clinician to respect the patient's faith and become more familiar with their belief system. Rosmarin and Pirutinsky (2020) evaluated whether Orthodox Jewish patients benefited more from treatment with therapists who shared their religion and found that the religious patients benefited equally from therapists who matched their religious affiliation and those who did not. Other research has suggested that nonreligious therapists are more effective at integrating S/R into psychotherapy than religiously affiliated clinicians (Propst et al., 1992; Rosmarin et al., 2021). One potential explanation for these latter findings is that it can be particularly meaningful to spiritual or religious patients when an unaffiliated clinician validates and seeks to understand S/R dimensions of life. Thus, therapists can be as effective whether or not they share their patient's S/R affiliation, and, perhaps, even more effective if they are not religiously inclined themselves.

KEY TECHNIQUES FOR TRAINEES TO LEARN

Functional Assessment of S/R

Given that S/R can be related to a person's psychological well-being in both adaptive and maladaptive ways, it is important (after obtaining consent) to conduct a functional analysis of S/R to examine how it may be relevant to the patient's presenting complaints. Broadly speaking, S/R can have positive and negative effects on symptoms. On the positive side, the patient may have spiritual resources that can be drawn upon to cope with their psychological difficulties. On the negative side, S/R can contribute to psychopathology in one of two ways. Some patients report S/R beliefs or practices that exacerbate maladaptive feelings (e.g., excessive guilt over not fully believing in God) or are a source of interpersonal conflict (e.g., feeling disconnected from one's S/R community). For others, psychological symptoms take on S/R themes, as seen in certain presentations of obsessive–compulsive disorder (OCD) in which obsessions and compulsions take on religious themes (i.e., scrupulosity). Notably, positive and negative effects of S/R on symptoms tend to be positively correlated with one another. Thus, many patients have both positive and negative effects of S/R.

The assessment of positive aspects of S/R can play out in several ways. Some patients immediately identify specific S/R resources that they use in their everyday lives; in this case, the therapist can take note and examine whether there are ways to incorporate those resources into treatment. Other patients may not identify such resources but mention some they have used in the past. In these cases, clinicians can assess interest in examining possible ways to incorporate such resources in treatment. For those patients who specifically do not want to draw on such resources, it is important to assess why: Is it because the patient is simply disinterested in discussing S/R issues in treatment? Or, perhaps, the patient might be experiencing spiritual struggles. In this case, the therapist might ask whether the patient would like to further explore such difficulties.

The literature suggests there are three main categories of spiritual struggles that patients may experience: intrapersonal, interpersonal, and divine (Pargament et al., 2005). Intrapersonal struggles are S/R-themed struggles that people have with themselves. This can include judging themselves harshly for not strictly adhering to one's S/R laws or customs or setting S/R standards for them that are impossible to fulfill. Interpersonal spiritual struggles, however, involve others in the faith community. This can include having altercations with S/R leaders or other group members, as well as grappling with perceived wrongdoings of clergy or other esteemed members of their faith community. Lastly, divine spiritual struggles are those that people have with the faith itself, such as questions about fairness (i.e., "How can terrible things happen to good people?"), doubting whether their S/R beliefs are even true, or, in more severe cases, struggling with a complete loss of faith. Often, patients present with more than one spiritual struggle, and, many times, one struggle can lead to another. For example, people who experience divine struggles often also experience intrapersonal struggles that follow because they blame themselves and have guilty feelings over their S/R doubts.

Spiritual symptoms are psychologically distressing symptoms that take on S/R themes, such as scrupulosity (often found in OCD), religious delusions (often found in schizophrenia), and hyperreligiosity (often found in bipolar disorder). When faced with spiritual symptoms, clinicians need to familiarize themselves with the patient's religion to determine whether their beliefs and practices are in line with their S/R group, or if they are symptoms of a mental disorder. Clinicians who are unfamiliar with the particular beliefs and practices of their patients' S/R groups may mistakenly identify spiritual symptoms as bona fide religious practice or vice versa. When it is difficult to distinguish between psychological symptoms and actual S/R systems, it is important to be open to consulting with S/R group leaders to get help in making such a determination.

Case Conceptualization

Following assessment, clinicians can incorporate the information they have gathered into a case conceptualization and treatment plan. There are many ways clinicians can draw upon spiritual resources and integrate S/R into CBT, including cognitive methods such as reframing and behavioral methods such as behavioral activation (see Chapter 8 in this volume for more information). However, incorporating S/R into therapy is complex and more appropriate for clinicians who have a strong foundation in this domain.

When spiritual struggles are present, the clinician may begin by validating such difficulties, just as they would validate any other struggle the patient may report. It is not the clinician's place to validate or invalidate the content of the struggle (e.g., saying, "God does not hate you"); rather, it is best to address the struggle itself, and the accompanying emotional distress (e.g., "It must be very painful to feel that God hates you"), and create opportunities for exploration in the session. For spiritual symptoms, it is important to provide psychoeducation by explaining that symptoms are not occurring because the patient is religious per se, but, rather, that religion colors the way in which such symptoms manifest.

WHAT CHARACTERISTICS MAKE FOR A GOOD TRAINING CASE?

For many people, S/R plays a large role in their mental health in both positive and negative ways. However, while more than half of patients are interested in addressing S/R in their treatment (Rose et al., 2001; Rosmarin et al., 2015), many perceive therapy as a secular enterprise and do not realize that they can raise S/R-related issues with their therapist. Thus, as we have mentioned, it is important to assess S/R with all patients. That said, training experiences in working with S/R issues are richer when some aspect of a patient's life is affected by S/R in the ways we have described previously.

Spiritual Resources

If a trainee is working with a patient who has become disengaged from their faith due to depression but remains interested in their S/R beliefs and practices, there is room for assessment of and a discussion about negative and positive reinforcement loops using behavioral activation and psychoeducation. Patients with depression often feel immobilized, which leads to refraining from engaging in religious activities. Although this might provide temporary relief, it, ultimately, furthers their feelings of guilt and hopelessness, which intensifies the feeling of immobilization. Thus, psychoeducation can help the patient understand and weaken this vicious cycle. At the same time, therapists can encourage depressed patients to include religious activities as part of behavioral activation. If a trainee is working with a patient suffering from generalized anxiety disorder, there might be opportunities to gain experience in helping them draw on their spiritual resources to cope with the anxiety. Patients with generalized anxiety disorder are often searching for an unrealistic level of control over life events and may find it helpful to use their trust in God (or other supernatural powers) to help alleviate some of their worry. Thus, the more spiritual resources that the patient brings to the table, the more experience a trainee can gain in utilizing them to help patients cope with their psychological distress.

Spiritual Struggles

If a trainee is working with a patient experiencing spiritual struggles, along with anxiety or depression associated with feeling guilty, ashamed, or scared of divine punishment, the trainee can practice validating such concerns without undermining the patient's S/R beliefs or practices. This can be challenging because trainees often feel an urge to jump in and help the patient by reassuring them that they have nothing to be afraid of or be anxious about divine punishment or intervention. However, when patients experience spiritual struggles, they need an opportunity to be listened to and explore their thoughts and feelings without being told what they should or should not believe. Similarly, if a patient expresses struggles regarding loss of faith, the trainee may have an urge to persuade the patient to explore ways of leaving their faith, or to reconnect with it (the direction of persuasion may depend on the trainee's own S/R affiliations or lack thereof). This, too, is inappropriate. Instead, the clinician should listen to the patient's struggles and provide an opportunity to discuss these struggles and contemplate next steps, including the options of consulting with clergy and reconnecting with or leaving the S/R group completely, without pushing for one approach over another.

Spiritual Symptoms

A trainee may work with a patient who presents with spiritual symptoms, such as religious-themed OCD, and who reports confusion regarding whether his excessive prayer is actual religious practice or part of OCD. The patient might even report they are considering reluctantly disengaging from religious activities because of it. This would be a great training opportunity for the clinician to provide psychoeducation and even incorporate the religious fears into treatment in the form of doing religiously informed exposures. Another good training opportunity would be a patient diagnosed with schizophrenia who presents with religious delusions. The trainee will be able to get practice dealing with spiritual symptoms by first differentiating between actual S/R beliefs associated with the patient's religious group and delusional ones, and, second, by providing psychoeducation and reassurance that the symptom was not caused by S/R; rather it is a psychological symptom and the patient's S/R just colored the way in which it manifested.

COMMON MISTAKES THAT TRAINEES MAKE AND HOW TO ADDRESS THEM

Some of the common mistakes that trainees make when addressing S/R in CBT include failing to assess for S/R, failing to appreciate its significance, and generally not giving this domain adequate attention. This may result from training programs lacking coverage of the importance of S/R in therapy. Over the last few years, some attention has been given to this problem in the United Kingdom, as the World Psychiatric Association added religion and spirituality to the Core Training Curriculum for Psychiatry (Moreira-Almeida et al., 2016; World Psychiatric Association, 2002). However, psychiatry and psychology training programs in the United States continue to lag behind in this area, which is why a majority of psychology students reported little to no training in how to assess and address religious issues in treatment (Rosmarin et al., 2013). Given the lack of training, it is not surprising that 36% of CBT clinicians were not fully comfortable addressing religious issues with clients (Rosmarin et al., 2013), and 50% of psychiatrists felt discouraged from discussing S/R with patients either because of insufficient training or out of concern about inadvertently offending patients (Curlin, Lawrence, et al., 2007). Amazingly, some psychiatrists even tried changing the subject when patients bring up S/R in treatment (Curlin, Lawrence, et al., 2007). Another contributing factor to the lack of attention to S/R is the disparity in S/R affiliation between clinicians and the clients they serve. Specifically, mental health clinicians report significantly lower levels of S/R than the general public (Delaney et al., 2007). Further, psychiatrists are less religious than physicians in other fields (Curlin, Odell, et al., 2007). However, given the prevalence of S/R in the general population and its widespread relevance to mental health issues, clinicians must assume that most of their patients will benefit from some discussion of their S/R and, therefore, make sure not to neglect this domain in treatment.

Another common mistake trainees make relates to values conflicts. Some clinicians (religious ones) can get carried away and view CBT as a way to evangelize. This is rare, given the culture of CBT in particular, and psychotherapy in general, but it does happen. Clinicians should focus on the clinical needs of the patient, rather than their own or their patient's spiritual needs. These are usually aligned, but, in some cases, they can conflict. For example, if a patient presents with depression and the clinician feels that behavioral activation is a suitable treatment approach, the clinician should explore behaviors that the patient would like to engage in to achieve pleasure and mastery, without attempting to convince the patient to specifically engage in S/R related activities. That said, it is certainly appropriate (and even encouraged) to point out S/R activities as possible options when they serve as spiritual resources.

It is also important for clinicians to learn how to respect patient's religious values, even when those values seem to conflict with their clinical needs. While it is fine to point out such conflicts to help patients make informed decisions, S/R is an aspect of diversity, and, as such, we feel clinicians should respect patients' choices. Clinicians should also be aware of their own biases and not let these influence therapeutic decision-making. For example, if a patient presents with religious guilt about masturbation, the clinician should not decide for the patient that masturbation is normal and developmentally appropriate or employ CBT techniques to help the patient see the clinician's point of view. Instead, the clinician should engage in values exploration and clarification with the patient (Eifert & Forsyth, 2005) and help them discover their beliefs about the subject before deciding how to address the issue. Often, just validating and clarifying the values conflict of a S/R related struggle is very helpful for patients (Pargament & Saunders, 2007).

Novice clinicians often struggle with how to handle spiritual struggles. Too frequently, trainees want to "put out the fire" by offering cognitive restructuring the second a patient voices spiritual struggles. For example, if a patient says, "God hates me," novice clinicians will knee-jerk into reasons why God loves them. However, in these cases, the more appropriate response is to simply provide an opportunity for the patient to explore their spiritual struggles. Clinicians will be surprised to see that patients often talk themselves out of struggles when they receive unconditional positive regard and validation. In fact, this concept is at the center of Rogerian psychotherapy (Rogers, 1951).

Finally, when treating patients with spiritual symptoms, it is important to clearly demarcate where S/R beliefs and practices end and where S/R symptoms begin. Clinicians need to be careful not to treat S/R symptoms as usual religious practice and also not to treat usual religious practice as S/R symptoms. Indeed, spiritual symptoms may resemble S/R practices to someone not familiar with the patient's particular religion. For example, a patient may present with compulsive handwashing before prayer. While this is a tradition found in many religions (Kiani & Saeidi, 2015), compulsive handwashing that causes distress and conflicts with one's values is not. However, clinicians who are unfamiliar with a patient's S/R beliefs and practices can easily mistake S/R symptoms for S/R practice. Rosmarin et al. (2010), for example, examined whether Jews' Orthodox affiliation was related to recognition of scrupulosity as OCD. They found that the non-Orthodox Jews were less likely to recognize scrupulosity as OCD than Orthodox ones, indicating that people are likely to underestimate spiritual symptoms when they do not have a frame of reference. It is also important to know what is considered usual religious practice for the patient and not to treat that as S/R symptoms.

For example, in the OCD case just described, the clinician needs to be careful not to treat a standard amount of S/R handwashing as an OCD symptom. It is especially important for patients and therapists to demarcate such lines before engaging in psychological treatments such as exposure therapy. Just like CBT clinicians would never do exposures with a virologist presenting with contamination OCD if we were not clear on what is and is not considered safe practice, similarly, clinicians must not engage in exposure therapy for S/R symptoms before they clarify what is and is not congruent with the patient's S/R beliefs and practices. It is worth noting that, sometimes, patients have spiritual symptoms, as well as spiritual struggles. For example, a patient can have religious-themed OCD (S/R symptom) and also feel disconnected from God (spiritual struggle) because they see their OCD as a form of divine punishment. This is where a dose of psychoeducation can be golden (i.e., sharing that OCD happens to religious and nonreligious people equally as much, but religious patients usually have more scrupulosity, and nonreligious ones have other, non-S/R, OCD symptoms).

ETHICAL ISSUES IN TREATMENT APPLICATION

As discussed previously, the primary reason that clinicians shy away from addressing S/R in treatment is a lack of training. However, some clinicians— even those who report being comfortable addressing S/R—pull back from this area due to ethical concerns. Some are concerned that S/R issues are more appropriate for clergy than for mental health clinicians. Others are concerned that they cannot be helpful unless they share the patient's S/R beliefs. Still others fear that viewing S/R concerns through a psychological lens may be perceived as invalidating the S/R worldview and that addressing spiritual struggles to help a patient with a psychological disorder denigrates S/R.

Regarding incorporating S/R in treatment, clinicians sometimes fear that encouraging S/R practice may be viewed as proselytism and that discouraging S/R practice can be interpreted as encouraging religious heresy. While all of these ethical concerns are valid and need to be addressed for clinicians to become more comfortable with assessing and incorporating S/R in therapy, it is even more ethically problematic not to address altogether. In fact, overlooking S/R domains is in direct conflict with the American Psychological Association's (2017) *Ethical Principles of Psychologists and Code of Conduct* (APA Ethics Code), Standard 2.01(b), Boundaries of Competence, which states the following:

> Where scientific or professional knowledge in the discipline of psychology establishes that an understanding of factors associated with . . . religion . . . is essential for effective implementation of their services or research, psychologists have to obtain the training, experience, consultation, or supervision necessary to ensure the competence of their services.

While well-intentioned, many clinicians unknowingly fail their patients as a result of lacking the training necessary to be competent in the S/R domain, which, likely, also affects many of their patient's mental health concerns. However, as the famous legal maxim goes, "ignorantia legis neminem excusat" ("ignorance of the law excuses no one"). Thus, it is important for supervisors to assess and address these concerns among trainees so that they do not stand in the way of providing comprehensive, quality care.

Supervisors can also help trainees distinguish between S/R issues that are unrelated to psychopathology (which would be more appropriate for clergy) and those that are, such as spiritual symptoms or struggles (which should be dealt with in therapy). While it is not the clinician's role to discourage specific religious practices for its own sake, it is helpful to assist patients in understanding the functional relationship between S/R and psychological symptoms and to point out spiritual struggles or symptoms that they have identified. Clinicians can then further process any difficulties and make necessary treatment recommendations.

Regarding using spiritual resources in treatment, supervisors can point out to trainees that clinicians are not there to encourage religious practice for its own sake. Rather, the clinician's role is to explore possible spiritual resources that can be drawn upon in treatment with their patients and to encourage patients to consider using them to help cope with psychological distress. Once these points are clear, trainees will likely understand that they can be effective regardless of their personal S/R affiliation (or lack thereof), as long that they can assess for the functional relationship between the patient's S/R and their symptoms, as well as explore spiritual resources together with the patient. Furthermore, examining this relationship and incorporating S/R into treatment (for patients who request that) do not devalue the sanctity of the S/R. If anything, they demonstrate to the patient that the clinician takes their S/R beliefs seriously and sees their value and meaning as they pertain to the patient.

COMMON OBSTACLES IN SUPERVISION AND WAYS OF OVERCOMING THEM

Effective supervision relies on the trainee being open minded, diversity focused, client focused, and understanding collaborative empiricism. It is also important that trainees do not bring into therapy any pro- or antireligious agendas. Proreligious agendas, for example, might lead to overemphasizing the role of spiritual resources and underestimating spiritual symptoms and struggles. Conversely, trainees with antireligious agendas may neglect to identify spiritual resources for their patients and may encourage patients with spiritual struggles or symptoms to abandon their faith as a way of ameliorating their emotional suffering. Therefore, supervisors should help trainees become aware of their biases and keep them in check when treating patients for whom S/R is relevant. Supervisors must also be aware of their own biases that can prevent trainees from bringing up S/R issues in supervision.

It is also helpful for beginning clinicians to supplement their training in the S/R domain since (as previously mentioned) many training programs provide little to no training in this area (Rosmarin et al., 2013). Useful resources include didactic workshops, reading, and, most important, in vivo work to get to a place of competence. It is worth noting that the art of integrating S/R into treatment goes well beyond this chapter, given that incorporating S/R into assessment and treatment requires nuance, knowledge, and a great deal of preparatory study (and practice under supervision) before it can be done competently.

CONCLUSION

Most Americans identify with some form of S/R. Furthermore, many patients express interest in addressing S/R in treatment. Yet, training programs provide almost no training in this area, and most clinicians feel underprepared when it come to the S/R domain. Therefore, it is often up to individual supervisors to supply training so that clinicians can be more comfortable and competent in assessing S/R and incorporating it in treatment when indicated. Assessment is a critical piece of clinical care because it provides the road map to treatment. Thus, it is important for trainees to learn about the different ways S/R can relate to patients' symptoms (in both positive and negative ways) and which specific aspects of S/R are important to assess. Given the considerable amount of training that CBT-oriented trainees usually receive regarding functional analysis, many already have the foundational tools necessary to be able to examine the relationship between S/R and presenting symptoms. It is just a matter of knowing what sort of questions to ask and what types of relationships to look for as a patient describes their S/R beliefs and practices. Readers are advised to use this chapter as a stepping stone in helping trainees to appreciate the relevance of S/R as it related to patients' mental health and to learn the basics of assessment when it comes to this aspect of patients' lives.

REFERENCES

American Psychological Association. (2017). *Ethical principles of psychologists and code of conduct* (2002, Amended June 1, 2010, and January 1, 2017). http://www.apa.org/ethics/code/index.aspx

Curlin, F. A., Lawrence, R. E., Odell, S., Chin, M. H., Lantos, J. D., Koenig, H. G., & Meador, K. G. (2007). Religion, spirituality, and medicine: Psychiatrists' and other physicians' differing observations, interpretations, and clinical approaches. *The American Journal of Psychiatry, 164*(12), 1825–1831. https://doi.org/10.1176/appi.ajp.2007.06122088

Curlin, F. A., Odell, S. V., Lawrence, R. E., Chin, M. H., Lantos, J. D., Meador, K. G., & Koenig, H. G. (2007). The relationship between psychiatry and religion among U.S. physicians. *Psychiatric Services, 58*(9), 1193–1198. https://doi.org/10.1176/ps.2007.58.9.1193

Delaney, H. D., Miller, W. R., & Bisonó, A. M. (2007). Religiosity and spirituality among psychologists: A survey of clinician members of the American Psychological Association. *Professional Psychology: Research and Practice, 38*(5), 538–546. https://doi.org/10.1037/0735-7028.38.5.538

Eifert, G. H., & Forsyth, J. P. (2005). *Acceptance and commitment therapy for anxiety disorders: A practitioner's treatment guide to using mindfulness, acceptance, and values-based behavior change.* New Harbinger Publications.

Gallup. (2011). *Religion.* http://www.gallup.com/poll/1690/religion.aspx

Hill, P. C., Pargament, K. I., Hood, R. W., McCullough, J. M. E., Swyers, J. P., Larson, D. B., & Zinnbauer, B. J. (2000). Conceptualizing religion and spirituality: Points of commonality, points of departure. *Journal for the Theory of Social Behaviour, 30*(1), 51–77. https://doi.org/10.1111/1468-5914.00119

Kiani, M. A., & Saeidi, M. (2015). Importance of hand hygiene in different religions. *Joint Commission Perspectives on Patient Safety, 3*, 1–2.

Marler, P. L., & Hadaway, C. K. (2002). "Being religious" or "being spiritual" in America: A zero-sum proposition? *Journal for the Scientific Study of Religion, 41*(2), 289–300. https://doi.org/10.1111/1468-5906.00117

Moreira-Almeida, A., Sharma, A., van Rensburg, B. J., Verhagen, P. J., & Cook, C. C. (2016). WPA position statement on spirituality and religion in psychiatry. *World Psychiatry, 15*(1), 87–88. https://doi.org/10.1002/wps.20304

Pargament, K. I., Murray-Swank, N. A., Magyar, G. M., & Ano, G. G. (2005). Spiritual struggle: A phenomenon of interest to psychology and religion. In W. R. Miller & H. D. Delaney (Eds.), *Judeo-Christian perspectives on psychology: Human nature, motivation, and change* (pp. 245–268). American Psychological Association. https://doi.org/10.1037/10859-013

Pargament, K. I., & Saunders, S. M. (2007). Introduction to the special issue on spirituality and psychotherapy. *Journal of Clinical Psychology, 63*(10), 903–907. https://doi.org/10.1002/jclp.20405

Pew Research Center. (2014a). *Attendance at religious services.* https://www.pewforum.org/religious-landscape-study/attendance-at-religious-services/

Pew Research Center. (2014b). *Frequency of prayer.* https://www.pewforum.org/religious-landscape-study/frequency-of-prayer/

Propst, L. R., Ostrom, R., Watkins, P., Dean, T., & Mashburn, D. (1992). Comparative efficacy of religious and nonreligious cognitive-behavioral therapy for the treatment of clinical depression in religious individuals. *Journal of Consulting and Clinical Psychology, 60*(1), 94–103. https://doi.org/10.1037/0022-006X.60.1.94

Rogers, C. R. (1951). *Client-centered therapy; Its current practice, implications, and theory.* Houghton Mifflin.

Rose, E. M., Westefeld, J. S., & Ansely, T. N. (2001). Spiritual issues in counseling: Clients' beliefs and preferences. *Journal of Counseling Psychology, 48*(1), 61–71. https://doi.org/10.1037/0022-0167.48.1.61

Rosmarin, D. H., Forester, B. P., Shassian, D. M., Webb, C. A., & Björgvinsson, T. (2015). Interest in spiritually integrated psychotherapy among acute psychiatric patients. *Journal of Consulting and Clinical Psychology, 83*(6), 1149–1153. https://doi.org/10.1037/ccp0000046

Rosmarin, D. H., Green, D., Pirutinsky, S., & McKay, D. (2013). Attitudes toward spirituality/religion among members of the Association for Behavioral and Cognitive Therapies. *Professional Psychology: Research and Practice, 44*(6), 424–433. https://doi.org/10.1037/a0035218

Rosmarin, D. H., & Pirutinsky, S. (2020). Do religious patients need religious psychotherapists? A naturalistic treatment matching study among Orthodox Jews. *Journal of Anxiety Disorders, 69*, 102170. https://doi.org/10.1016/j.janxdis.2019.102170

Rosmarin, D. H., Pirutinsky, S., & Siev, J. (2010). Recognition of scrupulosity and non-religious OCD by Orthodox and non-Orthodox Jews. *Journal of Social and Clinical Psychology, 29*(8), 930–944. https://doi.org/10.1521/jscp.2010.29.8.930

Rosmarin, D. H., Salcone, S., Harper, D. G., & Forester, B. (2021). Predictors of patients' responses to Spiritual Psychotherapy for Inpatient, Residential & Intensive Treatment (SPIRIT). *Psychiatric Services, 72*(5), 507–513. https://doi.org/10.1176/appi.ps.202000331

World Psychiatric Association. (2002). *Institutional program on the core training curriculum for psychiatry.*

18

Clinical Supervision in Delivering Cognitive Behavior Therapy Across Race, Ethnicity, and Culture

Monnica T. Williams and Joseph La Torre

As the United States becomes increasingly diverse racially, ethnically, and culturally, clinicians can expect to see increases in clients of color. These include people who may identify as African American, Hispanic American, Asian American, Native American, non-White internationals, or multiethnic individuals. People of color deserve care that is of equal quality to the care White clients receive, and it is an ethical duty as mental health providers to uphold this standard and put it into practice. Indeed, diversity is one of the principal domains of competence in supervisory skills as outlined by the American Psychological Association (APA; 2014) in its *Guidelines for Clinical Supervision in Health Service Psychology*, where diversity includes "race, ethnicity, culture, [and] national origin" (p. 11). Likewise, the APA (2017) *Multicultural Guidelines* exhort supervisors to model of culturally competent practices, as this plays a key role in helping students develop cultural competence.

At the same time, however, trainees of any ethnicity may have difficulty delivering proper treatment to diverse clients due to having learned cognitive behavior therapy (CBT) from a Western, White, Eurocentric perspective that may not always meet the needs of people of color (Leong & Kalibatseva, 2011). All therapists at some point will encounter clients who do not share their race, ethnicity, or culture. Yet many people know little to nothing about those who

The authors acknowledge Noor Sharif for assistance with clinical examples, Joel Lopez for help with reference materials, and Traleena Rouleau for developing the table for cultural issues in help-seeking.

https://doi.org/10.1037/0000314-019
Training and Supervision in Specialized Cognitive Behavior Therapy: Methods, Settings, and Populations, E. A. Storch, J. S. Abramowitz, and D. McKay (Editors)

are not like them. As such, trainees and supervisors alike must actively seek that knowledge for the good of all those they serve.

KEY CONCEPTS FOR TRAINEES TO LEARN

Trainees need to learn several key concepts when working with clients from culturally diverse communities. Clients of color may have varying levels of ethnic identity and acculturation, requiring different approaches, even between individuals from the same ethnic group (Chapman et al., 2018; Kim et al., 2001). All client assessments should consider race, ethnicity, and culture, which may strain CBT treatment approaches that were developed on Western samples and reflect predominantly Western values. Additionally, clients of color are more likely to be disadvantaged, and as such they will have fewer resources and more barriers to care (e.g., Leong & Kalibatseva, 2011). Disadvantage may be due to experiences of racism, current or historical, and racism in the lives of clients of color is stressful. To compound this, therapists may enact racism without realizing it (Constantine, 2007; Owen et al., 2014).

Ethnic Identity and Acculturation

Ethnic identity describes how people develop and experience a sense of belonging to their culture (Phinney, 1989). Traditions, customs, and feelings about one's heritage are important factors in ethnic identity development. Individuals progress through different stages as they learn to identify with their culture, come to understand the group customs and values, and ultimately comfortably identify with their ethnic group. Different models have been studied, and it is widely agreed that to achieve a strong sense of ethnic identity, people first go through a thorough process of exploration of their culture. This process has different stages, and the strength of an individual's ethnic identity will depend on the stage the person is in within the process (Phinney, 1989).

Ethnic identity can impact the rapport and trust between the therapist and a client of color, based on stage of identity development in the client (Graham-LoPresti et al., 2019). Most clients feel more comfortable discussing psychological problems with someone of the same ethnic and racial background, and they may answer questions about symptoms more accurately when matched (Smith & Trimble, 2016, Chapter 6). However, clients of color in an early stage of ethnic identity development may suffer from internalized racism, believing that White people are better and thus prefer a White therapist (Graham-LoPresti et al., 2019). Clients who are at a more advanced stage of ethnic identity development and those who are less acculturated may tend to prefer someone from their own ethnic group, and those who are secure in their identity development may prefer to be matched but still be comfortable with any good, culturally informed therapist. Alternatively, when pairing therapists and clients, supervisors must not assume that clients of color will always be more comfortable with a clinician from the same ethnocultural group as sometimes due to feelings of shame about mental health issues, speaking to a member from a different group may be preferable.

Race, Ethnicity, and Culture

Race, ethnicity, and culture form a critical basis of one's identity, and culture informs a person's values and worldview. *Race* may be characterized as the phenotypical expression of one's identity, while *ethnicity* can be thought of as being the expression of one's cultural identity. Race and ethnicity are both social constructions. However, ethnicity is a positive construct designed by specific cultural groups for their own benefit, whereas race is an inherently racist concept because it deliberately places people into castes based on their appearance and presumed ancestry (Williams, 2020). Therefore, people of color in America, Canada, or other Westernized countries may take pride in their race because it represents accomplishments and resilience in the face of continual oppression. Indeed, research indicates that people of color who are proud of their ethnic identity are better equipped to manage the stresses of racism (Williams et al., 2012).

In the context of CBT (and therapy more broadly), race, ethnicity, and culture are extremely important because they are intricately interwoven with one's life experiences. For example, members of marginalized ethnoracial groups may face discrimination on multiple levels due to their race, ethnicity, and culture. As such therapists must be prepared to confront these issues and speak openly about them with clients. Therefore, trainees and supervisors must work together to navigate these differences conscientiously if they are to provide adequate treatment to diverse, underrepresented, and underserved populations.

Empirically Supported Treatments May Not Be Universal

As previously noted, most CBT treatment approaches were developed on Western samples and reflect predominantly Western values. Moreover, some treatments were validated on homogeneous almost exclusively White samples or the demographics of treatment outcome study samples were not reported at all. For example, Mendoza et al. (2010) found that several randomized controlled trials of panic disorder failed to report any ethnoracial differences, and those that did used an overwhelmingly homogenous sample, which was on average 82.7% White ($n = 2,867$). Another study examining obsessive–compulsive disorder (OCD) randomized controlled trials from 1995 to 2008 found that samples ($n = 2,221$) were 91.5% White (Williams et al., 2010). Trials of eye movement desensitization and reprocessing have included almost no people of color at all (Grau et al., 2022). Therefore, trainees should understand that many treatments are not generalizable to people of color; as such, they may not work as intended and may need to be modified (e.g., Williams et al., 2014).

Clients of Color May Face Greater Barriers to Treatment

Trainees should appreciate that clients of color may experience more barriers to treatment than clients who are White due to lower income, racism, language, and immigrant status. Thus, it is not unusual for treatment to be temporarily derailed, for example, due to needing to take on more family obligations. Clinicians should therefore be understanding if treatment goals take longer to accomplish than expected based on manualized protocols. Trainees should also keep in mind that clients of color may be wary of seeking treatment because of shared cultural memory of medical abuses such as Tuskegee syphilis study of African Americans (Gamble, 1997). Worries of being discriminated against in treatment are well-founded and may include fears of receiving inadequate treatment, being misdiagnosed, confirming false stereotypes, having beliefs pathologized, or being labeled as severely mentally ill. Clients may have tried to handle issues on their own, only seeking therapy as a last resort, or drop out of treatment prematurely when symptoms start to abate. Barriers may also revolve around costs, difficulty getting time off work, inability to find a therapist in their own ethnic group, fears of being criticized by family for seeking out mental health care treatment, shame, transportation issues, fears of being involuntarily hospitalized, being treated unfairly due to racism, and language barriers (Williams et al., 2010).

Therapists may at times need to be allies for their clients of color. For example, if a client is a college student failing their classes due to poor mental health, it may be unreasonable to expect the client to be able to speak directly to their professor or other superiors for accommodations because many cultural groups highly respect teachers and consider having mental health challenges shameful. Also, students of color may be given less consideration in such circumstances due to racism and bias. Therapists may need to help advocate in such cases—for example, by directly assisting the client in making an appointment with the office of students with disabilities to have their classes dropped and expunged, making calls, writing letters, or even accompanying them to meetings.

Clients of Color May Experience Stress Due to Racism

Racism is widespread and can be extremely stressful to people of color. Berger and Sarnyai (2015) conducted a literature review showing that racial discrimination affects victims at a physiological level and in the brain appears to converge on the anterior cingulate cortex, leading to prefrontal cortex impairment exemplifying chronic social stress. This may lead to increases in cortisol and adrenaline, which both have the potential to place excessive stress on the body and can result in a number of health problems, such as rapid weight gain, muscle weakness, and diabetes. Psychologically speaking, racism can even lead to traumatization, and may merit a PTSD diagnosis (Williams, Metzger, et al., 2018; Williams, Printz, et al., 2018). Racial discrimination can cause other mental health problems in people of color as well, including anxiety, depression, substance use, eating disorders, and psychosis. Therefore, trainees should consider the additional stress caused by racialization in all aspects of the lives of their clients of color.

Therapists May Behave in Racist Ways Unintentionally

Although few therapists would consider themselves racists, they may enact racism without realizing it. For example, well-intentioned clinicians might say something that they believe is culturally relevant but is actually a misperception or generalization (e.g., Constantine, 2007). Stereotypical comments may also fall into this category of racism, referred to as *microaggressions* (Williams, 2020). When therapists act on these implicit biases, they also fail in providing proper care.

A student therapist once explained her approach to working with people of color by saying, "I don't see color." She thought that a denial of racial differences would increase trust within the therapeutic relationship. She didn't understand that to people of color "I don't see color" can mean "I don't see you." It means, "I don't understand, or choose not to acknowledge, the unique and oppressive experiences that contribute to your distress." This supervisee had good intentions, but she didn't see how harmful a colorblind approach can be in the therapy relationship (Parker et al., 2020).

Moreover, when therapists microaggress, it is not only threatening to the therapeutic alliance but also contributes to the client's stress. As such, clients are more likely to drop out or fail to follow treatment recommendations (Williams & Halstead, 2019). Therefore, therapists must understand the difference between actual cultural differences and pathological stereotypes that give rise to microaggressions.

KEY TECHNIQUES FOR TRAINEES TO LEARN

Some key techniques that trainees must learn to ensure they are delivering proper CBT treatment to clients from underrepresented groups include being aware of their own limitations and biases and working to correct errant beliefs by confronting them head on. Some ways trainees can do this include (a) having conversations with clients about race, ethnicity, and culture; (b) assessing the impact of racism through the use of validated instruments; (c) creating culturally informed case conceptualizations; and (d) integrating an antiracist framework in treatment.

Talking to Clients About Race, Ethnicity, and Culture

Trainees must learn how to have open dialogues about race, ethnicity, culture, and religion with clients, particularly those who identify as being members of a group different from the trainee. Most people of color, especially if they were born and raised in the United States, have been having conversations about racial issues since they were young (Priest et al., 2014). In contrast, most

White people are socialized not to talk about race and were taught growing up that being colorblind is how people show they are not racist (Underhill, 2018). As such, most White people have no practice talking about race, ethnicity, and culture and cannot do this well, either in day-to-day life or with clients (Sue et al., 2010). To correct this problem, trainees should practice these skills, identify areas of discomfort, and critically evaluate any implicit biases. Supervisors should encourage trainees to have race-related conversations with clients of color as often as possible, as appropriate.

Culturally Informed Case Conceptualization

Trainees and aspiring clinicians should be able to formulate culturally informed case conceptualizations, which make use of relevant demographic information to best understand and help the client. As outlined in the fifth edition of the *Diagnostic and Statistical Manual of Mental Disorders* (*DSM-5*; American Psychiatric Association, 2013), culturally informed conceptualizations will include an assessment and subsequent integration of several salient components of the client's life experience, including

> the values, orientations, knowledge and practices that individuals derive from membership in diverse social groups, aspects of one's background, developmental experiences, and current social contexts that may affect his or her perspective, such as geographical original, migration, language, religion, sexual orientation, or race/ethnicity, and the influence of family, friends, and other community members on the individual's illness experience. (p. 750)

Because modern Western psychiatry and clinical psychology are inherently Eurocentric schools of thought, not all clients may subscribe to these beliefs. Therapists must therefore be competent in incorporating an emic understanding of mental health problems into treatment (Graham-LoPresti et al., 2019). One way trainees can learn to do this is by making use of the *DSM-5* Cultural Formulation Interview (CFI). The CFI was developed as a concerted effort by the American Psychiatric Association to acknowledge and incorporate culturally predicated explanatory models into treatment. The interview emphasizes four main domains of assessment: (a) cultural definitions of the problem; (b) cultural perceptions of cause, context, and support; (c) cultural factors affecting self-coping and past help-seeking; and (d) cultural factors affecting current help-seeking. Table 18.1 includes some helpful cultural information about various ethnoracial groups and therapeutic considerations, with a focus on help-seeking for selected groups. (Turner et al., 2016; Williams, Chapman, et al., 2012).

Ultimately, culturally informed assessment and treatment rests upon a solid foundation of awareness, which helps to facilitate a process of recognizing each client's cultural context as equally valuable and places importance on working within clients' values and belief systems in all aspects of therapy (Graham-LoPresti et al., 2019). Therefore, supervisors should ensure that trainees obtain experience in making culturally informed case conceptualizations by practicing using approaches like the CFI with diverse clients at intake whenever possible.

TABLE 18.1. Examples of Help-Seeking Behaviors and Approaches in Selected Groups

Ethnic/racial group	Help-seeking behaviour	Integration by clinician
Asian	Family and social support may be preferred. Alternative healing methods (herbal medicine, acupuncture) may be favored. More likely to engage primary care. Collectivist coping strategies may be used. Avoidance of psychological services for fear of stigma. Reliance on religious sources of support.	If possible, involve important sources of support in treatment. Involve traditional healers. Acknowledge nature of somatic symptoms, consult with medical professionals, and incorporate a holistic approach to treatment. Respect that help-seeking may introduce familial conflict due to concerns over privacy and mutual support. Validate the difficulty associated with seeking services and provide psychoeducation on the damaging nature of stereotypes. Frame psychological services as a way to bolster personal strengths. Collaborate with religious leaders to support help-seeking within religious community and improve treatment outcome.
Hispanic/Latinx	Lack of service opportunities in rural areas, which may disproportionately affect Latinx migrant farm workers. More frequent engagement through primary care. May prefer to engage local ethnic sources of support. May engage *curanderos* (folk healers) and *sobadores* (masseurs). May believe in *fatalismo*, an understanding that God controls fate and that illnesses should be overcome individually. May prioritize *familismo* (family) and feel guilty about affecting the family through attending treatment. Value *respeto* (respect) in the family.	Offer psychological services through telehealth, create office spaces in rural areas, and travel to rural areas for sessions. Address somatic symptoms, consult with medical professionals, and integrate services within medical system. Consult with others from the client's cultural community (family, clergy) and involve them in treatment. Involve these healers in treatment and encourage the client to engage in culturally relevant treatment outside of therapy. Validate client's belief and seek to capitalize on client strengths to support their value of resilience.

(continues)

TABLE 18.1. Examples of Help-Seeking Behaviors and Approaches in Selected Groups (*Continued*)

Ethnic/racial group	Help-seeking behaviour	Integration by clinician
	Machismo (a Latino's duty to protect and financially support his family) may impact Latinos' comfort with treatment.	Frame treatment as an opportunity to become healthy to better support family.
	Marianismo (Latinas' duty to take care of the family and make personal sacrifices).	With child clients, respect the input of caregivers and frame them as leaders within the family unit.
		Discuss the client's understanding and adherence to gender roles and approach treatment as a chance to learn to better support family through improved mental health.
		Consider the appropriateness of group therapy of Latino men and Latina women to reduce stigma and openly discuss gender roles.
Black	May prefer internal sources of social support (family, friends, spiritual leaders).	Consult and involve important networks in treatment.
	Presence of stigma could inhibit clients from discussing symptoms outside of religious and familial circles.	Directly address stigma in treatment and collaborate and consult with cultural leaders to reduce stigma and increase comfort in treatment.
	Values of strength and resilience may discourage clients from seeking services due to stigma or shame.	Integrate values of strength and resilience into treatment and emphasize client strengths.
	Cultural mistrust toward White clinicians may discourage Black clients from seeking services in predominantly White service centers.	Acknowledge strength associated with seeking services in the face of potential stigma.
	Tendency to use emergency department services and access support only when symptoms are most severe.	Employ Black clinicians and staff, engage in racial and ethnic matching (if desired by the client), and openly discuss race within therapeutic dyads of differing races.
		Liaise with health care professionals and serve as a referral for medical institutions.
		Provide community psychoeducation about the importance of seeking services early.

TABLE 18.1. Examples of Help-Seeking Behaviors and Approaches in Selected Groups (*Continued*)

Ethnic/racial group	Help-seeking behaviour	Integration by clinician
Indigenous (American Indian/Alaska Native) in North America	Preference for less formal and more traditional sources of support and services offered on reservations.	If desired by client, offer treatment within reservation and involve informal sources of support in treatment.
	Engagement with spiritual activities to support mental health problems.	Consult with spiritual leaders in community to supplement treatment with valued spiritual approaches.
	Privacy concerns may prevent clients from seeking services.	Openly discuss concerns around confidentiality and thoroughly answer client questions.
	Stigma may deter clients from seeking services.	
	Westernized cognitive behavior therapy protocols may not align with Indigenous culture, tradition, and sources of knowledge and be reminiscent of colonization, prompting negative perceptions of mental health professionals.	Address fears of stigma and consider involving cultural leaders to further validate client's concerns.
		Explore the possibility of offering group therapy in which members of the cultural community openly discuss experiences with mental health struggles.
		Explore and integrate client's worldview and involve traditional healers.
		Emphasize client autonomy and ownership over treatment.
		Openly address ethnic differences between clinician and client and impact of history of colonization.
Middle Eastern	Clients may prefer relying on informal sources of support, including friends, elders, and family.	Involve these important sources of support in treatment.
	Clients may turn to traditional healers and religious leaders.	Consult and collaborate with these leaders to create an effective and culturally relevant treatment plan.
	Clients may prefer clinicians who have experience with religious rituals associated with Islam when approaching religious obsessions and compulsions.	If desired by client, employ clinicians who identify as Muslim or consult with imams to delineate difference between religious doctrine and symptomatology.
Indian	Men may be more likely than women to access services due to social structure hierarchies.	Conduct outreach work with Indian women to encourage service use and highlight available treatment options and coverage.
	Clients may wish to engage with religious services due to the mismatch between Westernized models and cultural beliefs.	Involve religious leaders and adapt treatment to integrate clients' beliefs.

Assessing for the Impact of Racism

Because racism can contribute to many negative mental health outcomes and cause barriers to treatment (Turner et al., 2016), supervisors should encourage trainees to assess the impact of racism in clients of color. Trainees can use the wide spectrum of validated assessments tools, especially if they are not yet sufficiently skilled to ask clients directly about their experiences with racism. Several self-report measures are useful for identifying problems such as micro-aggressions, including the Racial and Ethnic Microaggressions Scale (Nadal, 2011) and the Multiracial Microaggression Scale (Johnston & Nadal, 2010). The General Ethnic Discrimination Scale (Landrine et al., 2006) may be helpful for measuring frequency of ethnic discrimination throughout one's life and how it may be resulting in stress for the client. The Trauma Symptoms of Discrimination Scale (Williams, Printz, & DeLapp, 2018) is another instrument that can be used to measure distress caused specifically by discriminatory acts. The Racial Microaggressions in Counseling Scale (Constantine, 2007) may be useful for helping alert the supervisor to problems trainees may be having in properly interacting with their clients of color. For a more in-depth review of additional validated instruments, see Williams (2020).

In terms of clinician-administered interviews, the UConn Racial/Ethnic Stress and Trauma Survey (Williams, Metzger, et al., 2018) can help assess whether clients of color may be experiencing clinically significant levels of trauma or distress brought on by racism, as well as whether symptoms expressed may warrant a PTSD diagnosis (Williams, 2020). It is crucial for supervisors to ensure trainees understand the impact of racism on mental health and make space to discuss the client's experiences with discrimination. However, even if supervisors direct trainees to do so, they may avoid it due to fear of how the conversation could unfold, so follow-up is important.

Adapting CBT Treatments to Different Cultural Groups

As noted previously, CBT approaches emanate from a primarily Western perspective and therefore may not necessarily be entirely transferable or effective with other groups (Hays, 2009). Different cultures may also have differing culturally predicated explanatory models of psychopathology. For example, Fernández de la Cruz et al. (2016) demonstrated differences in perceived causes of OCD symptoms among different ethnoracial groups. More recently, however, studies examining treatment outcomes of CBT for people of color have been emerging and one study by Fernández de la Cruz et al. (2016) found that exposure and response prevention (ERP) for OCD was equally effective for White and non-White youth in the United Kingdom. At the same time, however, there were significant differences in attitudes and beliefs espoused by the different groups—namely, that participants of color tended to endorse fears of not saying the right thing, perhaps due to fear of harsh reprisals or being seen as unintelligent. This fear may be compounded by the fact that individuals from communities of color experience greater mental health stigma than White individuals (Williams et al., 2017). Ultimately, therapists must go beyond simply being able to recognize that CBT may be inadequate for certain groups and instead be able to modify and adapt treatment according to client needs. Trainees may need help from supervisors to do this effectively. Knowing how to modify a treatment generally takes more skill than simply recognizing it is inadequate.

Being an Antiracist Clinician

Since the murder of George Floyd, it has been said that we are in the midst of a new civil rights movement as the reality of racism moves into sharper focus (Strauss, 2020). As a result of this, several paradigm shifts have occurred, including a major revision in how we understand racism. Being nonracist is not enough to effectively treat people of color. Rather, clinicians and trainees alike must adopt an antiracist approach to ensure racialized clients receive the best treatment possible (Rosen et al., 2019). While people often think of racism as referring to "old-school racism," it is understood to mean both acts of racism that are unintentional or covert (e.g., microaggressions) and those that are intentional or overt (e.g., the use of racial slurs; Bartoli & Pyati, 2009; Williams, 2020). Trainees must recognize that racism may be enacted even when there is a lack of intention to be offensive or cause harm, and they should have a working knowledge of the different types of racism clients may experience (Rosen et al., 2019).

Supervisors should also help trainees learn to accept difficult feelings surrounding race rather than avoid them. One way to reduce avoidance is by assigning trainees a diversified caseload early on. Trainees should also be advised to be curious about their own stereotypes and biases and how to manage them. This can be facilitated through work that requires trainees to reflect on such issues, which will also allow them to participate actively in being part of the solution (Williams et al., 2022). Finally, trainees should also take risks to forge genuine relationships with people who are different and from diverse backgrounds, both in their professional and nonprofessional lives.

Despite all of this, trainees may still commit microaggressions or other insensitive acts, and so therapists should invite clients to let them know if anything like this ever occurs in session so that the therapist can initiate a repair.

WHAT CLIENT CHARACTERISTICS MAKE FOR A GOOD TRAINING CASE

The U.S. Census Bureau (2014) projected that by 2044, non-Hispanic Whites may no longer be the majority in the United States. As a result, trainees must prepare for an increasingly diverse clientele. Supervisors should encourage students to take on diverse clients and let them know that support is available as needed. Trainees and supervisors should also meet regularly to discuss culturally informed approaches to treatment as well as strategies for incorporating and integrating principles of multicultural therapy into CBT (Hays, 2009).

Racial Differences

Trainees need to gain experience treating clients from all racial groups because experiences of racism vary by racial category and skin tone. This is especially true for people with dark skin, who, as Keith and colleagues (2017) noted, are more likely to experience racial bias than are individuals who appear more White. This may also be true even if a group with darker skin has been in the United States for multiple generations while a new immigrant who appears lighter may simply be assumed to be White and therefore experience less discrimination. Furthermore, Sue et al. (2007) pointed out that it is not uncommon for someone to assume that just because a person has darker skin, they are not a true American and may be more criminally dangerous or less intelligent.

Ethnocultural Differences

Trainees must recognize that clients—especially clients of color—will have multiple layers of identity. In addition to one's socially constructed racial category and phenotypical characteristics, clients may also identify strongly with their ethnocultural group(s). This means that although a White person from New York City and a White person from Appalachia are both phenotypically and racially similar, their ethnicities may vary greatly. This is because racial categories are generally extremely broad, and races such as White may include groups with vastly different ethnocultural practices and backgrounds such as Italians, Germans, Portuguese, and Middle-Easterners. Similarly, the category of Black may include ethnicities from different regions of the world, including the Caribbean and Africa. People who are considered Asian may also, despite being of the same race, have tremendously different ethnoracial identities such as Chinese, Japanese, Korean, Thai, Cambodian, Vietnamese, Nepalese, Filipino, and Indian (Kim et al., 2001). Additionally, people of Filipino heritage may identify more closely with Hispanic cultural values than East Asian values. Individuals from these countries may also belong to ethnoracial minority groups such as ethnic Tibetans and Mongolians living within China whose traditional beliefs, practices, and cultures differ from the Han majority. Trainees should therefore learn about a client's ethnic group through a combination of asking the client and by doing their own study of the client's culture. The client should not be the sole educator of the therapist, but the therapist needs to learn from the client ways in which the client conforms or differs from their cultural norms.

Religious Differences

Religion is intricately linked to culture, and people express their faiths in many ways. For many people, their faith is what defines them as a person, and so a therapist cannot have a complete understanding of a person without some understanding of their spiritual beliefs. Trainees must recognize that there is a wide spectrum of religious traditions practiced in the world today, the majority of which espouse practices that are historically and culturally dissimilar from Judeo–Christian practices endorsed in the United States and Canada. Some traditions that trainees may encounter include Buddhism, Hinduism, Islam, Jainism, Sikhism, Shinto, Daoism, and Confucianism. Trainees must also be trained to respect clients who choose to incorporate into their worldview complementary and alternative medicines and traditional healing, such as yoga, astrology, and Voodoo (Moodley & Sutherland, 2010) as well as traditional Chinese medicine, meditation, acupuncture, herbalism, and shamanism. Increasing numbers of North Americans, especially the younger generations, are nonreligious, so it may be a struggle for such therapists to relate to the client's belief system. Chapter 17 in this volume provides more information on addressing religion and spirituality in supervision.

Sexual and Gender Minorities

Many people of color are also sexual or gender minorities. Taking the opportunity to work with people with intersectional identities is important, but the more stigmatized identities a person has, the more complex the issues are likely to be, due to the compounding effects of stigma (e.g., Wadsworth et al., 2020). Therefore, it might be best to start trainees with clients who have fewer stigmatized identities to gain experience and confidence, and then work up to those with many different stigmatized identities. One excellent resource for working with sexual or gender minority clients is Skinta (2020). See also Chapter 19 in this volume for more details on supervision and consultation in working with LGBTQ clients.

Immigrants and Refugees

When seeking mental health services, new immigrants and refugees may face several barriers, such as language, lack of knowledge of the public health systems, fears of deportation, misconceptions of mental illness, and financial hardship. Seeking psychotherapy is not uncommon among new immigrants and refugees; however, early termination rates are high, likely due to clinicians lacking cultural competency skills (e.g., Schlaudt et al., 2020). Refugees of color may have experienced a multiplicity of traumatic events, including working in concentration or labor camps for extensive periods of time, being subjected to ethnic cleansing, and being starved and tortured, as well as race-based trauma they may face when arriving in the United States, Canada, and Europe. If trainees have the opportunity to work with new immigrants and refugees, they should take it because it is important to learn how to work with these underserved groups.

English as a Second Language

Clients of color often come from diverse backgrounds and may not necessarily speak English as their native language. For many, English is a second language or may even be the third or fourth language one has learned. In addition, in some instances, clients may not have been afforded the opportunity to learn English in a formal educational setting and may therefore experience additional barriers to accessing proper treatment. When English is a client's second language, therapists should try their best to speak as clearly as possible. It is recommended that they steer clear of using highly complex vocabulary and instead tailor their language in a way that is easily comprehensible to the client without overadjusting. Also, if trainees are comfortable conversing in the native language of a client, it would be better to speak in this language as opposed to English. However, if the client cannot make themselves well-understood to the therapist, this is likely not a good training case. Although many clinics and hospitals make translators available, translated psychotherapy is substandard at best, and overall is not recommended. Rather than using a translator, it is advisable that a therapist be found who can communicate in the client's language. However, if interpreters must be used, this does provide an additional excellent training experience for supervisees.

Multicultural Families

Trainees may also take on clients who come from multicultural backgrounds, meaning that parents or close relatives may not all belong to the same ethno-cultural or ethnoracial group. For example, a client could be biracial with a Black mother and Native American father. In instances such as these, trainees must pay close attention to any conflicting views within the family and tailor treatment in a way that is culturally informed on both sides. This also means that when only some family members are White, the therapist may need to advocate for the non-White family members because they may be told their views are unimportant or secondary to the White person's understanding of the situation. For example, it is not uncommon for a client of color with one parent of color and one White parent to speak of experiences of racism and for the White parent to either disregard such statements or underestimate the severity of distress discrimination may be inducing (Johnston & Nadal, 2010). Ultimately, cases with multicultural elements are great learning experiences, but there are often a lot of moving parts involved, so they may be better suited for more advanced trainees.

COMMON MISTAKES TRAINEES MAKE AND HOW TO FIX THEM

It is common for trainees to make mistakes on their way toward cultural competency. In this section, we lay out the different kinds of mistakes they may make and how to address them.

Failure to Consider Non-Western Values and Worldviews

Clients may have priorities that therapists have not considered or are unaware of. If the client comes from a culture where respect is highly valued, they may hesitate to speak up and correct the therapist or steer the conversation in a different direction. Clients whose second language is English may have a difficult time communicating their value system, ideals, and worldview to the therapist. Therefore, trainees are encouraged to go beyond an etic assessment and try to understand the client's ethnocultural narrative. They may also ask the client directly what they would like to talk about during sessions and track improvement and changes together.

Pathologizing Cultural Differences

Many models of psychological wellness are based on Western values and worldviews. Without adequate knowledge and appreciation of different cultures, therapists risk pathologizing collectivistic cultural differences. Indeed, it is not uncommon for therapists to commit microaggressions by unknowingly making suggestions based on Western models of childrearing, family values, and morality (Williams, 2020). For example, it would be considered inappropriate for a therapist to encourage young adult clients to pursue their happiness independent of their family needs if they belong to a culture where children are expected to take care of their elderly or pay back their investments to their parents. In addition, in many cultures, it is expected that young adults live in intergenerational households until they are ready to get married, and moving out would be considered a family crisis. Thus, therapists must be able to conceptualize clients' problems in a greater context of societal and cultural norms.

Avoidance of Race, Ethnicity, and Culture

Because it is so easy to say the wrong thing, trainees may think it best to say nothing at all (Sue et al., 2010), but avoiding discussions about race, ethnicity, and culture is not a good idea. Clients may see avoidance as a sign of prejudice or lack of skill in interacting with people from other cultures. Further, clients may feel the therapist is not interested in important parts of their lives. Likewise, religion is an important part of culture that should not be ignored, but this is another area that therapists often feel uncomfortable discussing. The best way to fix this is through practice. As CBT therapists, we know that avoidance of feared stimuli only maintains the fear. Discomfort with these conversations can be conceptualized as a skills deficit that trainees can overcome through exposure. Engaging in conversations about race, ethnicity, and culture will ultimately reduce interracial anxieties and help to change cognitive distortions around race.

ETHICAL ISSUES

Mental health care is bound by a code of ethics, and it is our duty as psychologists to make sure we are upholding values that enable us to serve people as best we can. Some common ethical areas one must know how to navigate include working with clients of diverse backgrounds, different socioeconomic status, and clients with experiences of racial stress and trauma.

Working With Low-Income Clients

Some barriers that may significantly influence treatment may include those related to finances, particularly for low-income clients. In the United States, this may mean that the client does not have access to insurance that adequately covers behavioral health. In Canada, despite having universal health care, mental health may not be covered at all, and fees may be considered better allocated somewhere else such as for necessities such as food or transportation. In addition, low-income clients may not be able to afford their own car and may have to rely solely on public transportation or having a friend or family member bring them to therapy. Job demands may also be relevant because clients are not working while they are in therapy sessions and may lose needed income or not be given time off for appointments. Trainees should thus discuss how to best combat these barriers with their supervisors. Some examples include providing free initial consultations, having some evening or weekend hours, or offering reduced fee/sliding scale rates for clients who demonstrate financial hardship.

When to Refer Out a Client Due to Cultural Differences

Although cultural competency is something that can be learned, clinicians must have the discernment to recognize when clients should be referred out. This is because, at times, clients may come from a cultural perspective that is so vastly different from the therapist's that they may be ill-equipped to work with them. Rather than attempting to quickly become well-versed in the client's culture, it may be more effective—and overall more beneficial for the client—to be referred out to a clinician with the needed specialized skill set. This is especially true if the trainee and supervisor can locate a clinician with the necessary background relatively easily. But if a client is referred out for this reason, it should always be a warm handoff; the client must not be made to feel abandoned.

When a large cultural gap can be accommodated, trainees may still need to consult with others within the client's cultural community such as traditional healers, spiritual leaders, or clergy. Collaboration could include consulting healers through national forums, establishing working alliances as joint helping professionals, consulting confidentially on the client's case with the client's consent, and inviting healers to deliver training to trainees to enhance cultural competence (Pouchly, 2012). Ovuga and colleagues (1999) outlined two potential organizational systems for collaboration between traditional healers and clinicians in which clinicians and traditional healers could make referrals to each other or healers and clinicians could operate within the same service systems and receive joint training. One benefit of the latter system is that supervisors, trainees, and healers could all actively learn from each other. Ultimately, as the trainee's competence increases, they will be able to accommodate a wider array of cultural differences.

Accusations of Racism

It is important for therapists to be prepared for the possibility that a client of color may infer or accuse the therapist outright of being a racist. This may occur when the therapist commits a microaggression, such as stereotyping or making an assumption about the client's position on something due to their identity. Alternatively, it could be related to something the therapist does not do, such as act respectfully toward them. Although being accused of being racist will undoubtedly be upsetting for most therapist trainees, it is important for trainees to handle the situation in a way that prevents an escalation of hostilities. One way to do this is to open up a conversation around discrimination and racism by giving the client the chance to discuss the situation openly and freely without feeling that the therapist is upset or defensive because this could significantly impair the therapeutic alliance and may also leave the client with the impression that seeking out psychotherapy was a bad idea. In some cases, it may be appropriate for the supervisor to get involved directly to demonstrate to the client that the issue is being taken seriously.

COMMON OBSTACLES IN SUPERVISION AND WAYS OF OVERCOMING THEM

Several common obstacles may present themselves in the context of clinical supervision, such as lack of knowledge surrounding culture, ethnicity, and race and the presence of unaddressed implicit bias. Supervisors can overcome these obstacles with an approach centered on cultural competency.

Trainee Lacks Foundational Knowledge of Diversity Issues

Trainees may lack adequate foundational training in diversity issues. For example, although many graduate programs require various electives in different areas of psychology, not all require diversity training. Newly implemented standards around training by the APA (2014, 2015) and similar bodies of regulation have attempted to address this issue; however, the quality of such training varies. In addition, many students will not yet have had the needed coursework by the time they see their first client of color. In these cases, the supervisor may need to provide the trainee with supplementary reading to help bolster their knowledge (e.g., Turner et al., 2016; Williams, 2020; Williams et al., 2019). The trainee should also be encouraged to participate in an experiential antiracism workshop or other immersive activity (e.g., Bardone-Cone et al., 2016). Nonetheless, the range of clients such a trainee might see may be limited in this situation.

Supervisor Lacks Needed Diversity Knowledge

Many supervisors do not have current training in diversity issues. Consider that previous generations of psychologists received no diversity training at all, making them unprepared to teach diversity material to others. Further, early diversity education was focused on learning about norms for different ethnic groups, with little emphasis on the mental health impact of racism, implicit bias, cultural humility, or the importance of doing one's own internal anti-racism and anticolonialization work.

As a result, supervisors may not know how to identify or appropriately address racist actions committed by clients or others (Bartoli & Pyati, 2009). For example, one trainee sought support from their supervisor related to micro-aggressions and racist remarks committed by a client against another ethnic group. The supervisor said that these remarks were not relevant to address unless related to the client's presenting problem. This is incorrect because acts of verbal aggression should always be examined as important potential targets for clinical intervention (Williams, 2020). It is likely the client was causing harm to other people of color in their life as well—not just the thera-pist trainee (who deserved the support of her supervisor whether or not this was the case). Because the supervisor did not appreciate the importance and significance of the situation, the trainee felt pressured to continue working with the client, yet understandably remained highly uncomfortable in the presence of the client. Furthermore, the client never got offered any help related to the problematic behavior of perpetuating racism. The supervisor should have instructed the trainee in how to address the racist remarks during session.

This problem can extend beyond the therapy room because supervisors may not know how to address microaggressions or overt racism committed in a classroom or supervision group (Sue et al., 2009). As an example, a colleague in a supervision group committed a microaggression against a trainee of color, and the attending supervisor ignored it, pretending it did not happen. Several students were surprised this occurred and was not addressed, and the trainee of color felt shocked and humiliated. Because the act happened in the group, the supervisor should have addressed it in the group.

Supervisors themselves may commit microaggressions or even overt racism against trainees of color without awareness. For example, during a work-shop discussing multicultural clinical psychology and cultural competency, the only Black trainee in a clinical training program was asked to leave the room while the presenting supervisor discussed White privilege with the other (all White) students. This was because the supervisor did not want the rest of the White trainees to feel uncomfortable during this discussion while the Black trainee was present. The comfort and fragility of the White students was prioritized over the dignity and learning of the Black student. The super-visor should have prepared a lesson that could be taught to everyone in the group.

Failing to Address Cultural Issues With Trainees of Color

Supervisors working with trainees of color may fail to provide them with adequate or appropriate supervision around cultural and/or CBT issues. This can be a confusing landscape to navigate because trainees of color may know more than supervisors about some things but less about others. Trainees may know more about a client in their own ethnic group than a supervisor from a different ethnic group would know. However, there are two possible perils to this. First, a supervisor may fail to acknowledge a trainee's superior knowledge of a given cultural group and take a colorblind approach (ignoring or failing to ask the trainee). Supervisors may make the related assumption that a trainee's ethnic group is homogenous and therefore assume that a trainee will be able to work easily or seamlessly with clients from the same ethnic group. Second, the supervisor may assume the trainee knows better how to work with clients of color and fails to offer any useful supervision at all. Even if the trainee knows more about their own ethnic group, they still need to learn solid CBT skills. Supervisors should periodically check in with their trainees of color and ask them if their needs are being met surrounding these specific issues and how they can be supportive.

Supervisors may likewise assume that clients would rather work with therapists of their same ethnic background. Although this may be the case, supervisors should not make this assumption without checking with the client. For example, in one instance, a supervisor assigned a trainee a client from the same ethnic and religious group assuming that was what the client would prefer. In fact, the client did not want to work with a therapist from the same ethnic or religious background due to fears around being stigmatized or judged for not following cultural norms. Unfortunately, the client dropped out of therapy soon thereafter, and the supervisor failed to provide adequate support around this issue.

When supervisors lack the appropriate training and knowledge on how to provide appropriate supervision and support to trainees of color, it can be expected to increase stress and frustration in trainees who may then feel alone, unsupported, and poorly trained. As an example, one trainee sought support on how to work with clients as a Muslim woman who wears a headscarf given that clinical training espouses the idea of being a "blank slate" (i.e., a therapist's opinions, beliefs, life experiences, personal matters, etc. are not known to clients, are ambiguous, and should not be shared). However, for many trainees of color this is not possible as markers of their ethnicity, culture, and religious affiliation are visible. The supervisor did not know how to provide appropriate supervision around this topic and simply encouraged the trainee to seek support elsewhere (e.g., readings). The supervisor should have done the necessary work to gain the needed knowledge to understand the issues. In this case, the supervisor missed an opportunity for mutual learning and personal growth at the expense of the student and the student's clients. For more on working with trainees of color, see Oshin et al. (2019).

CONCLUSION

One must consider many important issues when working with trainees treating clients with diverse backgrounds or who may have diverse backgrounds themselves. Differences that factor into how treatment should be modified and adapted include racial, ethnic, cultural, and religious differences. To accommodate everyone, trainees and supervisors must work together to adopt best practices for culturally informed treatment. They must also be aware of the nuances that may be involved with working with clients of color, including potential barriers, such as mental health stigma, language differences, differing value systems, the possibility of committing microaggressions, and the impact discrimination and racism on clients. Even the best-prepared supervisors will need to continually update their knowledge to accommodate the rapidly evolving social and cultural landscape.

REFERENCES

American Psychiatric Association. (2013). *Diagnostic and statistical manual of mental disorders* (5th ed.). American Psychiatric Association.

American Psychological Association. (2014). *Guidelines for clinical supervision in health service psychology.* http://apa.org/about/policy/guidelines-supervision.pdf

American Psychological Association. (2015). *Preparing professional psychologists to serve a diverse public.* https://www.apa.org/ed/graduate/diversity-preparation

American Psychological Association. (2017). *Multicultural guidelines: An ecological approach to context, identity, and intersectionality.* http://www.apa.org/about/policy/multicultural-guidelines.pdf

Bardone-Cone, A. M., Calhoun, C. D., Fischer, M. S., Gaskin-Wasson, A. L., Jones, S. T., Schwartz, S. L., & Prinstein, M. J. (2016). Development and implementation of a diversity training sequence in a clinical psychology doctoral program. *Behavior Therapist, 39*(3), 65–75.

Bartoli, E., & Pyati, A. (2009). Addressing clients' racism and racial prejudice in individual psychotherapy: Therapeutic considerations. *Psychotherapy: Theory, Research, & Practice, 46*(2), 145–157. https://doi.org/10.1037/a0016023

Berger, M., & Sarnyai, Z. (2015). "More than skin deep": Stress neurobiology and mental health consequences of racial discrimination. *The International Journal on the Biology of Stress, 18*(1), 1–10. https://doi.org/10.3109/10253890.2014.989204

Chapman, L. K., DeLapp, R. C. T., & Williams, M. T. (2018). Impact of race, ethnicity, and culture on the expression and assessment of psychopathology. In D. C. Beidel & B. C. Frueh (Eds.), *Adult psychopathology and diagnosis* (8th ed., pp. 131–156). John Wiley & Sons.

Constantine, M. (2007). Racial microaggression against African American clients in cross-racial counseling relationships. *Journal of Counseling Psychology, 54*(1), 1–16. https://doi.org/10.1037/0022-0167.54.1.1

Fernández de la Cruz, L., Kolvenbach, S., Vidal-Ribas, P., Jassi, A., Llorens, M., Patel, N., Weinman, J., Hatch, S. L., Bhugra, D., & Mataix-Cols, D. (2016). Illness perception, help-seeking attitudes, and knowledge related to obsessive-compulsive disorder across different ethnic groups: A community survey. *Social Psychiatry and Psychiatric Epidemiology, 51*(3), 455–464. https://doi.org/10.1007/s00127-015-1144-9

Gamble, V. N. (1997). Under the shadow of Tuskegee: African Americans and health care. *American Journal of Public Health, 87*(11), 1773–1778. https://doi.org/10.2105/AJPH.87.11.1773

Graham-LoPresti, J., Williams, M. T., & Rosen, D. C. (2019). Culturally responsive assessment and diagnosis for clients of color. In M. T. Williams, D. C. Rosen, & J. W. Kanter (Eds.), *Eliminating race-based mental health disparities: Promoting equity and culturally responsive care across settings* (pp. 169–185). New Harbinger Books.

Grau, P. P., Kusch, M. M., Williams, M. T., Loyo, K. T., Zhang, X., Warner, R. C., & Wetterneck, C. T. (2022). A review of the inclusion of ethnoracial groups in empirically supported posttraumatic stress disorder treatment research. *Psychological Trauma: Theory, Research, Practice, and Policy, 14*(1), 55–65. https://doi.org/10.1037/tra0001108

Hays, P. A. (2009). Integrating evidence-based practice, cognitive–behavior therapy, and multicultural therapy: Ten steps for culturally competent practice. *Professional Psychology: Research and Practice, 40*(4), 354–360. https://doi.org/10.1037/a0016250

Johnston, M. P., & Nadal, K. L. (2010). Multiracial microaggressions: Exposing monoracism in everyday life and clinical practice. In D. W. Sue (Ed.), *Microaggressions and marginality: Manifestation, dynamics, and impact* (pp. 123–144). John Wiley & Sons, Inc.

Keith, V. M., Nguyen, A. W., Taylor, R. J., Mouzon, D. M., & Chatters, L. M. (2017). Microaggressions, discrimination, and phenotype among African Americans: A latent class analysis of the impact of skin tone and BMI. *Sociological Inquiry, 87*(2), 233–255. https://doi.org/10.1111/soin.12168

Kim, B. S. K., Yang, P. H., Atkinson, D. R., Wolfe, M. M., & Hong, S. (2001). Cultural value similarities and differences among Asian American ethnic groups. *Cultural Diversity & Ethnic Minority Psychology, 7*(4), 343–361. https://doi.org/10.1037/1099-9809.7.4.343

Landrine, H., Klonoff, E. A., Corral, I., Fernandez, S., & Roesch, S. (2006). Conceptualizing and measuring ethnic discrimination in health research. *Journal of Behavioral Medicine, 29*(1), 79–94. https://doi.org/10.1007/s10865-005-9029-0

Leong, F. T., & Kalibatseva, Z. (2011). Cross-cultural barriers to mental health services in the United States. *Cerebrum, 2011*, 5. https://www.ncbi.nlm.nih.gov/pmc/articles/PMC3574791/

Mendoza, D. B., Williams, M. T., Chapman, L. K., & Powers, M. (2012). Minority inclusion in randomized clinical trials of panic disorder. *Journal of Anxiety Disorders, 26*(5), 574–582. https://doi.org/10.1016/j.janxdis.2012.02.011

Moodley, R., & Sutherland, P. (2010). Psychic retreats in other places: Clients who seek healing with traditional healers and psychotherapists. *Counselling Psychology Quarterly, 23*(3), 267–282. https://doi.org/10.1080/09515070.2010.505748

Nadal, K. L. (2011). The Racial and Ethnic Microaggressions Scale (REMS): Construction, reliability, and validity. *Journal of Counseling Psychology, 58*(4), 470–480. https://doi.org/10.1037/a0025193

Oshin, L. A., Ching, T. H. W., & West, L. M. (2019). Supervising therapist trainees of color. In M. T. Williams, D. C. Rosen, & J. W. Kanter (Eds.), *Eliminating race-based mental health disparities: Promoting equity and culturally responsive care across settings* (pp. 187–201). New Harbinger Books.

Ovuga, E., Boardman, J., & Oluka, E. G. A. O. (1999). Traditional healers and mental illness in Uganda. *Psychiatric Bulletin, 23*(5), 276–279. https://doi.org/10.1192/pb.23.5.276

Owen, J., Tao, K. W., Imel, Z. E., Wampold, B. E., & Rodolfa, E. (2014). Addressing racial and ethnic microaggressions in therapy. *Professional Psychology: Research and Practice, 45*(4), 283–290. https://doi.org/10.1037/a0037420

Parker, G., Butler, S. K., Flynn, A., Young, D., Fisher, L., Williams, M., & Taylor, Z. (2020, September). Race and healing: Expanding the conversation. *Psychotherapy Networker.* https://www.psychotherapynetworker.org/magazine/article/2488/race-and-healing/

Phinney, J. (1989). Stages of ethnic identity development in minority group adolescents. *The Journal of Early Adolescence, 9*(1-2), 34–49. https://doi.org/10.1177/0272431689091004

Pouchly, C. A. (2012). A narrative review: Arguments for a collaborative approach in mental health between traditional healers and clinicians regarding spiritual beliefs. *Mental Health, Religion & Culture, 15*(1), 65–85. https://doi.org/10.1080/13674676.2011.553716

Priest, N., Walton, J., White, F., Kowal, E., Baker, A., & Paradies, Y. (2014). Understanding the complexities of ethnic-racial socialization processes for both minority and majority groups: A 30-year systematic review. *International Journal of Intercultural Relations, 43*(B), 139–155.

Rosen, D. C., Kanter, J. W., Villatte, M., Skinta, M. D., & Loudon, M. P. (2019). Becoming an antiracist White clinician. In M. T. Williams, D. C. Rosen, & J. W. Kanter (Eds.), *Eliminating race-based mental health disparities: Promoting equity and culturally responsive care across settings* (pp. 147–168). New Harbinger Books.

Schlaudt, V. A., Bosson, R., Williams, M. T., German, B., Hooper, L. M., Frazier, V., Carrico, R., & Ramirez, J. (2020). Traumatic experiences and mental health risk for refugees. *International Journal of Environmental Research and Public Health, 17*(6), 1943. https://doi.org/10.3390/ijerph17061943

Skinta, M. D. (2020). *Using contextual behavior therapy with sexual and gender minority clients: A practical guide to treatment.* Routledge. https://doi.org/10.4324/9780429030307

Smith, T. B., & Trimble, J. E. (2016). *Foundations of multicultural psychology: Research to inform effective practice.* American Psychological Association. https://doi.org/10.1037/14733-000

Strauss, V. (2020, June 6). "This is my generation's civil rights movement." *The Washington Post.* https://www.washingtonpost.com/education/2020/06/06/this-is-my-generations-civil-rights-movement/

Sue, D. W., Capodilupo, C. M., Torino, G. C., Bucceri, J. M., Holder, A. M., Nadal, K. L., & Esquilin, M. (2007). Racial microaggressions in everyday life: Implications for clinical practice. *American Psychologist, 62*(4), 271–286. https://doi.org/10.1037/0003-066X.62.4.271

Sue, D. W., Lin, A. I., Torino, G. C., Capodilupo, C. M., & Rivera, D. P. (2009). Racial microaggressions and difficult dialogues on race in the classroom. *Cultural Diversity & Ethnic Minority Psychology, 15*(2), 183–190. https://doi.org/10.1037/a0014191

Sue, D. W., Rivera, D. P., Capodilupo, C. M., Lin, A. I., & Torino, G. C. (2010). Racial dialogues and White trainee fears: Implications for education and training. *Cultural Diversity & Ethnic Minority Psychology, 16*(2), 206–213. https://doi.org/10.1037/a0016112

Turner, E. A., Cheng, H. L., Llamas, J. D., Tran, A. G., Hill, K. X., Fretts, J. M., & Mercado, A. (2016). Factors impacting the current trends in the use of outpatient psychiatric treatment among diverse ethnic groups. *Current Psychiatry Reviews, 12*(2), 199–220. https://doi.org/10.2174/1573400512666160216234524

Underhill, M. R. (2018). Parenting during Ferguson: Making sense of white parents' silence. *Ethnic and Racial Studies, 41*(11), 1934–1951. https://doi.org/10.1080/01419870.2017.1375132

U.S. Census Bureau. (2014). *Non-Hispanic Whites may no longer comprise over 50 percent of the U.S. population by 2044.* https://www.census.gov/content/dam/Census/newsroom/releases/2015/cb15-tps16_graphic.pdf

Wadsworth, L. P., Potluri, S., Schreck, M., & Hernandez-Vallant, A. (2020). Measurement and impacts of intersectionality on obsessive-compulsive disorder symptoms across intensive treatment. *The American Journal of Orthopsychiatry, 90*(4), 445–457. https://doi.org/10.1037/ort0000447

Williams, M., & Halstead, M. (2019). Racial microaggressions as barriers to treatment in clinical care. *Directions in Psychiatry, 39*(4), 265–280.

Williams, M., Powers, M., Yun, Y. G., & Foa, E. B. (2010). Minority representation in randomized controlled trials for obsessive-compulsive disorder. *Journal of Anxiety Disorders, 24*(2), 171–177.

Williams, M. T. (2020). *Managing microaggressions: Addressing everyday racism in therapeutic spaces.* Oxford University Press. https://doi.org/10.1093/med-psych/9780190875237.001.0001

Williams, M. T., Chapman, L. K., Wong, J., & Turkheimer, E. (2012). The role of ethnic identity in symptoms of anxiety and depression in African Americans. *Psychiatry Research, 199*(1), 31–36. https://doi.org/10.1016/j.psychres.2012.03.049

Williams, M. T., Faber, S. C., Nepton, A., & Ching, T. (2022). Racial justice allyship requires civil courage: Behavioral prescription for moral growth and change. *American Psychologist.* Advance onliine publication. https://doi.org/10.1037/amp0000940

Williams, M. T., Malcoun, E., Sawyer, B. A., Davis, D. M., Bahojb Nouri, L., & Bruce, S. L. (2014). Cultural adaptations of prolonged exposure therapy for treatment and prevention of posttraumatic stress disorder in African Americans. *PTSD and Treatment Considerations, 4*(2), 102–124. https://doi.org/10.3390/bs4020102

Williams, M. T., Metzger, I. W., Leins, C., & DeLapp, C. (2018). Assessing racial trauma within a *DSM-5* framework: The UConn Racial/Ethnic Stress & Trauma Survey. *Practice Innovations, 3*(4), 242–260. https://doi.org/10.1037/pri0000076

Williams, M. T., Printz, D. M. B., & DeLapp, R. C. T. (2018). Assessing racial trauma with the Trauma Symptoms of Discrimination Scale. *Psychology of Violence, 8*(6), 735–747. https://doi.org/10.1037/vio0000212

Williams, M. T., Rosen, D. C., & Kanter, J. W. (2019). *Eliminating race-based mental health disparities: Promoting equity and culturally responsive care across settings.* New Harbinger Books.

Williams, M. T., Sawyer, B., Ellsworth, M., Singh, R., & Tellawi, G. (2017). Obsessive-compulsive and related disorders in ethnoracial minorities: Attitudes, stigma, and barriers to treatment. In J. Abramowitz, D. McKay, & E. Storch (Eds.), *The Wiley handbook of obsessive-compulsive disorders* (pp. 847–872). John Wiley & Sons. https://doi.org/10.1002/9781118890233.ch48

19

Supervision and Consultation in the Delivery of Cognitive Behavior Therapy to LGBTQ Individuals

Audrey Harkness and John E. Pachankis

Lesbian, gay, bisexual, transgender, and queer (LGBTQ)–affirmative cognitive behavior therapy (CBT) is an evidence-based treatment approach that seeks to address the minority stress pathways that are hypothesized to contribute to the mental health disparities affecting LGBTQ individuals (Pachankis, 2015). *Minority stress* refers to the added stress that LGBTQ people experience due to internalized, interpersonal, and structural stigma directed toward LGBTQ people and communities, which in turn leads to elevated risk of mental health problems among LGBTQ people (Hatzenbuehler, 2009; Meyer, 2003). In perhaps the most prominent example (Pachankis et al., 2015; Pachankis, Mahon, et al., 2020), LGBTQ-affirmative CBT was created by adapting the Unified Protocol, an evidence-based cognitive behavioral treatment that takes a transdiagnostic approach to treating emotional disorders (Barlow et al., 2017). In this approach, the original Unified Protocol was adapted to specifically address the unique stressors (i.e., minority stress) that contribute to the mental health disparities affecting LGBTQ clients. A more comprehensive description of this treatment is provided elsewhere (Burton et al., 2019; Pachankis, 2014).

KEY CONCEPTS FOR TRAINEES TO LEARN

LGBTQ-affirmative CBT is guided by six overarching principles that are important for trainees to understand and integrate across their work with LGBTQ clients, regardless of the techniques they are implementing (Burton

https://doi.org/10.1037/0000314-020
Training and Supervision in Specialized Cognitive Behavior Therapy: Methods, Settings, and Populations, E. A. Storch, J. S. Abramowitz, and D. McKay (Editors)

et al., 2019; Pachankis, 2014). It is also important for supervisors to continually integrate these principles into supervision. As articulated in previous work (Pachankis & Goldfried, 2007), principle-based training promotes "complex clinical thinking" and helps trainees flexibly and effectively implement treatment manuals, including LGBTQ-affirmative CBT. The principles guiding LGBTQ-affirmative CBT practice, training, and supervision are discussed next.

Mental Health Symptoms Are a Normal Response to Minority Stress

In the context of early and ongoing experiences with minority stress, which may be overt or subtle, it is to be expected that LGBTQ people would experience mental health symptoms, such as depression and anxiety. However, LGBTQ clients may blame themselves for their mental health symptoms, having deeply internalized societal messages that LGBTQ people are inherently pathological or blameworthy. As such, it is important in working with LGBTQ clients to consider the role of stigma and discrimination in creating distress.

Minority Stress Teaches LGBTQ Clients Negative Lessons About Themselves That Can Be Unlearned

LGBTQ people are exposed to negative messages about what it means to be LGBTQ throughout the life course. Even if these messages are not as overt as anti-LGBTQ bullying, for example, or present in LGBTQ people's immediate social environments, subtle anti-LGBTQ messages are common (e.g., an LGBTQ student group being assigned to a suboptimal meeting space), as are anti-LGBTQ societal messages (e.g., legislative decisions about whether to protect LGBTQ workers). Therefore, all members of the LGBTQ community are exposed, in one form or another, to negative messages about LGBTQ people. These messages are powerful and can become internalized, worsening mental health outcomes. Therefore, it is important for LGBTQ clients to unlearn these powerful, negative lessons while capitalizing on any of the client's self-directed "unlearning" before treatment.

LGBTQ Clients Can Be Empowered to Communicate Assertively and Openly to Cope With the Unfair Effects of Minority Stress

Among the many powerful negative lessons that minority stress often teaches LGBTQ people is that their experiences, emotions, needs, wants, and preferences are not valid. For instance, sexual minority men who express emotions, violating traditional gender roles, may be dismissed for being "overly emotional" and confirming stereotypes of gay men. Others may have experienced lessons that their sexual orientation or gender identity is a "phase," another powerfully dismissive lesson. These experiences may teach LGBTQ clients to suppress their emotions and behave unassertively to protect themselves from the harms of not being taken seriously by others following genuine self-expression.

LGBTQ-affirmative CBT seeks to empower LGBTQ clients to communicate their experiences, emotions, needs, wants, and preferences assertively and openly.

LGBTQ People Have Unique Strengths

The LGBTQ community has a history of resilience and strength in the face of substantial barriers to health and wellness, including advocacy and activism, navigating the process of coming out, and building families of choice. As members of the LGBTQ community, LGBTQ clients are part of this history of resilience. Additionally, LGBTQ clients likely have their own specific examples of responding to minority stress with resilience and building unique strengths. LGBTQ-affirmative CBT takes a strengths-based approach by validating and building upon these strengths throughout treatment.

LGBTQ People's Sexuality Is Healthy

Another powerful, negative message that LGBTQ people often face is that there is something "wrong" or "unhealthy" about same-sex expressions of sexuality. Same-sex sexuality is a natural, healthy part of human sexuality, yet interpersonal and societal lessons can teach LGBTQ people to conceal, hide, or feel ashamed of their sexual desires and experiences, which can lead to self-fulfilling prophecies of dysregulated sexuality. LGBTQ-affirmative CBT affirms same-sex sexuality as healthy and natural.

Genuine, Supportive Relationships Are Central to LGBTQ People's Well-Being

Because of anti-LGBTQ stigma, LGBTQ people can face interpersonal rejection in many components of their lives, including from parents, family, friends, religious institutions, workplaces, and even from other LGBTQ people. Experiences of rejection, understandably, can lead to distress. Similarly, when social support networks are deteriorated by rejection, it is harder to cope with other sources of distress. Even for LGBTQ people who have experienced affirmation through their non-LGBTQ social network, including family and friends, it is important to have genuine relationships with other LGBTQ people who may provide a unique form of social support, including by providing a valid mirror of the LGBTQ experience. Therefore, a guiding principle of LGBTQ-affirmative CBT is to help LGBTQ clients build and maintain genuine and supportive relationships to foster positive mental health and coping.

KEY TECHNIQUES FOR TRAINEES TO LEARN

Many of the techniques for delivering LGBTQ-affirmative CBT will be familiar to trainees who have a background in CBT. The main distinguishing feature of these techniques is that they are tailored to address the minority stress that underlies many LGBTQ clients' distress (Burton et al., 2019; Pachankis, 2014). Therefore, we describe the tailored aspects of CBT techniques as they are applied in LGBTQ-affirmative CBT. When providing supervision and training on LGBTQ-affirmative CBT, we recommend emphasizing that these techniques are always informed by the treatment principles articulated earlier (Pachankis & Goldfried, 2007).

Psychoeducation About Minority Stress

Trainees will present the minority stress model as it relates to LGBTQ-affirmative CBT. For instance, trainees should be prepared to describe the following rationale, in their own words, for using an LGBTQ-affirmative CBT approach:

> LGBTQ individuals face mental health disparities that are not explained by individual deficits but rather by the extra stress that LGBTQ people have to deal with because of stigma and discrimination—a concept we call *minority stress*. Therefore, this treatment is designed to address those extra sources of stress to help LGBTQ clients experience optimal mental health and wellness within a society that is not always affirming.

Trainees should explore how the minority stress model applies to the client's life. This includes exploring the types of experiences that the client faced with respect to minority stress, including early, ongoing, overt, and subtle experiences of minority stress. To be prepared for such a conversation, it is helpful for trainees to have basic familiarity with potential sources of minority stress and the overall minority stress model. Hatzenbuehler (2009) and Meyer (2003) are potential sources for educating trainees on the minority stress model and minority stressors that contribute to mental health disparities.

Awareness and Acceptance of Emotional Reactions to Minority Stress

An essential skill for this treatment is to build the client's awareness and acceptance of their emotional reactions to minority stress. As noted previously, the first principle of this treatment is that emotional distress is a normal response to minority stress. Basic awareness and acceptance of one's emotional reactions to minority stress are necessary precursors to cognitive and behavioral skills training. As such, this technique focuses on building nonjudgmental present-focused emotional awareness and acceptance, aided by mindfulness exercises such as mindful breathing, body scans, and three-point checks. This technique also involves building awareness of the emotional impact of minority stress through a mood induction exercise in which the trainee guides the client through recalling a minority stress situation and inviting the client to experience their emotional reactions. Trainees need to be prepared to process this mood induction in session, followed by helping the client plan for independent mood inductions for home practice.

Challenge Minority Stress Cognitions

Restructuring maladaptive thinking and building cognitive flexibility is a common CBT technique (Barlow et al., 2017). In LGBTQ-affirmative CBT, we focus on teaching trainees to help clients restructure maladaptive minority stress cognitions. Because of the impact of minority stress, LGBTQ clients may develop automatic thinking patterns involving expectations of rejection and loneliness, internalized stigma, or contingent self-worth. It is important to help clients recognize these automatic thinking patterns as rooted in "thinking traps," such as jumping to conclusions or thinking the worst, and to build cognitive flexibility by challenging these minority stress cognitions. Socratic questioning, as in traditional CBT, can be used (e.g., "Is this definitely true?" "What is the worst thing that could happen?"), as well as tailored reappraisal strategies focused on minority stress (e.g., "Is it worth my energy to respond to this anti-LGBTQ comment?" "These people are ignorant," "Even though things are hard right now, hopefully they'll get better"; Madsen & Green, 2012). Importantly, LGBTQ-affirmative CBT recognizes the reality of minority stress and, rather than attempting to deny the unfair and often painful impact of such stress, helps clients build motivation to rework self-defeating cognitions rooted in minority stress to ultimately build mastery against such stress.

Decrease Emotional Avoidance in Relation to Minority Stress

The Unified Protocol describes *emotional behaviors* as those that individuals use to manage strong emotions, either by preventing emotions from becoming too intense or reducing the intensity of strong emotions (Barlow et al., 2017). For LGBTQ clients, early and ongoing experiences with minority stress can produce strong emotions. Emotional behaviors can be used to cope with the strong emotions produced by minority stress, which can become problematic if these emotional behaviors lead to negative long-term consequences (e.g., social isolation, self-silencing, denying one's own needs, feeling unable to cope with strong emotions). Therefore, LGBTQ-affirmative CBT focuses on countering emotional behaviors, including behavioral avoidance, cognitive avoidance, and safety signals. Trainees will explore with the client their emotional behaviors and the function of these behaviors with respect to their minority stress experiences. For example, a client may withdraw socially (emotional behavior) to avoid rejection or victimization. Trainees will work with the client to develop alternative, and of course safe, behaviors that counter their emotional behaviors in the context of minority stress. Toward the end of treatment, trainees will help their clients build an exposure hierarchy to help them plan for continued emotion experiments in which they counter emotional behaviors in response to minority stress, continuing beyond treatment. Importantly, LGBTQ-affirmative CBT does not encourage exposure to actual experiences of victimization or discrimination but rather to the stressful internal sequelae of such events (e.g., internalized stigma, rumination, social isolation).

Assertiveness Training

Many LGBTQ people learn that they do not have the right to express their personal needs, wants, or desires due to invalidating interpersonal experiences and denial of personal rights afforded to others. These invalidating experiences can lead to unassertiveness, a specific type of emotional behavior. Unassertiveness reduces short-term discomfort but can have great long-term personal costs to LGBTQ clients (e.g., HIV acquisition as a result of not asserting condom use or increasing levels of social anxiety due to unassertive avoidance). Therefore, a key component of LGBTQ-affirmative CBT is assertiveness training. Trainees will begin by defining assertiveness, discussing with their client the impact of minority stress on their assertive behavior and the way that unassertiveness can function as an emotional behavior. Trainees will introduce the "Assertiveness Bill of Rights," (Alberti & Emmons, 2017), which emphasizes core rights that all people have but that minority stress experiences can interfere with believing (e.g., "the right to say 'no' without feeling guilty," "the right to have and express my own feelings and opinions"). Assertiveness training concludes with in-session role plays, therapist feedback on verbal and nonverbal behaviors, and planning for ongoing assertiveness practice between sessions.

Self-Affirmation Exercise

As another LGBTQ-affirmative CBT technique, trainees can complete a self-affirmation exercise with their clients, which is intended to consolidate treatment gains and foster resilience to minority stress. This exercise is informed by prior work showing that brief self-affirmation writing exercises foster the long-term resilience of marginalized groups (Pachankis, Williams, et al., 2020; Walton et al., 2015). Trainees will ask clients to read a vignette of an LGBTQ person navigating a minority stress situation, and then invite the client to write a letter to that individual, describing their own experiences with minority stress, how they have handled it, and how skills from this treatment have helped. The purpose of this "saying is believing" exercise is for clients to consolidate their treatment gains and resilience to minority stress.

CLIENT CHARACTERISTICS IN IDEAL TRAINING CASES

When choosing a training case for LGBTQ-affirmative CBT, it is important to consider which clients may benefit the most from such a treatment. Next, we describe, based on our clinical experience and prior research, which client characteristics are ideal for a training case.

LGBTQ-affirmative CBT is guided by the minority stress model, which suggests that minority stress drives mental health disparities among LGBTQ people. Although this treatment can be used with any LGBTQ client regardless of the degree to which the minority stress model may resonate with them, we have found that those clients whose life experiences align more strongly with the minority stress model tend to benefit more from this treatment. Additionally, less experienced trainees may find that LGBTQ-affirmative CBT is not as complex to deliver to clients who identify more strongly with the minority stress model, making these clients particularly effective training cases. For example, LGBTQ clients who can identify their early and ongoing minority stress experiences and locate the origins of their distress in these experiences may provide an easier opportunity for trainees to see how to apply LGBTQ-affirmative CBT. With more experience, it can be helpful for trainees to progress toward implementing this treatment with clients who may not as readily identify as strongly with the minority stress model, which involves more complex clinical thinking and implementation of treatment.

This recommendation is reinforced by empirical findings. For instance, Millar and colleagues (2016) found that sexual minority men who reported greater internalized homonegativity (i.e., implicitly measured internalized negative beliefs about sexual minority people) benefitted more from LGBTQ-affirmative CBT than those with less internalized homonegativity. In other words, those who, before treatment, implicitly indicated stronger associations between sexual minorities and something "wrong" or "bad" showed greater reductions in depression, anxiety, alcohol use, and sexual risk behavior than those who began treatment with more positive associations about sexual minorities. Another study similarly found that internalized stigma affected the benefits that young men derived from a behavioral HIV prevention and relationship education program for young male couples (Feinstein et al., 2018). These findings concur with our clinical experiences that ideal training cases may be those clients who experience greater internalized sexual orientation and gender identity stigma, as well as a greater sense that minority stress is a driver of their mental health concerns.

Despite this, we believe that any LGBTQ client could benefit from LGBTQ-affirmative CBT because it is adaptable to an individual's presenting concerns and the drivers of their mental health concerns. As we describe further in the next section, a common mistake in implementing this treatment is to push the minority stress model excessively or to attribute a client's distress only to minority stress when this may not accurately follow the case conceptualization. Trainees therefore should receive training on carefully presenting the minority stress model at the level that fits their case conceptualization. Careful supervision is needed for trainees who are beginning to learn to implement LGBTQ-affirmative CBT, particularly when delivering it to those clients whose experiences do not initially align as strongly with the minority stress model.

COMMON MISTAKES AND HOW TO ADDRESS THEM

Next, we describe common missteps and guidance for supervising trainees to avoid them. These include (a) assuming the client's presenting problem is related to their sexual orientation or gender identity, (b) pushing clients to come out, (c) disaffirming a client's minority stress experiences, and (d) not using an intersectional lens to understand minority stress.

Assuming the Presenting Problem Is Related to Sexual Orientation or Gender Identity

Although this treatment approach is guided by the minority stress model, it is a mistake to assume that LGBTQ client's presenting problems are always directly related to their sexual orientation or gender identity. First, it is important for trainees to understand that simply having a sexual or gender minority identity does not drive mental health disparities among LGBTQ communities; minority stress does. It is important that trainees are clear with clients about this distinction and repeatedly emphasize this throughout treatment. More broadly, however, minority stress may not always drive a client's presenting concerns. As with all people, a variety of stressors can lead to distress among LGBTQ clients, and it is important not to dismiss LGBTQ individuals' distress that is unrelated to sexual orientation or gender identity. In previous research, LGBTQ clients reported that it was unhelpful for therapists to inappropriately focus on their sexual orientation or gender identity (Israel et al., 2008). Shelton and Delgado-Romero (2011) found that one of the most common microaggressions that LGBTQ clients experience in therapy is when the therapist assumed that sexual orientation drove all the client's presenting concerns. LGBTQ participants described experiences in therapy in which their therapist brought up their sexual orientation identity in a way that was disconnected from their own presenting concerns or felt abrupt or oversimplified. It is essential for supervisors to help trainees learn how to integrate the minority stress model into LGBTQ-affirmative treatment while also appreciating the many other potential influences on LGBTQ clients'—and indeed all people's—mental health.

Pushing Clients to Come Out

Another common mistake that well-meaning trainees make is to prematurely push clients to disclose their sexual orientation or gender identity to others. For most LGBTQ people, experiences of the closet and coming out represent primary developmental challenges and sources of resilience not commonly experienced by the general population. For some LGBTQ clients, coming out to family, friends, coworkers, or others may be a primary treatment goal, which is highly amenable to LGBTQ-affirmative CBT. However, trainees are cautioned against pushing clients to come out and failing to recognize the functional role of the closet. Concealing one's sexual or gender minority identity may facilitate protection against stigma and discrimination while potentially exacerbating mental health concerns and stress (Pachankis et al., 2020). Clients in disaffirming environments may be accurately assessing that it would be physically or psychologically unsafe to be out as LGBTQ in their current social environment. Other clients may simply determine that the benefits of presenting and living heterosexually outweigh the benefits of being out. On the other hand, coming out can lead to positive mental health effects, such as increased connection with LGBTQ peers and a sense of genuineness or autonomy. Coming out is a stressful process, with data showing that sexual minority men who recently came out are more likely to be depressed or anxious than men who are closeted (Pachankis et al., 2015). For women, the reverse pattern was found to be true, with recently out women less likely to be depressed than women who were closeted. These findings suggest the importance of helping trainees work with their clients to assess the costs and benefits of coming out, which may depend on individual, contextual, and cultural factors. We have found that balancing an appreciation of the potentially functional role of the closet, while also not colluding with anti-LGBTQ bias, can be a helpful focus of supervision because trainees may find it challenging to work with clients who do not wish to be fully out.

It is essential for trainees to be trained in and use an intersectional lens as they apply LGBTQ-affirmative CBT. As articulated by Kimberlé Crenshaw (1989), *intersectionality* refers to interlocking systems of oppression, through which stress, discrimination, and stigma are amplified at the intersections of multiple marginalized identities. LGBTQ clients do not all experience equivalent stigma and discrimination. Sexual minority stress intersects with and is shaped by other forms of minority stress, based on racial/ethnic identity, religious identity, socioeconomic status, immigration status, ability status, and many other components of identity. Each of these aspects of identity are inseparable from LGBTQ clients' sexual orientation and gender identities. Inattention to and dismissiveness of intersectionality in therapy has been shown to worsen LGBTQ clients' experiences of therapy (Berke et al., 2016). Similarly, the American Psychological Association (APA) *Guidelines for Psychological Practice With Lesbian, Gay, and Bisexual Clients* (2012) and the *APA Multicultural Guidelines* (2017) articulate the need for clinicians to adopt an intersectional lens. Supervisors may find it helpful to spend time in supervision exploring the meaning and application of intersectionality theory while trainees prepare case conceptualizations and treatment plans, as well as while reviewing recordings of therapy sessions.

Disaffirming Minority Stress Experiences

Another common mistake is for well-meaning trainees to inadvertently disaffirm LGBTQ clients' experiences of minority stress when implementing cognitive restructuring, emotional experiments, and assertiveness exercises. The purpose of building cognitive flexibility in response to minority stress is to help LGBTQ clients accurately assess their current context and unlearn the powerful, negative lessons that early and ongoing minority stress experiences have taught. However, it is critical that trainees learn to work with clients to disentangle real, ongoing threats from automatic thinking patterns that stem from earlier minority stress experiences. For instance, it would be unhelpful and disaffirming, as well as a misapplication of the cognitive structuring technique, for a therapist to push an LGBTQ client whose parents have stated they would never allow their child to be gay and live in their home to try to "build cognitive flexibility" by encouraging the client to restructure the thought "It is not safe to come out to my parents because I will be kicked out." This thought is an accurate assessment of their environment, and the client's emotional pain should be validated as they recognize this real threat. Similarly, emotion experiments and assertiveness exercises need to be designed while appreciating the potential dangers within LGBTQ clients' lives. It is unhelpful, and potentially harmful, for trainees to push their clients to enter situations that could introduce physical danger. Careful supervision and training can help trainees appreciate the real impact of anti-LGBTQ violence on LGBTQ clients' lives to ensure they deliver treatment in a way that promotes client safety.

ETHICAL ISSUES

A key ethical issue in delivering LGBTQ-affirmative CBT is whether LGBTQ clients do in fact need a unique treatment (Pachankis, 2018). Clearly, psychotherapy for LGBTQ clients should be affirming (APA, 2012), but what is less established is the degree to which a specific LGBTQ-affirmative treatment model is needed for LGBTQ clients. CBT is well-documented as an evidence-based treatment for depression, anxiety, substance use, and many other psychological concerns (Stewart & Chambless, 2009). Although LGBTQ clients are presumably included in many of these prior trials of CBT, LGBTQ identity status has often not been collected or reported in these trials, creating unanswered questions regarding the degree to which LGBTQ clients benefit from these established treatments, compared with heterosexual and cisgender clients (Heck et al., 2017; Pachankis, 2018). This gap in scientific knowledge makes it impossible to know whether tailored CBT treatments are, in fact, required to attain equivalent treatment outcomes for LGBTQ clients. As the scientific literature grows regarding the degree to which LGBTQ clients benefit from standard CBT compared with LGBTQ-affirmative CBT, supervisors and trainees will gain additional information about the degree to which a tailored treatment is needed for LGBTQ clients, as well as whether there are certain LGBTQ clients (e.g., those with greater experiences with stigma) who stand to benefit more from a tailored versus standard version of CBT.

Another ethical question in the application of LGBTQ-affirmative CBT is whether there are limits to the applicability of the treatment based on a client's presenting concerns and level of psychological distress. Consistent with the Unified Protocol, from which this treatment was adapted, LGBTQ-affirmative CBT is intended to be transdiagnostic, addressing the shared underlying drivers of psychological disorders rather than specific symptoms associated with different psychological disorders (Barlow et al., 2017). In our experience, most LGBTQ clients' presenting concerns have been addressable using LGBTQ-affirmative CBT. Similarly, Barlow and Farchione's (2017) edited text on the applications of the Unified Protocol articulates its ability to be applied to a variety of problems, including posttraumatic stress disorder, suicidal thoughts and behaviors, and complex cases with high comorbidity. We, too, have had success working with LGBTQ clients with these presenting concerns using LGBTQ-affirmative CBT. However, with some clients with severe trauma symptoms, we have found it useful to integrate grounding exercises, particularly following the mood induction exercise, to help clients feel centered following such an exercise (Scheer et al., in press). We encourage supervisors to work with trainees to learn what types of mood inductions may be appropriate with clients who have severe trauma symptoms. Similarly, although many of the skills from this treatment can be used with clients who are experiencing suicidal ideation, we encourage supervisors to work with trainees to learn how to appropriately assess suicidal risk and respond with appropriate modifications to the treatment protocol when needed in the context of an acute crisis.

COMMON OBSTACLES IN SUPERVISION AND HOW TO ADDRESS THEM

We have found several supervision topics to be helpful in offsetting obstacles to trainees delivering LGBTQ-affirmative CBT effectively. Some of these topics trainees often bring to supervision; for others, trainees may not bring them to supervision, but they are still important to explore. In fact, they may be especially important to explore if trainees are not raising these topics in supervision. We describe each topic next.

When Therapists Are Not Members of the LGBTQ Community

One challenge that trainees, particularly those who do not identify as a part of the LGBTQ community, sometimes raise is how to affirm LGBTQ clients when the therapist is not a member of the community. LGBTQ individuals are more likely to present to therapy than their heterosexual/cisgender peers (Cochran et al., 2003). Every trainee is likely to work with an LGBTQ client at some point in their training, regardless of their own identity or interest in working with LGBTQ clients. Therefore, it is important to support all trainees, regardless of their personal identity, to affirm LGBTQ clients. It should not be assumed that trainees have LGBTQ-affirming views or are able to effectively communicate these views to their clients because all trainees have all grown up in a society that stigmatizes LGBTQ people. As such, even well-intentioned trainees may "make mistakes" in therapy, saying words that unintentionally offend, making inaccurate assumptions about LGBTQ clients, and other disaffirming behaviors (Shelton & Delgado-Romero, 2011). Supervision should be a space in which trainees can both explore and be held accountable for these behaviors, to grow and learn while ensuring their clients are receiving affirming treatment.

The point brings us to the Multicultural Orientation Framework, an extension of the multicultural competence model, which explores how cultural processes in therapy impact treatment outcomes (Owen et al., 2011). The Multicultural Orientation Framework includes three key concepts that are important for trainees to learn: (a) *cultural humility*, which refers to being attuned and open to the client's own experiences of their cultural identity, rather than imposing the therapist's own understanding or perspective; (b) *cultural opportunities*, which are the points in therapy where a client's cultural identity and experiences can be authentically and respectfully explored; and (c) *cultural comfort*, which refers to the ease with which therapists are able to engage in conversations about client's cultural identities, an ease that develops with training and experience. Supervisors can help trainees practice cultural humility while delivering LGBTQ-affirmative CBT, capitalizing on and creating opportunities to discuss clients' cultural contexts and how they shape their minority stress experiences, and build comfort in talking with clients about their cultural identities and minority stress experiences. Unfortunately, therapeutic alliance ruptures caused by microaggressions in treatment (i.e., identity-related ruptures) are common and associated with worse treatment outcomes (Hook et al., 2016). However, clients who experience such a rupture in therapy but perceive their therapist to have greater cultural humility are less likely to show these worsened treatment outcomes (Davis et al., 2016; Owen et al., 2016). These findings suggest the importance of helping trainees implement LGBTQ-affirmative CBT from a place of cultural humility to ensure that in situations where identity-based ruptures occur, they are prepared to repair the therapeutic relationship, learn from the mistake, and continue supporting the client toward their treatment goals.

Attending to Intersectionality

Another common supervision topic is the multiple axes of identity that clients exist within, beyond their LGBTQ identities. There are several training models to help trainees conceptualize a client's multifaceted aspects of identity which can be used in supervision, such as the ADDRESSING framework (Hays, 2007). The ADDRESSING framework provides guidance to explore multidimensional cultural identities, including age, disabilities, religion, ethnicity, socioeconomic status, sexual orientation, indigenous heritage, national origin, and gender. This, and other frameworks, can help trainees understand how multidimensional aspects of clients' identities shape their experiences of sexual minority stress. We have found that sometimes trainees learning this treatment approach are focused on being LGBTQ-affirmative while forgetting that other components of identity also shape clients' experiences of being LGBTQ and their overall selves. Therefore, we encourage supervisors to consistently work with trainees on exploring clients' multiple aspects of identity in therapy, and for supervision to be inclusive of minority stress experiences that may exist along multiple axes of identity.

Addressing Client Identity Conflict

A final challenge is navigating the delivery of this treatment when an LGBTQ client is experiencing conflict about their LGBTQ identity. Trainees with LGBTQ-affirmative views may find it challenging to balance their own views of how a client "should" manage their LGBTQ identity, including in the context of other important identities or values. For instance, when working with a client who possesses an identity centered around a religion that propels negative messages about LGBTQ people, many trainees might believe that the logical treatment goal is to help the client to forgo their religious identity to affirm their LGBTQ identity. Despite this well-meaning trainee wanting the client to feel affirmed as an LGBTQ person, this approach may not fully appreciate the client's important religious identity. Beckstead and Israel (2007) identified potential sources of conflict about sexual orientation, including internalized stigma from a heterosexist society, cultural conflicts, religious conflicts, and political conflicts. They recommended (a) ensuring that ethical principles to "do no harm" are followed when working with clients experiencing conflict about their sexual orientation, (b) maintaining an LGBTQ-affirmative stance by avoiding collusion with anti-LGBTQ beliefs, (c) providing empathy for the conflict while also helping the client address misinformation about LGBTQ people, (d) not assuming that a client's LGBTQ identity is their most central identity, and (e) collaborating with the client to establish treatment goals and plans. A full review of their recommendations is beyond the scope of this chapter; therefore, we refer the reader to their original recommendations for a more comprehensive review. These recommendations may also be a useful reading to integrate into supervision and training, particularly for trainees who are working with LGBTQ clients experiencing conflict about their identities.

CONCLUSION

We present here some basic information on LGBTQ-affirmative CBT and approaches to supervising trainees who are learning to deliver this treatment. This chapter is meant as an introduction, not a comprehensive review of LGBTQ-affirmative CBT. For trainees and supervisors seeking to learn more about the full treatment, we refer to our therapist guide and client workbook of LGBTQ-affirmative CBT (Pachankis et al., in press-a, in press-b) as well as a compendium of evidence-based practices as applied to LGBTQ clients (Pachankis & Safren, 2019). Our goal is for this introduction to provide supervisors with guidance for discussing important topics related to delivering LGBTQ-affirmative CBT to ensure that LGBTQ clients receive the best possible care.

REFERENCES

Alberti, R., & Emmons, M. (2017). *Your perfect right: Assertiveness and equity in your life and relationships* (10th ed., rev.). Impact Publishers.

American Psychological Association. (2012). Guidelines for psychological practice with lesbian, gay, and bisexual clients. *American Psychologist, 67*(1), 10–42. https://doi.org/10.1037/a0024659

American Psychological Association. (2017). *Multicultural guidelines: An ecological approach to context, identity, and intersectionality.* https://www.apa.org/about/policy/multicultural-guidelines.pdf

Barlow, D. H., & Farchione, T. (Eds.). (2017). *Applications of the unified protocol for transdiagnostic treatment of emotional disorders.* Oxford University Press. https://doi.org/10.1093/med-psych/9780190686017.003.0012

Barlow, D. H., Farchione, T. J., Sauer-Zavala, S., Latin, H. M., Ellard, K. K., Bullis, J. R., Bentley, K. H., Boettcher, H. T., & Cassiello-Robbins, C. (2017). *Unified protocol for transdiagnostic treatment of emotional disorders: Therapist guide* (2nd ed.). Oxford University Press.

Beckstead, L., & Israel, T. (2007). Affirmative counseling and psychotherapy focused on issues related to sexual orientation conflicts. In K. J. Bieschke, R. M. Perez, & K. A. DeBord (Eds.), *Handbook of counseling and psychotherapy with lesbian, gay, bisexual, and transgender clients* (2nd ed., pp. 221–244). American Psychological Association. https://doi.org/10.1037/11482-009

Berke, D. S., Maples-Keller, J. L., & Richards, P. (2016). LGBTQ perceptions of psychotherapy: A consensual qualitative analysis. *Professional Psychology: Research and Practice, 47*(6), 373–382. https://doi.org/10.1037/pro0000099

Burton, C. L., Wang, K., & Pachankis, J. E. (2019). Psychotherapy for the spectrum of sexual minority stress: Application and technique of the ESTEEM treatment model. *Cognitive and Behavioral Practice, 26*(2), 285–299. https://doi.org/10.1016/j.cbpra.2017.05.001

Cochran, S. D., Mays, V. M., & Sullivan, J. G. (2003). Prevalence of mental disorders, psychological distress, and mental health services use among lesbian, gay, and bisexual adults in the United States. *Journal of Consulting and Clinical Psychology, 71*(1), 53–61. https://doi.org/10.1037/0022-006X.71.1.53

Crenshaw, K. (1989). Demarginalizing the intersection of race and sex: A Black feminist critique of antidiscrimination doctrine, feminist theory and antiracist politics. *University of Chicago Legal Forum, 1989*, 139–168.

Davis, D. E., DeBlaere, C., Brubaker, K., Owen, J., Jordan, T. A., Hook, J. N., & Tongeren, D. R. V. (2016). Microaggressions and perceptions of cultural humility in counseling. *Journal of Counseling and Development, 94*(4), 483–493. https://doi.org/10.1002/jcad.12107

Feinstein, B. A., Bettin, E., Swann, G., Macapagal, K., Whitton, S. W., & Newcomb, M. E. (2018). The influence of internalized stigma on the efficacy of an HIV prevention and relationship education program for young male couples. *AIDS and Behavior, 22*(12), 3847–3858. https://doi.org/10.1007/s10461-018-2093-6

Hatzenbuehler, M. L. (2009). How does sexual minority stigma "get under the skin"? A psychological mediation framework. *Psychological Bulletin, 135*(5), 707–730. https://doi.org/10.1037/a0016441

Hays, P. A. (2007). *Addressing cultural complexities in practice: Assessment, diagnosis, and therapy* (2nd ed.). American Psychological Association.

Heck, N. C., Mirabito, L. A., LeMaire, K., Livingston, N. A., & Flentje, A. (2017). Omitted data in randomized controlled trials for anxiety and depression: A systematic review of the inclusion of sexual orientation and gender identity. *Journal of Consulting and Clinical Psychology, 85*(1), 72–76. https://doi.org/10.1037/ccp0000123

Hook, J. N., Farrell, J. E., Davis, D. E., DeBlaere, C., Van Tongeren, D. R., & Utsey, S. O. (2016). Cultural humility and racial microaggressions in counseling. *Journal of Counseling Psychology, 63*(3), 269–277. https://doi.org/10.1037/cou0000114

Israel, T., Gorcheva, R., Burnes, T. R., & Walther, W. A. (2008). Helpful and unhelpful therapy experiences of LGBT clients. *Psychotherapy Research, 18*(3), 294–305. https://doi.org/10.1080/10503300701506920

Madsen, P. W. B., & Green, R.-J. (2012). Gay adolescent males' effective coping with discrimination: A qualitative study. *Journal of LGBT Issues in Counseling, 6*(2), 139–155. https://doi.org/10.1080/15538605.2012.678188

Meyer, I. H. (2003). Prejudice, social stress, and mental health in lesbian, gay, and bisexual populations: Conceptual issues and research evidence. *Psychological Bulletin, 129*(5), 674–697. https://doi.org/10.1037/0033-2909.129.5.674

Millar, B. M., Wang, K., & Pachankis, J. E. (2016). The moderating role of internalized homonegativity on the efficacy of LGB-affirmative psychotherapy: Results from a randomized controlled trial with young adult gay and bisexual men. *Journal of Consulting and Clinical Psychology, 84*(7), 565–570. https://doi.org/10.1037/ccp0000113

Owen, J., Tao, K. W., Drinane, J. M., Hook, J., Davis, D. E., & Kune, N. F. (2016). Client perceptions of therapists' multicultural orientation: Cultural (missed) opportunities and cultural humility. *Professional Psychology: Research and Practice, 47*(1), 30–37. https://doi.org/10.1037/pro0000046

Owen, J. J., Tao, K., Leach, M. M., & Rodolfa, E. (2011). Clients' perceptions of their psychotherapists' multicultural orientation. *Psychotherapy: Theory, Research, & Practice, 48*(3), 274–282. https://doi.org/10.1037/a0022065

Pachankis, J. E. (2014). Uncovering clinical principles and techniques to address minority stress, mental health, and related health risks among gay and bisexual men. *Clinical Psychology, 21*(4), 313–330. https://doi.org/10.1111/cpsp.12078

Pachankis, J. E. (2015). A transdiagnostic minority stress treatment approach for gay and bisexual men's syndemic health conditions. *Archives of Sexual Behavior, 44*(7), 1843–1860. https://doi.org/10.1007/s10508-015-0480-x

Pachankis, J. E. (2018). The scientific pursuit of sexual and gender minority mental health treatments: Toward evidence-based affirmative practice. *American Psychologist, 73*(9), 1207–1219. https://doi.org/10.1037/amp0000357

Pachankis, J. E., Cochran, S. D., & Mays, V. M. (2015). The mental health of sexual minority adults in and out of the closet: A population-based study. *Journal of Consulting and Clinical Psychology, 83*(5), 890–901. https://doi.org/10.1037/ccp0000047

Pachankis, J. E., & Goldfried, M. R. (2007). An integrative, principle-based approach to psychotherapy. In S. G. Hofmann & J. L. Weinberger (Eds.), *The art and science of psychotherapy* (pp. 49–68). Taylor & Francis.

Pachankis, J. E., Harkness, A., Jackson, S. D., & Safren, S. A. (in press-a). *Transdiagnostic LGBTQ-affirmative cognitive-behavioral therapy: Therapist guide.* Oxford University Press.

Pachankis, J. E., Jackson, S. D., Harkness, A., & Safren, S. A. (in press-b). *Transdiagnostic LGBTQ-affirmative cognitive-behavioral therapy: Workbook.* Oxford University Press.

Pachankis, J. E., Mahon, C. P., Jackson, S. D., Fetzner, B. K., & Bränström, R. (2020). Sexual orientation concealment and mental health: A conceptual and meta-analytic review. *Psychological Bulletin, 146*(10), 831–871. https://doi.org/10.1037/bul0000271

Pachankis, J. E., & Safren, S. A. (Eds.). (2019). *Handbook of evidence-based mental health practice with sexual and gender minorities.* Oxford University Press. https://doi.org/10.1093/med-psych/9780190669300.001.0001

Pachankis, J. E., Williams, S. L., Behari, K., Job, S., McConocha, E., & Chaudoir, S. R. (2020). Brief online interventions for LGBTQ young adult mental and behavioral health: A randomized controlled trial in a high-stigma, low-resource context. *Journal of Consulting and Clinical Psychology, 88*(5), 429–444.

Scheer, J. R., Clark, K. A., McConocha, E., Wang, K., & Pachankis, J. E. (in press). Toward evidence-based therapy for sexual minority women: Voices from community members and treatment providers. *Cognitive and Behavioral Practice.*

Shelton, K., & Delgado-Romero, E. A. (2011). Sexual orientation microaggressions: The experience of lesbian, gay, bisexual, and queer clients in psychotherapy. *Journal of Counseling Psychology, 58*(2), 210–221. https://doi.org/10.1037/a0022251

Stewart, R. E., & Chambless, D. L. (2009). Cognitive-behavioral therapy for adult anxiety disorders in clinical practice: A meta-analysis of effectiveness studies. *Journal of Consulting and Clinical Psychology, 77*(4), 595–606. https://doi.org/10.1037/a0016032

Walton, G. M., Logel, C., Peach, J. M., Spencer, S. J., & Zanna, M. P. (2015). Two brief interventions to mitigate a "chilly climate" transform women's experience, relationships, and achievement in engineering. *Journal of Educational Psychology, 107*(2), 468–485. https://doi.org/10.1037/a0037461

20

Training and Supervision of Cognitive Behavioral Couple Therapy

Danielle M. Weber and Donald H. Baucom

In contrast to individual cognitive behavior therapy (CBT), which targets individual distress, cognitive behavioral couple therapy (CBCT) typically targets distress in a relationship. Although couples can present to therapy with different specific concerns, couples experiencing relationship distress are generally characterized by more negatives and fewer positives relative to happy couples. One way this manifests is in how partners behave—that is, many distressed relationships exhibit frequent exchanges of negative behaviors, such as hostile exchanges that lead to escalating conflict, and fewer positive activities, which can make the relationship feel devitalized. Along with these behaviors, these distressed couples can also experience higher levels of negative emotion and fewer positive emotions; likewise, each partner may think more negatively and less positively about the relationship. To address this relationship distress, the goal of couple therapies such as CBCT becomes how to optimize couple functioning through reduction of any destructive negative patterns and enhancing opportunities for positives in the relationship.

Although distressed couples are characterized by common themes, they vary greatly in what factors created and maintain their distress. Treatment, therefore, needs to identify the relevant factors for a given couple and then tailor interventions to target those areas. To facilitate identification of the factors relevant for a couple, CBCT proposes a model to guide therapists to consider the different factors that contribute to couple functioning. Given that couples vary widely, CBCT is not a manualized treatment but instead is a principle-driven approach in which the treatment plan flows from the

https://doi.org/10.1037/0000314-021
Training and Supervision in Specialized Cognitive Behavior Therapy: Methods, Settings, and Populations, E. A. Storch, J. S. Abramowitz, and D. McKay (Editors)

specific conceptualization of the couple. On the basis of this conceptualization, interventions focal to behaviors, emotions, and cognitions naturally follow. Next, we briefly discuss the CBCT approach; for further detail, see Baucom et al. (2020).

KEY CONCEPTS FOR TRAINEES TO LEARN

The CBCT model integrates components of individual CBT with relationship science. First, consistent with individual CBT, the CBCT model examines the importance of behaviors, emotions, and cognitions. In isolation, each person will experience behaviors, emotions, and cognitions that are interrelated. Moreover, these experiences occur between partners (e.g., one partner reacts behaviorally to the other's emotions). Additionally, these behaviors, emotions, and cognitions may be responses to the broader environment. Therefore, the role of behaviors, emotions, and cognitions becomes complicated when examining a unit comprising multiple individuals within a broader environment. Thus, the CBCT model adopts a contextual approach by exploring factors at the level of (a) each individual, (b) the couple, and (c) the environment.

First, at the *individual* level, it is important to attend to what each partner contributes to the relationship. That is, if partners are experiencing individual challenges (e.g., mental health difficulties), this will affect the relationship (e.g., Whisman, 2019). Additionally, relationship difficulties can arise even if each partner is healthy, such as when partners have differences in their needs (e.g., one is planful and the other is spontaneous). Thus, each partner will impact the couple as a whole. Next, the couple is more than the sum of the separate partners (Baucom et al., 2020). Couples must define boundaries to determine what is unique to the relationship; if these boundaries are ill-defined and disrupted (e.g., infidelity), difficulties can occur. Moreover, once boundaries are defined, couples must learn how to operate within the relationship. For example, couples must adopt ways to communicate; notably, communication difficulties are a common reason for couples to seek therapy. Finally, the couple does not exist in a vacuum but lives within a physical and social environment. The couple's environment can provide resources (e.g., a local family who offers to babysit) and also sources of stress (e.g., losing a job).

In sum, the CBCT approach explores behaviors, emotions, and cognitions within a contextual model. On the basis of a therapist's conceptualization of the relevant factors for a couple, interventions can target behaviors, emotions, and cognitions that can apply at the individual, couple, or environmental level. These interventions are briefly explicated next.

KEY TECHNIQUES FOR TRAINEES TO LEARN

First, behavioral interventions target specific behaviors exchanged within the couple. One primary behavioral intervention is using *communication skills training* to promote effective communication. The therapist teaches the couple guidelines for communication and provides structure so that they can practice these skills with the therapist's assistance. Additionally, the therapist might promote specific behavioral changes in partners' daily lives. *Guided behavior change* might be used, in which the therapist provides rationale and invites ideas from the couple about changes in a particular area of life. These interventions can apply at any level of context. An example of this intervention at the environmental level would be guiding a same-sex couple in how they respond if they encounter discrimination, including planning how they support each other and respond in a way that is consistent with their values and desire for safety.

Next, emotional interventions are designed to promote better understanding of and, at times, alteration of emotions within the couple. A couple-level intervention to address emotions would involve the therapist teaching each partner how to share and receive emotional expressions in the context of their communication. Using components of communication skills training focal to emotional expression, the therapist can teach the partner who is speaking to share emotions genuinely in a way that the other partner can receive, while teaching the listening partner to accept the emotions of the other partner.

Finally, cognitive interventions target one or both partners' thoughts within the relationship. Psychoeducation is one intervention that employs the therapist as an expert to help dispel myths. Importantly, directly challenging cognitions as used in individual CBT can feel threatening in the context of a partner; that is, the other partner may "agree" with the therapist's comments about the other person's "distorted thinking," which can make the partner feel attacked. Instead, the therapist can adopt a technique called *guided discovery* geared toward understanding one or both partner's beliefs using nonconfrontational language. For example, the therapist may use guided discovery to explore a partner's individual perspective in the presence of the other partner, so each partner can gain a deeper understanding of their own individual needs.

The model and interventions just described principally address *what* the therapist is doing to target these distress-maintaining patterns. Additionally, it is also important to consider *how* the therapist intervenes. Consistent with individual CBT, a CBCT therapist adopts a collaborative approach by soliciting feedback from the couple to jointly create the conceptualization and treatment plan. Beyond this and other nonspecific skills general to all CBT, CBCT therapists uniquely must foster a therapeutic environment in which both partners feel encouraged to change. This requires providing warmth and structure to make sure that efforts from both partners are attended to and reinforced. The interventions reviewed earlier require the therapist to provide a compelling rationale and the skills necessary for couples to bring about changes in their relationships; however, couples will only make these changes in the context of a trusting relationship in which they feel free to make suggestions and attempts at change that are respected by the other partner and the therapist.

To recap, the CBCT model adopts a contextual approach to conceptualize factors that influence couple functioning. The model integrates conceptual foundations of individual CBT with the contextual complexity of relationship science. According to the needs of the couple, interventions target cognitions, emotions, and behaviors at these various contextual levels in a trusting environment that promotes optimal change. It is this theoretical foundation that is essential for all trainees in the CBCT approach to understand before seeing their first cases.

CLIENT CHARACTERISTICS IN IDEAL TRAINING CASES

Given the complexity of the CBCT model, it is important that therapists are assigned cases that facilitate their understanding of the core model. Notably, some concerns that couples raise require additional, tailored attention. These concerns include issues such as prominent physical or mental health difficulties and a history of infidelity or intimate partner violence (IPV). First, if a partner experiences prominent physical or mental health difficulties, a principal concern might be how to manage the condition in addition to relationship distress. Next, if a couple experiences infidelity or IPV, the couple may require a high degree of structure to manage dysregulated behaviors and emotions (e.g., safety planning, managing interference from the outside person participating in the affair) as well as tailored psychoeducation to address specific concerns related to these experiences. Notably, interventions have expanded the CBCT model to address each of these unique considerations (e.g., for interventions focal to psychopathology, see Baucom et al., 2020; for physical health, see Fischer et al., 2016; for infidelity, see Baucom et al., 2017; for IPV, see Epstein et al., 2015). However, these cases should be reserved for advanced trainees who have a firm grasp of the CBCT model and wish to enhance their training with model expansions.

COMMON CHALLENGES IN CBCT AND HOW TO ADDRESS THEM

Once they begin to practice CBCT with their first couples, training therapists commonly experience challenges in implementing the interventions previously discussed. Thus, supervisors must be attentive to these challenges to enhance the therapist's abilities. These challenges commonly arise in each of the intervention categories presented previously—that is, when intervening to address couples' behaviors, emotions, and cognitions.

Reducing Disruptive Behavior

Therapists frequently struggle with the interventions necessary to reduce a couple's disruptive behaviors, including problematic communication. As discussed previously, behavioral interventions include teaching the couple communication skills and providing structure so that the couple can practice these skills. In individual CBT, the therapy room provides an opportunity for a client to learn a skill outside the context in which a stressor is experienced (i.e., their daily lives). In contrast, in couple therapy, the source of stress (i.e., the other partner) is present in the therapy room. Thus, the therapy room can itself be a context in which disruptive behavior presents, often derailing the focus of the session. The therapist likely entered the session with a particular agenda and intervention in mind; therefore, if these disruptive behaviors emerge in session, the therapist must decide whether they will intervene on these behaviors more directly or return to the previous agenda. On one hand, for couples with problematic communication, observing disruptive patterns in the moment provides a convenient entry for intervention. However, if the therapist falls into a pattern of only responding to what is immediately present in session, they may fail to address important underlying or ongoing concerns. Therefore, it might be important not to follow every "lead" but to follow the predetermined agenda for the session. At the same time, there are instances in which ignoring these patterns in the moment may preclude effective interventions, such as when couples are still focused on negative interactions and are not attending to new session material. In our experience, therapists commonly struggle with making a clinically informed decision about what to do next at these important choice points.

To address this common challenge, the supervisor can help the therapist hone their decision-making abilities regarding how to direct sessions in the context of disruptive behaviors. The supervisor can help the therapist consider different situations and how they might respond, including weighing the pros and cons of different interventions. Through viewing session recordings, the supervisor can highlight moments in sessions where the therapist might have made one of these decisions and clarify the factors that were at play for the therapist. The supervisor can encourage the therapist to keep in mind the overall treatment plan and the desired goal for a given session. Thus, if the therapist is prone to responding to what is immediately present in the moment, the supervisor might ask them to reflect on whether these disruptive behaviors relate to broader themes in the case conceptualization. If so, the supervisor would help the therapist understand how the therapist can integrate the intervention on this present behavior into the plan for that session. If the behaviors present are not related to broader themes and seem to be a distraction from the more primary issues, the supervisor may help the therapist think through how to respond in a way that can contain the pattern and then transition back to the original clinical target. After the supervisor's intervention to help therapists consider different situations and what factors would contribute to their in-session treatment decisions, the supervisor can help therapists think about how they would actively pursue one of these routes based on their informed decision making.

Even after therapists decide on a given path for a session, they are commonly challenged by how to successfully manage it in the context of such disruptive behaviors. That is, if a therapist does not impose sufficient structure, a highly conflictual couple can quickly escalate in session. The supervisor should work with the therapist on how to structure sessions to (a) prevent disruptions from occurring in the first place and (b) respond adequately to disruptions to regain control of the session. First, the supervisor can help the therapist role-play language to use in session that can set expectations for what the therapist is seeking. For instance, the supervisor can help the therapist think of ways to ask questions to solicit input from one partner at a time to impose structure so that the partner who is not being addressed is less likely to interject. If teaching a skill, the supervisor can help the therapist consider ways to tailor instructions to attend to what might be especially important for each partner to keep in mind to minimize disruptions. Next, the supervisor can help the therapist respond in the context of disruptions that do occur, such as by stopping a problematic interaction and redirecting the session. Notably, some therapists may feel uncomfortable interrupting clients, which results in the therapist allowing an unhelpful interaction to continue in session. The supervisor can help the therapist explore their discomfort and provide psychoeducation about why interruption is necessary to socialize couples to the structure of couple therapy needed to bring about behavior change.

Addressing Emotions

Along with disruptive behaviors, distressed couples also frequently experience difficult emotions that the therapist will have to learn to address. During these instances when emotions are heightened, the therapist must be able to intervene on the emotions themselves. One common challenge therapists experience here involves the therapist's own emotional reaction to the emotions in the room. Although individual therapists will also have to contend with negative emotions, these emotions are rarely instigated by a source of stress in the therapy room; in contrast, emotions in couple therapy are often more presently directed at the partner. Moreover, these emotions reported by partners can be hostile in nature, which may be less common in individual therapy settings. If therapists feel overwhelmed by these escalating negative emotions between partners, they may struggle to implement effective interventions.

If a therapist experiences this common challenge of contending with their own emotional reactions, supervisors can work with them on how to make sense of and use their own emotions in session. It is important for supervisors to assess the therapist's capacity to tolerate intense emotions in sessions. If the therapist becomes overwhelmed by the emotional content of sessions to the point that intervening is difficult, the supervisor can intervene by validating their emotional reaction as well as explore ways for the therapist to regulate their emotions during sessions. The supervisor might then help the therapist by role playing different interventions to enhance their comfort intervening even in emotional contexts. In instances where the therapist is having an emotional reaction but it is not getting in the way of interventions, the supervisor might help the therapist think about how their own emotions can be useful to inform their intervention strategy. That is, in certain contexts, the therapist's expressing emotion in response to a highly emotional context can enhance the therapeutic relationship. Moreover, modeling emotional expression can be beneficial for partners who are highly emotionally avoidant. Thus, the supervisor can work with the therapist about how to use their emotions adaptively in session in a way that feels safe and manageable to the therapist.

Addressing Cognitions

Therapists also often encounter challenges when intervening with cognitions. Frequently, partners in distressed relationships are divided in their thinking, in that each commonly sees the other person as worthy of blame for difficulties in the relationship. As a result, they can lack motivation to make changes in their own behavior to benefit the relationship. One of the goals for the couple is to see their difficulties through a relational rather than individual lens; that is, the therapist tries to frame the difficulties as one for the couple as a whole, which then builds the foundation for couple-level change. Although therapists are trained to view concerns through this relational lens, thinking this way in session can be challenging; when a challenging clinical situation arises that taxes the therapist's ability to think clearly, the tendency is to default to what feels most natural.

In a fast-paced interaction, it is easy for therapists to attend to the most immediate concern addressed by one partner; in doing so, however, the therapist is only reacting to what is immediately present rather than seeing the "big picture" of the couple dynamic as a whole. Thus, the therapist is not able to teach the couple about the relational nature of their challenges because the therapist is only viewing the dynamic as a series of individual concerns. Moreover, because many training therapists have a foundation in individual therapy approaches, the default may be to respond to these concerns with individual interventions. This can result in the therapist intervening on one partner's cognitions while the other partner observes, which leads to the partner receiving the intervention to feel targeted, the other partner to feel ignored, and the underlying difficulty (a relationship process) remaining unaddressed. Thus, one primary challenge for beginning therapists intervening on cognitions is their own tendency to think in an individual as opposed to couple perspective.

If the therapist is struggling to adopt this couple perspective, the supervisor can work with them to strengthen this way of thinking and to implement it in the therapy room. If the therapist is struggling with their foundational grasp of the relational perspective and relational interventions overall, the supervisor can provide psychoeducation and examples to help consolidate learning of this relational model. Alternatively, the therapist may demonstrate a core understanding of the relational perspective but find it challenging to implement in the context of a challenging clinical context. The supervisor can then use a more targeted approach, perhaps involving the use of video review, to show moments within sessions that the therapist found challenging. The supervisor can ask the therapist to explain how they were understanding the situation, as well as identify alternative ways that the therapist could respond that are more consistent with a relational approach. Thus, one approach is for the supervisor to use cognitive interventions to strengthen the therapist's ability to think in a relational perspective. Once this understanding is achieved, the supervisor can intervene to improve the therapist's abilities to conduct these couple-level interventions in the moment.

Nonspecific Therapeutic Skills

Beyond these specific interventions to address behaviors, emotions, and cognitions, therapists may also struggle with the nonspecific skills of how to implement these interventions in a way that fosters collaboration among the partners. For instance, if partners adopt a blaming, critical attitude toward each other, the therapist might feel pulled to react to the couple or one partner in particular with frustration. This frustration could manifest in therapist interventions that feel brusque and punish the couple for their less effective efforts. If the therapist is struggling with creating a collaborative and warm relationship with the couple, the supervisor can intervene to explore the therapist's internal reaction to the couple.

In summary, training therapists can experience challenges when intervening on couples' behaviors, emotions, and cognitions while engaging in nonspecific therapeutic skills. With appropriate supervision in place, therapists can gain competence in how they engage with these challenging clinical situations.

ETHICAL ISSUES IN TREATMENT APPLICATION

Along with challenges when intervening on major clinical targets, training therapists also can struggle managing important ethical issues encountered in couple therapy. Beyond general ethical issues that occur across all types of therapy, one consideration that is unique to couple therapy involves the consideration of who is the client. In individual therapy, the individual is the only potential focus. In couple therapy, the couple as a unit is considered to be the client, which implies that the focus of therapy should be the joint goals of the couple as a unit. However, the CBCT model also emphasizes the importance of each separate partner and the broader environment. Therefore, even if the couple is the client, the needs of each individual and the environment merit attention. Importantly, there may be times that the needs of one partner or a member of the broader social environment (e.g., a child) conflict with the goal of the couple overall. In these instances, the therapist must decide how to prioritize the most important clinical targets while being respectful of all parties' needs. Therefore, unlike in individual therapy where the focus can be primarily on one client, in couple therapy there are multiple potential foci that receive different weights depending on the couple, an issue often brought to supervision.

Identifying Treatment Targets

For training therapists in particular, it can feel challenging to identify the most important treatment targets among the many important needs presented by the individuals, the couple, and the environment. As noted previously, in challenging clinical contexts, therapists can commonly default to their own belief systems and experiences in relationships. For instance, a therapist might observe a mixed-gender couple that practices traditional gendered division of roles in the household; the therapist, who personally values more egalitarian division of roles, may encourage the couple to change this pattern based on the belief that this traditional division of roles is harmful or out of sync with current norms.

In attending to the needs of the couple as well as the individual and environment, it is critical that supervisors teach therapists that decisions about clinical targets not be made on personal reactions but be based on principles provided by the CBCT model. First, therapists must keep in mind the general principles of what typically is adaptive in relationships. More negative and fewer positive behaviors, emotions, and cognitions typically characterize distressed relationships. Thus, if the therapist observes such patterns in the couple, these patterns can be flagged as potential targets. However, second, it is critical to consider the broad context within which these patterns occur. That is, couples exist within cultures and value-systems that make certain patterns more or less acceptable or adaptive for a given couple. In the example just given, a couple might live within a culture where traditional gender roles are valued. Thus, if the therapist decides to intervene based simply on their own personal beliefs, they might ignore the extent to which these behaviors are rooted within the couple's personal belief systems.

It is, however, not simply the case that if something is acceptable within a given culture, then it is necessarily adaptive for the couple. Most importantly, along with considering the principles of what typically works in relationships and the broad context, the therapist must be attentive to how functional such patterns are for the couple. That is, the supervisor should help the therapist evaluate how such patterns are affecting the couple, each partner, and the environment. In the previous example, the therapist might notice that the female partner is exhibiting signs of depression; after further assessment, the therapist might conclude that the female partner does not feel like she has agency, which has led her to feel powerless or a loss of control. Thus, even though the couple has not identified their traditional gender roles as an area needing change, the therapist might nevertheless point out the specific consequence of this pattern in their relationship for the well-being of the female partner in particular. Depending on the information from this evaluation for a given couple, the particular weight of focus on either partner, the couple, or environment might shift.

Confidentiality

The particular weighting of these factors also influences how therapists handle the issue of confidentiality. In individual therapy, the bounds of confidentiality are explicit. However, in couple therapy, confidentiality inherently becomes more complicated. That is, there are instances in which one partner might communicate something to the therapist and ask that the information not be shared with the other partner. Some practicing therapists may adopt broad rules, such as rules that prioritize the couple (i.e., a "no secrets" policy wherein anything disclosed in confidence would then be told to the other partner) or the individual (i.e., the therapist keeps all private disclosures secret from the other partner). However, we believe that the specific approach must be tailored based on the weighting of the well-being of the individual, couple, or environment. For instance, a therapist might generally have implemented a policy that whatever is shared by one partner is to be shared in a couple context as well. However, a partner may disclose to the therapist that they are concerned about their safety because of IPV. Because one partner is at risk for harm and raising this concern around the other partner could enhance this risk, the therapist might keep this disclosure confidential and decide how to proceed in a way that maximizes the safety of that partner.

Given the complexity of considering the needs of each partner, the couple as a whole, and the broader environment simultaneously, therapists commonly struggle with such ethical issues. The supervisor can provide support by helping the therapist return to the broader principles inherent in CBCT to take a tailored approach when such issues ethical issues arise.

APPROACH TO TRAINING AND SUPERVISION

For therapists to engage thoughtfully with these clinical challenges while implementing the CBCT approach, supervisors must structure the training and supervision in a way that maximizes learning. One viable training and supervision structure for CBCT that we have implemented in various contexts is briefly outlined next; for further details, see Baucom and Boeding (2013). The sequence includes several core components: (a) teaching the CBCT theoretical model and its research base, (b) teaching the core interventions with structured practice to enhance learning, and, finally, (c) developing therapists treating clinical cases with ongoing supervision. Given the complexity of the model, we believe it is important that trainees gain sufficient conceptual understanding and practice with interventions before seeing couples clinically. Although this initial training might sound obvious, our experience in many training contexts is that therapists in training enter a new clinical context and immediately begin seeing clients with little explicit initial training incorporated in the process. Because many programs do not include training in couple therapy, it is important to provide such training before clinical services are implemented. Thus, it is important to overcome the myth that couple therapy is the same as individual therapy—simply with two clients in the room.

The first two components of teaching the model and intervention strategies are integrated and typically span 1 to 2 months of weekly 2.5-hour didactic training sessions when implemented in a graduate student training clinic.

This can also be adapted into a 5-day workshop in a more intensive format, but the details reviewed next are specific to the training clinic model. In this initial phase of teaching, the supervisor/trainer aims to create a similar atmosphere to what therapists create in session with couples; that is, the supervisor teaches from a place of expertise within a collaborative, supportive environment. The supervisor teaches the content (e.g., the role of behavior, cognitions, emotions, and couple interaction patterns in relationships) in a presentation format while incorporating group discussion. In these discussions, the supervisor tries to instill understanding of the principles inherent in the approach while encouraging each therapist to integrate that understanding into their own therapeutic style. As a group, the therapists in training also watch video demonstrations and live role plays of the supervisor/trainer as therapist with discussion to help trainees form exemplars of how interventions could be implemented. Moreover, therapists form groups of three to role play different intervention techniques with live feedback from the supervisor/trainer.

Following the didactic phase of training, couple cases are screened and assigned to therapists in training. Therapists record sessions, and these recordings are viewed by the supervisor. Although one function of supervision is for therapists to provide their own perspective about a session, therapists may be attentive to some aspects of sessions but not others. Therefore, it is important for the supervisor to watch recordings of sessions when feasible. By watching sessions, supervisors can provide not only global perspectives about a couple or the therapist based on therapist report but also provide specific feedback based on what is observed within session. Importantly, one challenge implementing this approach is the time demand this places on supervisors. In our experience, this supervisor workload can be reduced by (a) a limited number of therapists, (b) therapists seeing a limited number of couples, or (c) having multiple supervisors, depending on the clinical context and demands. Broad discussion of cases, treatment plans, and roadblocks are valuable, and when supplemented by in-depth discussion of specific sessions observed by the supervisor, supervision can be optimized.

Once therapists begin to see cases, supervision can be delivered in a combination of group and individual formats that serve different purposes. First, group supervision comprises supervisors and all or a subset of therapists. Therapists take turns presenting cases and requesting feedback. Group supervision functions to (a) help the therapist presenting a case receive feedback from multiple sources and (b) help all therapists learn through observing different therapists and couples beyond the therapist's own personal experience. The therapist who is presenting can ask broad questions based on brief case summaries or ask more specific questions after showing clips from sessions. These questions can focus on the couple, such as a specific dynamic or the treatment plan, or on the therapist, including the therapist's intervention or personal reactions to the couple. The supervisor's role in group supervision is to ensure that a therapist's needs are being met while ensuring an educational experience for the entire group of therapists, including those who are not presenting. A common challenge for the supervisor is establishing a strong group dynamic to avoid group supervision from becoming individual supervision with spectators present. Notably, this challenge is one that applies to group supervision of any therapy and is not specific to group supervision in CBCT.

Along with weekly or regular group supervision, therapists receive individual supervision biweekly or according to what time frame fits the setting. Individual supervision functions to address the tailored needs of the individual therapist. Because this time is devoted entirely to one therapist, this affords greater opportunity to explore their couples and own personal development in depth. Moreover, a one-on-one setting allows discussion of any concerns about clinical work that would feel less comfortable to address in a group context. The supervisor should attend to the therapist's strengths and help hone the therapist's self-awareness of their abilities, just as the therapist does with the couple as they increasingly learn new skills.

Within these individual supervision sessions, there is also a focus on the therapist's specific work with couples as well as the therapist's broad developmental trajectory as a couple therapist. In considering the developmental function of supervision, we have encountered a unique challenge that may differ from other settings. As noted, many couple therapy trainees are not beginning therapists; rather, many trainees have had individual therapy experience, perhaps even years of individual therapy experience. This difference in the starting point of trainees creates a unique challenge for individual supervision.

In contrast to a beginning therapist who may still be formulating their own self-awareness of their abilities, a therapist experienced in individual therapy may enter the couple therapy training experience with some confidence in their general therapeutic skills. After beginning couple therapy, however, therapists can respond in two ways. First, therapists may be shocked at how "new" the sensation seems and feel strongly reminded of what it was like to be a beginning therapist. Experienced individual therapists have referred to this abrupt change in confidence as feeling "deskilled" and may experience a loss of confidence in their abilities. It is important for supervisors to normalize feeling overwhelmed by a new approach to therapy and help therapists incorporate their multiple clinical skills into this new context. Second, therapists may feel so confident and comfortable with individual therapy that they are less open to supervision and constructive feedback. In such circumstances, we have found it productive to emphasize a collaborative, collegial perspective that demonstrates genuine respect for the therapist's skills and experiences with an emphasis of building on those and expanding them in a dyadic context. Thus, a perspective of lifelong therapist growth and enhancement that involves embracing new and challenging clinical experiences with the inherent discomfort that arises from such experiences can go a long way to creating an optimal supervision experience for both new and experienced clinicians engaging in couple therapy for the first time.

CONCLUSION

The rich complexity of couples' lives requires a conceptual model that captures the nuance of the factors that can contribute to relationship distress as well as interventions that can be flexibly adapted to address the most pressing clinical targets. We believe the principles and interventions provided by the CBCT approach can greatly benefit not only the couple as a unit but also each individual partner and the broader environment. However, because of the inherent complexity of conceptualizing and intervening on relational phenomena, beginning couple therapists commonly experience challenges in this approach. For instance, in the context of spontaneous, disruptive exchanges between partners, therapists may default to focusing only on the most immediately present, individual concern rather than considering the "big picture." Therefore, we believe that it is essential for beginning CBCT therapists to receive a structure of support including (a) didactics devoted to the CBCT model, (b) structured practice to enhance learning of intervention strategies, and (c) ongoing group and individual supervision tailored to the beginning therapist's needs. As the therapist aims to do with their couples in therapy, the supervisor creates a warm and collaborative environment in which the therapist can optimally grow in their skills and development as a couple therapist, both for the benefit of the therapist and the couples assigned to their care.

REFERENCES

Baucom, D. H., & Boeding, S. (2013). The role of theory and research in the practice of cognitive-behavioral couple therapy: If you build it, they will come. *Behavior Therapy*, *44*(4), 592–602. https://doi.org/10.1016/j.beth.2012.12.004

Baucom, D. H., Fischer, M. S., Corrie, S., Worrell, M., & Boeding, S. E. (2020). *Treating relationship distress and psychopathology in couples: A cognitive-behavioural approach*. Routledge.

Baucom, D. H., Pentel, K. Z., Gordon, K. C., & Snyder, D. K. (2017). An integrative approach to treating infidelity in couples. In J. Fitzgerald (Ed.), *Foundations for couples' therapy: Research for the real world* (pp. 206–215). Routledge/Taylor & Francis Group. https://doi.org/10.4324/9781315678610-21

Epstein, N. B., Werlinich, C. A., & LaTaillade, J. J. (2015). Couple therapy for partner aggression. In A. S. Gurman, J. L. Lebow, & D. K. Snyder (Eds.), *Clinical handbook of couple therapy* (pp. 389–411). Guilford Press.

Fischer, M. S., Baucom, D. H., & Cohen, M. J. (2016). Cognitive-behavioral couple therapies: Review of the evidence for the treatment of relationship distress, psychopathology, and chronic health conditions. *Family Process*, *55*(3), 423–442. https://doi.org/10.1111/famp.12227

Whisman, M. A. (2019). Psychopathology and couple and family functioning. In B. H. Fiese, M. Celano, K. Deater-Deckard, E. N. Jouriles, & M. A. Whisman (Eds.), *APA handbook of contemporary family psychology: Applications and broad impact of family psychology* (Vol. 2, pp. 3–20). American Psychological Association. https://doi.org/10.1037/0000100-001

21

Supervision of Cognitive Behavioral Therapy for Substance Use Disorders

Paige Morrison, Jessica Spofford, and Mercedes Carswell

There is a dearth of research examining clinical supervision outcomes, and when narrowed to cognitive behavior therapy (CBT) and further to CBT for substance use disorders (CBT-SUD), this number becomes even smaller (Alfonsson et al., 2020; Burrow-Sánchez et al., 2020). In the few cases in which it was studied, the methodology is often flawed (Alfonsson et al., 2020). Recently, there has been a broad push to standardize supervision, including that of CBT, through the development of theory-based, behaviorally anchored core competencies and the use of psychometrically sound objective measurements (Alfonsson et al., 2020; DeMarce et al., 2021; Thwaites et al., 2015). To further complicate the picture, many American counseling and clinical psychology doctoral programs do not provide formalized supervision training (Shallcross et al., 2010). One study found fewer than 20% of psychologists providing supervision received formalized supervision training (Peake et al., 2002). Hadjistavropoulos et al. (2010) found that only 25% of Canadian professional psychology doctoral programs required extensive formalized supervision training. Despite the lack of formalized, structured, clinical supervision training, many psychologists report having to supervise trainees (Shallcross et al., 2010).

The literature also indicates a small percentage of psychologists have received training in substance use disorders (SUD), even though psychologists are likely to encounter patients with substance misuse (Burrow-Sánchez et al., 2020; Substance Abuse and Mental Health Services Administration [SAMHSA], 2018).

https://doi.org/10.1037/0000314-022
Training and Supervision in Specialized Cognitive Behavior Therapy: Methods, Settings, and Populations, E. A. Storch, J. S. Abramowitz, and D. McKay (Editors)

Dimoff et al. (2017) found that almost half of accredited clinical psychology doctoral programs lacked SUD training and only about one third of programs have one or more faculty with SUD interest or at least one SUD-specific treatment clinic. This lack of SUD training is contrasted with the continued struggle of Americans with SUD and the ever-rising numbers of overdose deaths (Dimoff et al., 2017; Lipari & Van Horn, 2017). In a recent survey of substance use among Americans aged 12 years old or older, more than 140 million endorsed alcohol use within the past month, with 67 million of those endorsing binge drinking; more than 61 million endorsed tobacco use; and more than 30 million reported illegal substance use or prescription opioid abuse (SAMHSA, 2018).

These statistics point to a clear deficit: There is a demand for clinical supervision in SUD treatment given the increasing rate of SUD among Americans, yet there is an extensive lack of formalized supervision and SUD-specific training. The challenge in providing appropriate supervision is further exacerbated by the minimal research available on CBT-SUD–specific supervision. This creates a need to increase literature discussing CBT-SUD supervision, SUD training among psychologists, and formalized supervision training among counseling and clinical psychology doctoral students. This chapter expands on approaches and considerations in providing CBT-SUD supervision.

KEY CONCEPTS FOR TRAINEES TO LEARN

There are several overarching concepts a supervisor may teach or review with their trainees, including the cognitive behavioral model for treating SUDs, differentiation between skills exposure and skill mastery, and the role of cravings and urges within SUDs. The concepts reviewed in this section provide a foundation to support skill development and case conceptualization.

Cognitive Behavioral Model for Treating Substance Use Disorders

It is important to assess trainees' level of experience with the CBT model to determine their preparedness to apply the model within an SUD population. Early in training, supervisors should aid trainees in ascertaining the etiology and maintenance of a patient's substance use via a "biopsychosocial" approach. From the biopsychosocial perspective, supervisees collaborate with the patient and supervisor to identify environmental impacts (e.g., community norms, availability), potential reinforcers (e.g., the experience of social reinforcement or avoidance of anxiety), emotions that increase the likelihood of alcohol use, and the expectancies patients may have developed about their substance use—for example, "This will be more enjoyable with a drink," "I can't get through this pain without using" (Longabaugh & Morgenstern, 1999; Rotgers, 2003). Key components of a CBT-SUD treatment focus on interventions to enhance self-efficacy, develop coping skills, and reduce patients' positive substance-related expectancies (Moos, 2007). Through theoretical understanding, trainees will develop the ability to identify which CBT intervention or approach may best suit a patient's needs.

The beginning of supervision can be a good time to use parallel practices with supervisees to aid in developing their understanding of core concepts. Supervisors should develop a full conceptualization with supervisees and may consider incorporating a worksheet to facilitate the learning process. Table 21.1 shows a sample treatment planning document for trainees to help choose interventions by synthesizing patient information within the CBT model.

Exposure Versus Mastery

CBT-SUD has a multitude of interventions allowing for greater individualization of care. Trainees might become overwhelmed when having to determine which interventions to use and the depth in which to teach them to their patient. Furthermore, as a time-limited and goal-focused treatment, it is important for supervisees to develop confidence in their choice of interventions. Skill mastery is a main goal of CBT for SUD (Barry, 1999). A focus of supervision should be on patients' development of and mastery over a select group of skills tailored to their specific substance use goals rather than a brief exposure to an overflowing "toolbox." A multisession approach should be taken with skill-building because mastery of a CBT skill is likely to take more than one session, as well as ongoing patient practice (DeMarce et al., 2021). The skills chosen for mastery should be based on the collaborative and empowerment focus of CBT. The CBT-SUD supervisor can provide additional support as the trainee and patient work together to narrow down the options of skills based on the patient's identified needs (DeMarce et al., 2020).

Supervisors can further reinforce the focus on mastery through modeling. When new CBT interventions are taught to supervisees, more than one supervision meeting should be allotted to cover the skill. Trainees should be assigned homework to practice the intervention, and upon return to supervision, homework will be reviewed and trainee summaries of the intervention should be elicited. The structure mirrors the skill training process in CBT-SUD (Carroll,

TABLE 21.1. Determining Interventions in Cognitive Behavioral Therapy for Substance Use Disorders

Key information	Etiology or maintenance?	Underlying theory or framework	Proposed intervention
"I just get so angry, and drinking will calm me down."	Both	Positive expectancies	Coping skills (anger management)
			Five-column thought record
"All my friends drink and drink more than me."	Maintenance	Social reinforcement	Refusal skills
		Social norms	Provide evidence, normative data
			Social skills

1998; DeMarce et al., 2020; Rotgers, 2003). Similarly, role plays or direct practice of interventions can be completed in supervision to develop mastery while preparing trainees for role plays in their therapy session. Trainees are asked to collaborate in identifying interventions to be learned and applied in session. In later stages of supervision, autonomy should be given to supervisees to choose and implement interventions with supervisors taking a consultant role.

Urges and Cravings

Urges and cravings to use a substance are unique to and common in treating SUD. Understanding the etiology, impact, and treatment of these specific symptoms can be inadvertently minimized by supervisors as a basic component of the model and one of the more common symptoms of SUD. Trainees new to the field should be given the time to cultivate an understanding of cravings and urges to be better prepared to aid patients in coping with them.

In CBT, urges and cravings are considered antecedents of high-risk or substance-using situations. They increase a patient's vulnerability to return to substance use (Larimer et al., 1999). Within the CBT framework, urges and cravings develop via classical conditioning, where cues in the environment or within oneself become associated with strong desires to resume substance use (Rotgers, 2003). After working on case conceptualization and treatment planning, supervisors should take time with trainees to share recent literature about cravings and urges within the domains of behavioral conditioning, neurochemistry, and treatment outcomes to aid the supervisee in fitting the concept into the larger biopsychosocial context of CBT. Choosing literature that matches treatment settings, the substance of choice, or patient diversity factors can be pivotal in developing CBT-SUD competence.

KEY TECHNIQUES FOR TRAINEES TO LEARN

Supervisors facilitate their trainees' transition from understanding basic CBT-SUD concepts to integrating the concepts into treatment, a process requiring the development of a variety of therapeutic techniques. This section outlines specific techniques that are essential to the implementation of CBT-SUD. Techniques include treatment planning and measurement-based care, as well as, as noted by McHugh and colleagues (2010), the four key components of functional analysis, cognitive and motivational strategies, shifting contingencies, and skill training.

Treatment Planning and Measurement-Based Care

CBT-SUD, like general CBT models, emphasizes individualization and identification of goals (McHugh et al., 2010). Creating a unique substance-related treatment plan is a main focus of the initial CBT-SUD sessions (Carroll, 1998;

DeMarce et al., 2020). CBT-SUD is a broad intervention that allows for flexibility in the means by which SUD is targeted. It does not require the patient to be abstinent from any substances to enter or successfully complete care. Supervisees should learn to explore beyond abstinence goals, increasing their comfort in discussing harm reduction or maintenance. Functional analysis, which is discussed later, may help supervisees draw links between goals that might appear unrelated to substance use (e.g., decreasing depression or anxiety, increasing activities). As supervisors, it is important to aid trainees in creating goals that the patient and trainee understand, agree to, and can measure over time. Measurable goals can aid in the identification of instances of return to substance use, patient progress, and skill and intervention selection. Building a solid treatment plan, with measurable objectives, can also aid in the core psychotherapy components of collaboration, rapport building, and empowerment. Supervisors can create training plans with supervisees in an environment and implementation that also expresses the model's values. Further along in patient care, supervision might include practicing treatment plan development via open-ended questions, reviewing previously created plans with trainees, and critiquing plans.

Clinical assessment measures and measurement-based care are key components of treatment planning (DeMarce et al., 2021); allowing supervisees to track changes in patients over time, adjust treatment as needed, and share progress with patients. Learning how to select appropriate measures will allow trainees to effectively monitor progress and personalize treatment (Scott & Lewis, 2015). Supervisors may take time in supervision to review clinical measures appropriate for an SUD population. Using measurement-based care can help supervisees use CBT-SUD, without undermining their self-efficacy. Supervisors should prepare trainees to use consumption or severity measures (e.g., Brief Addictions Monitor; Cacciola et al., 2013); life quality, satisfaction, or function measures (e.g., World Health Organization Quality of Life-BREF; The WHOQOL Group, 1998); and related symptom measures (e.g., Beck Anxiety Inventory; Beck & Steer, 1993; DeMarce et al., 2020; Scott & Lewis, 2015). The options for measures, like CBT-SUD skills, might seem daunting to a trainee. Supervisors work with trainees to master a few measures in multiple domains to enhance care outcomes. Supervisees should be empowered to support their ongoing treatment plans through the clinical data, and supervisors can normalize shifting the treatment plan based on changes in the data. Of note, although supervision is inherently evaluative, clinical measures should not be used to evaluate a trainee's effectiveness as a provider unless significant data are ignored or clinically indicated adjustments are not implemented.

Components of CBT-SUD

Four specific components of effective CBT-SUD were identified by McHugh et al. (2010): functional analysis, cognitive and motivational strategies, shifting contingencies, and skill training.

Functional Analysis

Functional analysis is a common component of an initial clinical interview. In treating SUDs from this model, trainees must learn to ask patients about high-risk situations or triggers (DeMarce et al., 2020; McHugh et al., 2010). Carroll (1998) suggested trainees learn to focus on identifying social, environmental, emotional, cognitive, and physical triggers to use. Additionally, preexisting skills and strengths should be identified, as well as obstacles and difficulties (Carroll, 1998). By identifying these factors, the functional analysis provides a more complex understanding of the patient's substance use. Combined with the clinical measures discussed previously, a functional analysis also allows for enhanced case conceptualization and treatment plans.

Motivational and Cognitive Strategies

Early in treatment and in supervision, trainees may need to assess or enhance their patients' level of motivation to make a change in their substance use. Motivational interviewing (MI) skills are paramount to successful engagement in CBT-SUD throughout care. Supervisors may want to teach trainees the four processes of MI—engaging, focusing, evoking, and planning—as well as the MI core skills—asking open-ended questions, affirming, reflecting, and summarizing (Miller & Rollnick, 2013). Supervisors might also review the foundational cognitive strategies, including cognitive restructuring, mindfulness, and psychoeducation (Carroll, 1998; DeMarce et al., 2020; McHugh et al., 2010).

Shifting Contingencies

During treatment, trainees should be prepared to help patients determine how treatment goal achievement or maintenance of success will be rewarded. Contingency management components can be considered, together with helping trainees notice and communicate about subtler, naturally occurring rewards (McHugh et al., 2010).

Skills Training

Development of coping skills is one of the "active ingredients" (McHugh et al., 2010) within CBT-SUD. As discussed earlier, skills training should be focused on mastery (Barry, 1999). SUD-specific coping skills for mastery include the development of a patient coping plan, urge surfing, scheduling, and alternative activity planning, and urge monitoring.

PATIENT CHARACTERISTICS AND CASE SELECTION

Beginning clinicians may find comfort in using their newly acquired CBT-SUD skills with less challenging cases (Dobson & Shaw, 1993). Although CBT-SUD training cases ideally should be fairly straightforward, external factors, such as clinic demands and available referrals, may not allow the supervisee that comfort. Perris (1993) warned of a potential case selection pitfall when less experienced clinicians take on cases with severe symptomatology at a stage when they need to develop their technical skills. He recommended that supervisees select multiple cases to discuss in supervision before making a definitive case disposition with the supervisor. It also becomes imperative that supervisors consider the potential complications and treatment adaptations required for more complex training cases to ensure thoughtful, effective supervision for supervisees working with more demanding cases. For example, McHugh et al. (2010) identified multiple challenges that can hinder a CBT intervention, including cognitive deficits, low levels of literacy, acute medical concerns, and significant psychosocial stressors. The authors suggested clinicians meet these challenges by guiding the treatment with a comprehensive case conceptualization, based on a solid functional analysis, while maintaining flexibility with treatment components. The CBT-SUD supervisor can use the supervision session to explore potential adaptations, finding alternative ways to review handouts and complete thought records for patients with literary limitations (e.g., using visual resources to explain concepts, allow audio-recording of thought record entries) or modifying the session structure for patients with cognitive deficits (e.g., shortened session length to allow for difficulties with attention; repetition of significant points with concrete, patient-specific examples to assist with memory).

A patient's choice of substance may also factor into CBT-SUD case selection. The CBT-SUD learning experience may be enhanced by cases who display positive treatment effects over the course of the intervention. Although CBT has proven effective in treating abuse of various substances (Dutra et al., 2008; Farronato et al., 2013; Magill & Ray, 2009), a meta-analysis of controlled CBT trials concluded that the treatment effects were strongest when used with marijuana users (Magill & Ray, 2009). Further, Dutra and colleagues (2008) found that the psychosocial interventions for SUD were least efficacious for patients with polysubstance use. When considering training cases, a supervisor might choose to guide a supervisee toward a case presenting with cannabis use disorder while avoiding patients who meet criteria for multiple SUDs.

The clinical setting in which the intervention will be offered can influence case selection. Treatment delivered in an outpatient clinic implies that the training case's presentation is consistent with the American Society of Addiction Medicine (ASAM) criteria (Mee-Lee et al., 2013) for an outpatient level of care. For example, patients undergoing severe withdrawal, suffering with medical conditions that require intense medical monitoring, or who have comorbid psychiatric conditions that require acute stabilization (e.g., acute suicidal ideation, active psychosis, significant neurocognitive impairment) would not be an appropriate training case in an outpatient clinic. Supervisors and supervisees can assess the CBT-SUD referral using ASAM criteria (Mee-Lee et al., 2013) and consult further with the referral source to ensure appropriateness for their level of care. Of note, study samples in a heavily cited CBT-SUD efficacy meta-analysis contained exclusionary criteria for suicidal or homicidal ideation and active psychosis (Magill & Ray, 2009). Supervisors may consider similar exclusionary criteria when selecting training cases because CBT-SUD effectiveness is not as well-researched for patients with these severe symptoms.

As noted earlier, the flexibility of a CBT-SUD intervention allows for use with patients who may have moderation goals instead of more traditional abstinence goals. Treatment goals may influence case selection because, in our experience, modification goals can be challenging for clinicians learning CBT-SUD. Modification goals require a clear personal limit for substance consumption and an adapted conceptualization of relapse or return to use. In an extensive meta-analysis of CBT-SUD treatment efficacy, Magill and colleagues (2019) noted that an emphasis on relapse prevention in CBT suggests the intervention is compatible with patients who have a goal of maintaining abstinence. It is plausible that novice CBT-SUD supervisees will find more educational benefit from working with training cases who voice a goal of abstinence and can connect with the relapse-prevention components of the intervention.

COMMON TRAINEE MISTAKES IN CBT-SUD AND HOW TO OVERCOME THEM

When learning new treatments and interventions, trainees will inevitably make mistakes. Supervisors can be proactive, managing and often preventing errors with awareness of and vigilance for common mistakes in supervision and clinical practice. In this section, we explore common mistakes, their causes, and offer mitigating techniques for supervisors to use in their practice.

Moving Too Quickly Into Skill-Building

In a manualized CBT-SUD treatment, there might also be a strong pull for trainees to move quickly into skill-building, increase patient self-efficacy and provide tools to reach treatment goals. Many patients seeking SUD care may experience hazardous or life-threatening levels of substance use. For supervisees, the move to skill building might be perceived as another stopping point between life and death. However, strategy selection and skills training are the final task of CBT-SUD (Rotgers, 2003). CBT-SUD is not equivalent to coping skills training. A strong therapeutic alliance that is safe and accepting, combined with a strengthened motivation to change, makes CBT-SUD effective (DeMarce et al., 2020; Rotgers, 2003). In a review of treatment manual use to augment technical skill, Lambert and Ogles (1997) found that therapists may focus primarily on the technique to the detriment of relational aspects of their work, becoming less supportive and more defensive. If a supervisee displays a fixation on skill acquisition from the CBT-SUD manual, the supervisor may choose to allot time in supervision to explore how relational factors influence the therapeutic alliance and treatment outcomes.

Teaching supervisees to engage in rapport building, collaboration, and the creation of a commitment to change early in treatment will help them master CBT-SUD. Supervisors can do this by incorporating MI interventions as a component of CBT-SUD. The emphasis on empathy, equality, and goal orientation in MI (McHugh et al., 2010) merges well with the main components of CBT-SUD.

Further, role play in supervision can be a powerful way to help increase the use of open questions, affirmations, reflections, and summaries to increase change talk (Miller & Rollnick, 2013). For example, role plays with "ambivalent patients" can help supervisees become more comfortable with discord and correct their righting reflexes.

Agenda-Setting Errors

Agenda setting is a key component of traditional CBT approaches (Wright et al., 2002). In CBT-SUD treatment manuals, it is a recommended component that helps set structure and goals for each session (Carroll, 1998; DeMarce et al., 2020). Mastery of agenda setting can be especially useful for trainees because CBT-SUD can take a broad approach to session content, including substance use, cooccurring diagnoses, the inclusion of family members, homework review, skill building, and other interventions. Agenda setting models the structured foundation of CBT-SUD while countering the chaotic nature of active substance use and early recovery. Drug-related cognitive changes can create a challenge for clinicians helping patients with SUDs to develop healthy coping strategies (Gould, 2010). Agenda setting and scheduling can help manage these deficits.

Missing Agenda

Trainees may not include agenda setting in their sessions. Supervisors can help develop this skill by modeling it. Supervision can start with an agenda and end with an assessment of the success of the set agenda. Over time, agenda setting should move from a supervisor-led process to more a collaborative process and later a supervisee-led agenda, modeling the progression in therapy.

Underdeveloped Agenda

An underdeveloped agenda may leave the trainee unsure of what to do with the session time and leave patients without an understanding of what will be completed in the session. When trainees leave out specific agenda items, patients may be unsure how to collaborate or what to add to an agenda. Supervisors may wish to provide specific guidance on session structure such as the 20/20/20 rule developed by Carroll (1998) in which the first 20 minutes is dedicated to current concerns, functioning, and substance use and cravings. The second 20 minutes focuses on skill introduction and discussion. The 20 minutes at the end of session is allotted for collaboration and development of practice assignments and problem-solving potential barriers. The supervisor may also invite supervisees to observe agenda setting in one of their sessions.

Too Much on the Agenda

With a time-limited treatment of generally 12 to 16 sessions, trainees can feel pressured to load each session. Supervisors can aid trainees in prioritizing interventions based on patient's needs and treatment goals. This may also be a good time to review mastery versus exposure, working with supervisees to adapt and change agenda fullness and to encourage them to seek patient feedback and evaluate their performance week to week. Creating space for more autonomy in supervision agenda setting may create a space of practice and skill development.

Homework Errors

Often, difficulties arise around issues related to home assignments; trainees fail to attend to emotions related to noncompletion of patients' home assignment, rushed discussion of the home assignment at the end of session, not starting the home assignment during session, giving the assignment in a too-direct manner rather than collaboratively, not reviewing the home assignment during the following session, and delivering insufficient rationale about home assignments (DeMarce et al., 2020; Haarhoff & Kazantzis, 2007). CBT-SUD supervisors can problem-solve with supervisees as the home assignment errors occur. One way to approach home assignment noncompletion is through use of Socratic questioning to explore the patient's motivation and their own rationale or reasoning (DeMarce et al., 2020). When these errors do occur, it results in the patient lacking desired modeled behavior or not completely understanding its function, and this increases the likelihood of noncompletion of the home assignment for follow-up session (DeMarce et al., 2020). Haarhoff and Kazantzis (2007) suggested mitigating some of these common home assignment mistakes by helping the trainee develop a plan: (a) focus on ideas for homework early on during treatment planning and motivation building phase when there are less obvious things to assign, (b) share with supervisee and eventually patient the importance of and reasons for home assignments, and (c) identify common home assignments based on skills taught in session. Additionally, supervision can enhance competence here by creating a home assignment for the supervisee from the first session and supervisor self-assigned home assignments (e.g., finding articles, examples, or preparing for the next week). Lastly, discussion of the trainee's beliefs and emotions experienced in response to a patient's presentation or behavior (i.e., noncompletion of home assignment) during supervision can assist trainees in developing awareness of their emotions and beliefs within the therapeutic relationship, facilitating development of metacompetence (Davis et al., 2015; Haarhoff & Kazantzis, 2007; Thwaites et al., 2015).

Language and Stigma

Trainees can begin CBT-SUD cases with unknown bias- or stigma-influenced language choices. Supervisors need to be aware of how the trainee's language is used within the SUD subject area. Common labels used in treatment, such as *addict*, *alcoholic*, or *relapse*, are seen as stigmatizing among many people in recovery and their families (Ashford et al., 2019). CBT-SUD supervision should involve discussion of the sociopolitical history of stigma in SUD, its continued pervasiveness, and factors facilitating ongoing stigma, such as language, individual beliefs and bias (including among providers; see Foster & Onyeukwu, 2003; Howard & Holmshaw, 2010; McHugh et al., 2010), policies, criminalization of SUD, and structural barriers (Alexander, 2012; Broyles et al., 2014; McGinty et al., 2018). Supervisors should also discuss ways supervisors can decrease stigma within the therapy relationship (i.e., using recovery-based language, examining and addressing implicit bias, using empathy and narratives; for elaboration of techniques, see Broyles et al., 2014; McGinty et al., 2018).

Underprepared for Return to Use

Within the CBT-SUD model, a return to use is considered a part of the recovery process. It is initiated by a high-risk situation, followed by lack of adequate coping, decreased self-efficacy, engagement in positive expectancies, and potential or ongoing use (Barry, 1999). During a training case, there may be times when a patient has not mastered or acquired the skills necessary to cope with a high-risk situation or has yet to learn how to manage positive expectancies and will return to use. Trainees new to SUD treatment may feel unprepared for patient setbacks; return to use often occurs without the supervisee predicting its occurrence. Role playing return-to-use scenarios in supervision can increase trainee self-confidence in managing the situation within the CBT-SUD model. Supervisors should also prepare trainees to discuss abstinence violation effects (Barry, 1999) and have several available resources or worksheets to use should a return to use occur. Skill development focused on the ability to identify a return to use or increase use compared with the patient goal (strongly related to treatment planning), addressing return to use in a nonjudgmental and supportive way, engaging in an updated functional analysis, and assess patient motivation (DeMarce et al., 2020) before a return to use can help with preparedness and expanding existing skills into a challenging situation.

ETHICAL ISSUES IN TREATMENT APPLICATION FOR SUPERVISION OF CBT-SUD

The American Psychological Association's (2017) *Ethical Principles of Psychologists and Code of Conduct* states, "Psychologists evaluate students and supervisees on the basis of their actual performance on relevant and established program requirements" (Standard 7.02, Mandatory Individual or Group Therapy) and "psychologists who delegate work to . . . supervisees . . . take reasonable steps to . . . see that such persons perform these services competently" (Standard 2.05, Delegation of Work to Others). These Standards indicate that the ethical delivery of supervision requires psychologists to provide clinical training using empirically established discipline competencies and this extends to supervising CBT-SUD cases.

Practicing ethical supervision includes evaluating trainee competency using preidentified, standardized, operationally defined, behaviorally anchored competency ratings through observation of the trainee. Empirical literature indicates areas of competencies to assess for and cover in CBT-SUD clinical supervision can vary but generally include the 19 competencies listed in Exhibit 21.1 (Alfonsson et al., 2020; DeMarce et al., 2021; Gnys et al., 2014; Prasko et al., 2011).

Use of evidence-based guidelines, while incorporating ethical codes and adhering to identified competencies solidified by peer-reviewed research, increases the likelihood clinical supervision is provided by ethical means (Borders, 2014). Ellis and colleagues (2014) expanded Ellis's (2001) problematic supervision construct by formulating 10 criteria the supervisor must meet to provide "minimally adequate supervision." These criteria include proper credentials, appropriate knowledge and skills, consent for supervision, frequency and duration of supervision, monitoring of cases, providing ethical feedback, investment in supervisee's growth, attention to diversity issues, appropriate maintenance of confidentiality and attention to power differentials. They further noted that when a supervisor fails to meet these 10 criteria, supervision becomes problematic and falls into one of two categories: "bad supervision" and "harmful supervision." Poor supervision is a failure to monitor quality of care and serve as a gatekeeper to the profession (Ellis et al., 2014, p. 439). Also, the supervisor shows a "lack of investment" in supervision as evidenced by lack of timely feedback, inattention to trainees' concerns, and no focus on supervisee professional growth (p. 436). Harmful supervision results in "psychological, emotional, and/or physical harm or trauma to the supervisee" (p. 440) and clear violations of ethics and standards of care and practice. Ellis et al. (2014) found a large percentage of supervisees, either currently or in the past as having received inadequate supervision (50.9%) or harmful supervision (96.3%). Up to one third of supervisory ethical concerns have been related to feedback issues (Goodyear, 2014). Feedback is also an important competency in CBT-SUD implementation (Gnys et al., 2014) and supervision (DeMarce et al., 2021).

EXHIBIT 21.1

Competencies to Assess

1. Assessment of presenting problem
2. Orientation to CBT
3. Affirmation/self-efficacy
4. Explore/elicit feelings
5. Review of previous home assignment
6. Coping skills training
7. New home assignment
8. Elicit cognitions
9. Setting the agenda
10. Role play
11. Feedback
12. Guided discovery
13. Reflective statements and summaries
14. Eliciting behaviors
15. Therapeutic relationship
16. Past high-risk situations
17. Potential future high-risk situations
18. Resumed substance use
19. Explore cravings and urges

Note. CBT = cognitive behavior therapy.

Other problematic supervision practices include power differentials and multicultural issues, both of which are important considerations in CBT-SUD supervision. Specifically, psychologists commonly fail to acknowledge or initiate conversations about the inherent power differential within the supervisory relationship as well as the racial or ethnic dynamics between trainee and supervisor (Ellis et al., 2014; Pieterse, 2018; see also Chapter 18, this volume). In 2017–2018, 65% of doctoral degree completions were White students (National Center for Education Statistics, 2019). From 1976 to 2016, there was an increase in doctoral degree conferrals among racial and ethnic minority students (Perez-Felkner et al., 2020). Data suggest that the likelihood of a White supervisor having a racial or ethnic minority predoctoral or postdoctoral supervisees is increasing (Pieterse, 2018; Upshaw et al., 2020).

CBT-SUD supervisors should be prepared to initiate power-related conversations with the supervisee in an authentic and supportive manner. This will allow the supervisor to model for the supervisee use of CBT-SUD competencies including the focus on relationship and interpersonal effectiveness skills, increasing self-efficacy (Alfonsson et al., 2020; Goodyear, 2014; Shallcross et al., 2010), and micro skills such as self-reflection (Davis et al., 2015; Thwaites et al., 2015). If psychologists fail to discuss these variables in the training relationship, it may be experienced as a microaggression by the supervisee and result in stunted self-efficacy, and the supervisee may feel silenced (Pieterse, 2018; Upshaw et al., 2020). Such failure on the part of the supervisor may also be considered unethical (Borders, 2014; Pieterse, 2018; Upshaw et al., 2020).

It is also important for multicultural conversations to occur between the trainee and patient to better understand the patient's experiences. Currently, 40% of SUD admissions are racial and ethnic minority patients who are at increased risk for poor outcomes (Saloner & Lê Cook, 2013). When conducting the initial assessment within CBT-SUD, just as they assess for other adverse life experiences, so too should the trainee assess for racial or ethnic trauma, its impact on the patient (e.g., assumptions or beliefs in response to such events, experience of internalized racism as a result), and its impact on emotions, and incorporate the information gathered into the case conceptualization (DeMarce et al., 2021; Pieterse, 2018).

OBSTACLES WHEN PROVIDING SUPERVISION IN CBT-SUD

Adequate time designated for training can be a considerable obstacle in supervision. It is not uncommon for supervisors to take on supervisory responsibilities while managing their own clinical, academic, and administrative duties. Supervisors may find it difficult to manage competing supervision priorities in the time-limited supervision session. Consistent with the design of CBT-based interventions, employing a mutually agreed-on agenda in the CBT supervision session allows supervisees to get the most out of each supervision session, adequately covering clinical material and creating optimal learning experiences (Newman & Kaplan, 2016, Chapter 3). As noted earlier, agenda setting in the supervision session also models the skill supervisees are asked to use with their training cases. Liese and Alford (1998) offered guidance on the structure of a CBT supervision session: checking in, setting the agenda, bridging from the previous supervision session, enquiring about previously supervised cases, reviewing homework, prioritizing of agenda items, discussing an individual (recorded) case, using direct instruction and guided discovery, using standardized supervision instruments, assigning relevant homework, and summarizing and eliciting feedback from the supervisee. Supervisors may choose to incorporate this structure into their own work, use the proposed session organization in other relevant literature (Gordon, 2012; Liese & Beck, 1997), or create their own standard agenda for the supervision session.

Another potential impediment in supervision is a discrepancy between the focus of the supervision session and the supervisee's educational needs. Clinicians learning CBT-SUD may enter supervision with varying levels of familiarity with the intervention and the patient population. It is essential for the supervisor to consider the supervisee's level of experience when determining the focus of supervision (Perris, 1993). In conducting CBT supervision, the primary goal is to guide the supervisee's adaptation of CBT philosophy in treatment to facilitate the patient's recovery, with a secondary goal of teaching specific techniques (Pretorius, 2006); the supervisor initially prioritizes acquisition and application of CBT philosophy over acquisition of skills and techniques. With manualized CBT-SUD treatments, there may be a temptation to focus early supervision sessions on learning the skills covered in the initial sessions of the intervention. However, novice CBT-SUD therapists may benefit from early supervision sessions that review how their patient's perception of a situation, emotions, and behaviors are interconnected and work to sustain the SUD, taking time to formulate a strong CBT case conceptualization. A supervisor also cannot assume previous exposure to CBT negates the need for supplementary training. A clinician with prior training in CBT may not have experience working with SUD and require additional training on the disease course, symptomatology, common psychosocial stressors secondary to SUD (e.g., homelessness, legal challenges, social isolation), and unique challenges faced by patients with SUD (e.g., post–acute withdrawal syndrome, building a sober support network). Notably, the focus of supervision may change over time, with attention to technical skills early in the supervisory course moving to an emphasis on the therapists' own impact on the therapeutic process (Perris, 1993). Supervisors are encouraged to continually assess the educational needs of their supervisees and focus on more advanced technical and relational components of CBT-SUD as supervision progresses.

The extent of a supervisor's training in supervision, or lack thereof, may also be a barrier to providing supervision. Personal experience as a supervisee and competence as psychotherapist does not guarantee competence as a supervisor (Knapp et al., 2017, Chapter 14). Supervisors can conduct a self-assessment of their own training needs and develop a plan to address any deficits. Becoming a competent supervisor is a lifelong, cumulative, developmental process (Falender et al., 2004). Supervisors may consider continuing education courses on best practices in supervision, regularly reviewing relevant literature on supervision, and peer consultation about supervision with other CBT supervisors as methods to build competence.

CONCLUSION

CBT-SUD supervisors should feel prepared to provide supervision to diverse trainees with diverse caseloads. By taking a developmental approach to supervision, supervisors can guide clinicians selecting appropriate cases to learn how to apply the cognitive behavioral model to the treatment of SUD, develop skills mastery, and understand urges and cravings all while overcoming common novice CBT-SUD errors. Trainees should depart CBT-SUD supervision with a mastery of techniques, the capacity to apply measurement-based care, and the ability to integrate personal and diversity factors to their clinical work. Supervisors may aim to accomplish these goals through ethical supervision, embodying the values of CBT-SUD including empowerment and rapport building, and continuing their own education for developing supervision competence. Despite low rates of supervision and SUD training in early psychologist education, we hope this chapter provides a basis for supervisors to reduce this gap with their supervisees and within their own clinical practice.

REFERENCES

Alexander, M. (2012). *The new Jim Crow: Mass incarceration in the age of colorblindness.* The New Press.

Alfonsson, S., Lundgren, T., & Andersson, G. (2020). Clinical supervision in cognitive behavior therapy improves therapists' competence: A single-case experimental pilot study. *Cognitive Behaviour Therapy, 49*(5), 425–438. https://doi.org/10.1080/16506073. 2020.1737571

American Psychological Association. (2017). *Ethical principles of psychologists and code of conduct* (2002, amended effective June 1, 2010, and January 1, 2017). https://www. apa.org/ethics/code/

Ashford, R. D., Brown, A., & Curtis, B. (2019). Expanding language choices to reduce stigma: A Delphi study of positive and negative terms in substance use and recovery. *Health Education, 119*(1), 51–62. https://doi.org/10.1108/HE-03-2018-0017

Barry, K. L. (1999). *Tip 34: Brief intervention and brief therapies for substance abuse: Treatment Improvement Protocol (TIP) Series 34.* Center for Substance Abuse Treatment.

Beck, A. T., & Steer, R. A. (1993). *Manual for the Beck Anxiety Inventory.* Psychological Corporation.

Borders, L. D. (2014). Best practices in clinical supervision: Another step in delineating effective supervision practice. *American Journal of Psychotherapy, 68*(2), 151–162. https://doi.org/10.1176/appi.psychotherapy.2014.68.2.151

Broyles, L. M., Binswanger, I. A., Jenkins, J. A., Finnell, D. S., Faseru, B., Cavaiola, A., Pugatch, M., & Gordon, A. J. (2014). Confronting inadvertent stigma and pejorative language in addiction scholarship: A recognition and response. *Substance Abuse, 35*(3), 217–221. https://doi.org/10.1080/08897077.2014.930372

Burrow-Sánchez, J. J., Martin, J. L., & Taylor, J. M. (2020). The need for training psychologists in substance use disorders. *Training and Education in Professional Psychology, 14*(1), 8–18. https://doi.org/10.1037/tep0000262

Cacciola, J. S., Alterman, A. I., Dephilippis, D., Drapkin, M. L., Valadez, C., Jr., Fala, N. C., Oslin, D., & McKay, J. R. (2013). Development and initial evaluation of the Brief Addiction Monitor (BAM). *Journal of Substance Abuse Treatment, 44*(3), 256–263. https://doi.org/10.1016/j.jsat.2012.07.013

Carroll, K. M. (1998). *A cognitive behavioral approach: Treating cocaine addiction* (NIH Publication No. 984308). National Institute on Drug Abuse.

Davis, M. L., Thwaites, R., Freeston, M. H., & Bennett-Levy, J. (2015). A measurable impact of a self-practice/self-reflection programme on the therapeutic skills of experienced cognitive-behavioural therapists. *Clinical Psychology & Psychotherapy, 22*(2), 176–184. https://doi.org/10.1002/cpp.1884

DeMarce, J. M., Gnys, M., Raffa, S. D., & Karlin, B. E. (2020). *Cognitive behavioral therapy for substance use disorders among veterans: Therapist manual* (Rev. ed.). U.S. Department of Veterans Affairs.

DeMarce, J. M., Gnys, M., Raffa, S. D., Kumpula, M., & Karlin, B. E. (2021). Dissemination of cognitive behavioral therapy for substance use disorders in the Department of Veterans Affairs Health Care System: Description and evaluation of veteran outcomes. *Substance Abuse, 42*(2), 168–174. 10.1080/08897077.2019.1674238

Dimoff, J. D., Sayette, M. A., & Norcross, J. C. (2017). Addiction training in clinical psychology: Are we keeping up with the rising epidemic? *American Psychologist, 72*(7), 689–695. https://doi.org/10.1037/amp0000140

Dobson, K. S., & Shaw, B. F. (1993). The training of cognitive therapists: What have we learned from treatment manuals? *Psychotherapy: Theory, Research, & Practice, 30*(4), 573–577. https://doi.org/10.1037/0033-3204.30.4.573

Dutra, L., Stathopoulou, G., Basden, S. L., Leyro, T. M., Powers, M. B., & Otto, M. W. (2008). A meta-analytic review of psychosocial interventions for substance use disorders. *The American Journal of Psychiatry, 165*(2), 179–187. https://doi.org/10.1176/appi.ajp.2007.06111851

Ellis, M. V. (2001). Harmful supervision, a cause for alarm: Comment on Gray et al. (2001) and Nelson and Friedlander (2001). *Journal of Counseling Psychology, 48*(4), 401–406. https://doi.org/10.1037/0022-0167.48.4.401

Ellis, M. V., Berger, L., Hanus, A. E., Ayala, E. E., Swords, B. A., & Siembor, M. (2014). Inadequate and harmful clinical supervision: Testing a revised framework and assessing occurrence. *The Counseling Psychologist, 42*(4), 434–472. https://doi.org/10.1177/0011000013508656

Falender, C. A., Cornish, J. A., Goodyear, R., Hatcher, R., Kaslow, N. J., Leventhal, G., Shafranske, E., Sigmon, S. T., Stoltenberg, C., & Grus, C. (2004). Defining competencies in psychology supervision: A consensus statement. *Journal of Clinical Psychology, 60*(7), 771–785. https://doi.org/10.1002/jclp.20013

Farronato, N. S., Dürsteler-MacFarland, K. M., Wiesbeck, G. A., & Petitjean, S. A. (2013). A systematic review comparing cognitive-behavioral therapy and contingency management for cocaine dependence. *Journal of Addictive Diseases, 32*(3), 274–287. https://doi.org/10.1080/10550887.2013.824328

Foster, J. H., & Onyeukwu, C. (2003). The attitudes of forensic nurses to substance using service users. *Journal of Psychiatric and Mental Health Nursing, 10*(5), 578–584. https://doi.org/10.1046/j.1365-2850.2003.00663.x

Gordon, P. K. (2012). Ten steps to cognitive behavioural supervision. *Cognitive Behaviour Therapist, 5*(4), 71–82. https://doi.org/10.1017/S1754470X12000050

Gnys, M., DeMarce, J. M., Raffa, S. D., & Karlin, B. E. (2014). *Cognitive Behavioral Therapy for Substance Use Disorders Rating Scale.* Department of Veterans Affairs.

Goodyear, R. (2014). Supervision as pedagogy: Attending to its essential instructional and learning processes. *The Clinical Supervisor, 33*(1), 82–99. https://doi.org/10.1080/07325223.2014.918914

Gould, T. J. (2010). Addiction and cognition. *Addiction Science & Clinical Practice, 5*(2), 4–14.

Haarhoff, B., & Kazantzis, N. (2007). How to supervise the use of homework in cognitive behavior therapy: The role of trainee therapist beliefs. *Cognitive and Behavioral Practice, 14*(3), 325–332. https://doi.org/10.1016/j.cbpra.2006.08.004

Hadjistavropoulos, H., Kehler, M., & Hadjistavropoulos, T. (2010). Training graduate students to be clinical supervisors: A survey of Canadian professional psychology programmes. *Canadian Psychology, 51*(3), 206–212. https://doi.org/10.1037/a0020197

Howard, V., & Holmshaw, J. (2010). Inpatient staff perceptions in providing care to individuals with co-occurring mental health problems and illicit substance use. *Journal of Psychiatric and Mental Health Nursing, 17*(10), 862–872. https://doi.org/10.1111/j.1365-2850.2010.01620.x

Knapp, S. J., VandeCreek, L. D., & Fingerhut, R. (2017). *Practical ethics for psychologists: A positive approach* (3rd ed.). American Psychological Association. https://doi.org/10.1037/0000036-000

Lambert, M. J., & Ogles, B. M. (1997). The effectiveness of psychotherapy supervision. In C. E. Watkins, Jr. (Ed.), *Handbook of psychotherapy supervision* (pp. 421–446). John Wiley & Sons, Inc.

Larimer, M. E., Palmer, R. S., & Marlatt, G. A. (1999). Relapse prevention: An overview of Marlatt's cognitive-behavioral model. *Alcohol Research & Health, 23*(2), 151–160.

Liese, B. S., & Alford, B. A. (1998). Recent advances in cognitive therapy supervision. *Journal of Cognitive Therapy: An International Quarterly, 12*, 91–94.

Liese, B. S., & Beck, J. S. (1997). Cognitive therapy supervision. In C. E. Watkins, Jr. (Ed.), *Handbook of psychotherapy supervision* (pp. 114–133). John Wiley & Sons, Inc.

Lipari, R. N., & Van Horn, S. L. (2017). Trends in substance use disorders among adults aged 18 or older. In *The CBHSQ Report* (pp. 1–10). Substance Abuse and Mental Health Services Administration.

Longabaugh, R., & Morgenstern, J. (1999). Cognitive-behavioral coping-skills therapy for alcohol dependence: Current status and future directions. *Alcohol Research & Health, 23*(2), 78–85.

Magill, M., Ray, L., Kiluk, B., Hoadley, A., Bernstein, M., Tonigan, J. S., & Carroll, K. (2019). A meta-analysis of cognitive-behavioral therapy for alcohol or other drug use disorders: Treatment efficacy by contrast condition. *Journal of Consulting and Clinical Psychology, 87*(12), 1093–1105. https://doi.org/10.1037/ccp0000447

Magill, M., & Ray, L. A. (2009). Cognitive-behavioral treatment with adult alcohol and illicit drug users: A meta-analysis of randomized controlled trials. *Journal of Studies on Alcohol and Drugs, 70*(4), 516–527. https://doi.org/10.15288/jsad.2009.70.516

McGinty, E., Pescosolido, B., Kennedy-Hendricks, A., & Barry, C. L. (2018). Communication strategies to counter stigma and improve mental illness and substance use disorder policy. *Psychiatric Services, 69*(2), 136–146. https://doi.org/10.1176/appi.ps.201700076

McHugh, R. K., Hearon, B. A., & Otto, M. W. (2010). Cognitive behavioral therapy for substance use disorders. *The Psychiatric Clinics of North America, 33*(3), 511–525. https://doi.org/10.1016/j.psc.2010.04.012

Mee-Lee, D., Shulman, G. D., Fishman, M. J., Gastfriend, D. R., & Miller, M. M. (Eds.). (2013). *The ASAM criteria: Treatment criteria for addictive, substance-related, and co-occurring conditions* (3rd ed.). The Change Companies.

Miller, W. R., & Rollnick, S. (2013). *Motivational interviewing: Helping people change* (3rd ed.). Guilford Press.

Moos, R. H. (2007). Theory-based active ingredients of effective treatments for substance use disorders. *Drug and Alcohol Dependence, 88*(2-3), 109–121. https://doi.org/10.1016/j.drugalcdep.2006.10.010

National Center for Education Statistics. (2019). *Doctor's degrees conferred by postsecondary institutions, by race/ethnicity and sex of student: Selected years, 1976–77 through 2017–18.* https://nces.ed.gov/programs/digest/d19/tables/dt19_324.20.asp

Newman, C. F., & Kaplan, D. A. (2016). *Supervision essentials for cognitive-behavioral therapy.* American Psychological Association. https://doi.org/10.1037/14950-000

Peake, T. H., Nussbaum, B. D., & Tindell, S. D. (2002). Clinical and counseling supervision references: Trends and needs. *Psychotherapy: Theory, Research, & Practice, 39*(1), 114–125. https://doi.org/10.1037/0033-3204.39.1.114

Perez-Felkner, L., Ford, J. R., Zhao, T., Anthony, M., Harrison, J. A., & Rahming, S. G. (2020). Basic needs insecurity among doctoral students: What it looks like and how to address it. *About Campus, 24*(6), 18–24. https://doi.org/10.1177/1086482219899649

Perris, C. (1993). Stumbling blocks in the supervision of cognitive psychotherapy. *Journal of Clinical Psychology and Psychotherapy, 1*(1), 29–43. https://doi.org/10.1002/cpp.5640010106

Pieterse, A. L. (2018). Attending to racial trauma in clinical supervision: Enhancing client and supervisee outcomes. *The Clinical Supervisor, 37*(1), 204–220. https://doi.org/10.1080/07325223.2018.1443304

Prasko, J., Vyskocilová, J., Mozny, P., Novotny, M., & Slepecky, M. (2011). Therapist and supervisor competencies in cognitive behavioural therapy. *Neuroendocrinology Letters, 32*(6), 781–789.

Pretorius, W. M. (2006). Cognitive behavioural therapy supervision: Recommended practice. *Behavioural and Cognitive Psychotherapy, 34*(04), 413–420. https://doi.org/10.1017/S1352465806002876

Rotgers, F. (2003). Cognitive-behavioral theories of substance abuse. In F. Rotgers, J. Morgenstern, & S. T. Walters (Eds.), *Treating substance abuse: Theory and technique* (pp. 166–189). The Guilford Press.

Saloner, B., & Lê Cook, B. (2013). Blacks and Hispanics are less likely than whites to complete addiction treatment, largely due to socioeconomic factors. *Health Affairs, 32*(1), 135–145. https://doi.org/10.1377/hlthaff.2011.0983

Scott, K., & Lewis, C. C. (2015). Using measurement-based care to enhance any treatment. *Cognitive and Behavioral Practice, 22*(1), 49–59. https://doi.org/10.1016/j.cbpra.2014.01.010

Shallcross, R. L., Johnson, W. B., & Lincoln, S. H. (2010). Supervision. In J. C. Thomas & M. Hersen (Eds.), *Handbook of clinical psychology competencies* (pp. 501–548). Springer. https://doi.org/10.1007/978-0-387-09757-2_19

Substance Abuse and Mental Health Services Administration. (2018). *Key substance use and mental health indicators in the United States: Results from the 2017 National Survey on Drug Use and Health* (HHS Publication No. SMA 18–5068, NSDUH Series H-53). https://www.samhsa.gov/data/nsduh/reports-detailed-tables-2017-NSDUH

Thwaites, R., Cairns, L., Bennett-Levy, J., Johnston, L., Lowrie, R., Robinson, A., Turner, M., Haarhoff, B., & Perry, H. (2015). Developing metacompetence in low intensity cognitive-behavioural therapy (CBT) interventions: Evaluating a self-practice/self-reflection programme for experienced low intensity CBT practitioners. *Australian Psychologist, 50*(5), 311–321. https://doi.org/10.1111/ap.12151

Upshaw, N. C., Lewis, D. E., & Nelson, A. L. (2020). Cultural humility in action: Reflective and process-oriented supervision with Black trainees. *Training and Education in Professional Psychology, 14*(4), 277–284. 10.1037/tep0000284

The WHOQOL Group. (1998). Development of the World Health Organization WHOQOL-BREF Quality of Life Assessment. *Psychological Medicine, 28*(3), 551–558. https://doi.org/10.1017/S0033291798006667

Wright, B., Williams, C., & Garland, A. (2002). Using the Five Areas cognitive-behavioural therapy model with psychiatric patients. *Advances in Psychiatric Treatment, 8*(4), 307–315. https://doi.org/10.1192/apt.8.4.307

INDEX

ABOUT THE EDITORS

Eric A. Storch, PhD, is a professor and McIngvale Presidential Endowed Chair in the Department of Psychiatry and Behavioral Sciences at Baylor College of Medicine (BCM). He serves as vice chair and head of psychology and codirects the obsessive–compulsive disorder (OCD) program at BCM. Dr. Storch specializes in the nature, assessment, and treatment of childhood and adult OCD, anxiety disorders, and anxiety among youth with autism. He has received multiple grants from the National Institutes of Health to investigate treatment efficacy, mechanisms of action, genetics, neuroethics, and how to enhance outcomes for those struggling with these conditions.

Jonathan (Jon) S. Abramowitz, PhD, is a professor and clinical psychologist in the Department of Psychology and Neuroscience at the University of North Carolina at Chapel Hill. He received his PhD at the University of Memphis. Dr. Abramowitz's research and clinical work focuses on obsessive–compulsive disorder (OCD) and anxiety disorders, including fears and phobias, health anxiety, and panic attacks. He has authored over 300 scientific publications and 20 books, which have been translated into several languages. He served as president of the Association for Behavioral and Cognitive Therapies and as editor or associate editor of several academic journals. Dr. Abramowitz has received wide recognition for his scholarly work and contributions.

Dean McKay, PhD, ABPP, is a professor in the Department of Psychology, Fordham University; past-president (2018) of the Society for a Science of Clinical Psychology; and past-president (2013–2014) of the Association for Behavioral and Cognitive Therapies. Dr. McKay is board certified by the American Board of Professional Psychology in both cognitive behavioral and clinical psychology. He has edited or coedited 21 books and published over 300 journal articles and book chapters. He is also on the Scientific Advisory Board of the International Obsessive Compulsive Disorder Foundation and the Scientific Council of the Anxiety and Depression Association of America. He is also a member of the Psychology of Pandemics Workgroup, an international consortium of researchers examining stress-related problems associated with pandemics that was formed in February 2020. Dr. McKay is a fellow of the American Psychological Association, Association for Psychological Science, and Association for Behavioral and Cognitive Therapies. His research has been primarily in anxiety disorders and obsessive–compulsive disorder, the role of disgust in psychopathology, and misophonia (selective sound sensitivity), as well as professional issues in the delivery of evidence-based interventions.